Informatik aktuell

Reihe herausgegeben von

Gesellschaft für Informatik e.V. (GI)

Bonn, Deutschland

Ziel der Reihe ist die möglichst schnelle und weite Verbreitung neuer Forschungs- und Entwicklungsergebnisse, zusammenfassender Übersichtsberichte über den Stand eines Gebietes und von Materialien und Texten zur Weiterbildung. In erster Linie werden Tagungsberichte von Fachtagungen der Gesellschaft für Informatik veröffentlicht, die regelmäßig, oft in Zusammenarbeit mit anderen wissenschaftlichen Gesellschaften, von den Fachausschüssen der Gesellschaft für Informatik veranstaltet werden. Die Auswahl der Vorträge erfolgt im allgemeinen durch international zusammengesetzte Programmkomitees.

Weitere Bände in der Reihe http://www.springer.com/series/2872

Christoph Palm · Thomas M. Deserno ·
Heinz Handels · Andreas Maier ·
Klaus Maier-Hein · Thomas Tolxdorff
(Hrsg.)

Bildverarbeitung für die Medizin 2021

Proceedings, German Workshop
on Medical Image Computing,
Regensburg, March 7–9, 2021

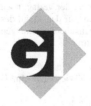

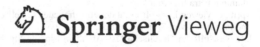

Hrsg.

Christoph Palm🆔
Fakultät für Informatik und Mathematik
Ostbayerische Technische Hochschule
Regensburg
Regensburg, Deutschland

Thomas M. Deserno
Peter L. Reichertz Institut für Medizinische
Informatik der TU Braunschweig und der
Medizinischen Hochschule Hannover
Braunschweig, Deutschland

Heinz Handels
Institut für Medizinische Informatik
Universität zu Lübeck
Lübeck, Deutschland

Andreas Maier🆔
Lehrstuhl für Mustererkennung
Friedrich-Alexander-Universität
Erlangen, Deutschland

Klaus Maier-Hein
Medical Image Computing, E230
Deutsches Krebsforschungszentrum
(DKFZ)
Heidelberg, Deutschland

Thomas Tolxdorff
Institut für Medizinische Informatik
Charité – Universitätsmedizin Berlin
Berlin, Deutschland

ISSN 1431-472X
Informatik aktuell
ISBN 978-3-658-33197-9   ISBN 978-3-658-33198-6   (eBook)
https://doi.org/10.1007/978-3-658-33198-6

Die Deutsche Nationalbibliothek verzeichnet diese Publikation in der Deutschen Nationalbibliografie; detaillierte bibliografische Daten sind im Internet über http://dnb.d-nb.de abrufbar.

Planung: Petra Steinmüller
Springer Vieweg ist ein Imprint der eingetragenen Gesellschaft Springer Fachmedien Wiesbaden GmbH und ist ein Teil von Springer Nature.
Die Anschrift der Gesellschaft ist: Abraham-Lincoln-Str. 46, 65189 Wiesbaden, Germany

Bildverarbeitung für die Medizin 2021

Veranstalter

ReMIC	Regensburg Medical Image Computing
	Ostbayerische Technische Hochschule Regensburg
	(OTH Regensburg)

Unterstützende Fachgesellschaften

BVMI	Berufsverband Medizinischer Informatiker
CURAC	Computer- und Roboterassistierte Chirurgie
DAGM	Deutsche Arbeitsgemeinschaft für Mustererkennung
DGBMT	Fachgruppe Medizinische Informatik der
	Deutschen Gesellschaft für Biomedizinische Technik im
	Verband Deutscher Elektrotechniker
GI	Gesellschaft für Informatik – Fachbereich Informatik
	in den Lebenswissenschaften
GMDS	Gesellschaft für Medizinische Informatik,
	Biometrie und Epidemiologie
IEEE	Joint Chapter Engineering in Medicine and Biology,
	German Section

Tagungsvorsitz

Prof. Dr. rer. nat. Christoph Palm
Regensburg Medical Image Computing (ReMIC)
Ostbayerische Technische Hochschule Regensburg (OTH Regensburg)

Tagungsbüro

Dr. med. Alexander Leis, Simone Böttger, Sümeyye R. Yildiran

Anschrift:	OTH Regensburg, Galgenbergstr. 30, 93051 Regensburg
Email:	orga-2021@bvm-workshop.org
Web:	https://bvm-workshop.org

Lokale BVM-Organisation

Simone Böttger, Dr. Alexander Leis, Leonard Klausmann, Robert Mendel, Prof. Dr. Christoph Palm (Leitung), David Rauber, Sümeyye R. Yildiran und weitere Mitarbeiter*innen des ReMIC der OTH Regensburg.

Verteilte BVM-Organisation

Begutachtung	Heinz Handels und Jan-Hinrich Wrage – Institut für Medizinische Informatik, Universität zu Lübeck
Mailingliste	Klaus Maier-Hein, André Klein und Jens Petersen – Abteilung Medizinische Bildverarbeitung, Deutsches Krebsforschungszentrum (DKFZ) Heidelberg
Special Issue	Andreas Maier – Lehrstuhl für Mustererkennung, Friedrich-Alexander Universität Erlangen-Nürnberg
Sponsoring	Thomas Tolxdorff und Thorsten Schaaf – Institut für Medizinische Informatik, Charité-Universitätsmedizin Berlin
Tagungsband	Thomas M. Deserno, Michael Völcker, Madlen Uick, Nick Igelbrink und Nico Stautmeister – Peter L. Reichertz Institut für Medizinische Informatik (PLRI), Technische Universität Braunschweig und Medizinische Hochschule Hannover
Web & News	Christoph Palm, Leonard Klausmann, Alexander Leis und Sümeyye R. Yildiran – Regensburg Medical Image Computing (ReMIC), Ostbayerische Technische Hochschule Regensburg

BVM-Komitee

Prof. Dr. Thomas M. Deserno, Peter L. Reichertz Institut für Medizinische Informatik (PLRI), Technische Universität Braunschweig und Medizinische Hochschule Hannover

Prof. Dr. Heinz Handels, Institut für Medizinische Informatik, Universität zu Lübeck

Prof. Dr. Andreas Maier, Lehrstuhl für Mustererkennung, Friedrich-Alexander-Universität Erlangen-Nürnberg

Prof. Dr. Klaus Maier-Hein, Abteilung Medizinische Bildverarbeitung, Deutsches Krebsforschungszentrum Heidelberg

Prof. Dr. Christoph Palm, Regensburg Medical Image Computing (ReMIC), Ostbayerische Technische Hochschule Regensburg

Prof. Dr. Thomas Tolxdorff, Institut für Medizinische Informatik, Charité–Universitätsmedizin Berlin

Programmkomitee

Jürgen Braun, Charité-Universitätsmedizin Berlin
Thorsten Buzug, Universität zu Lübeck
Thomas M. Deserno, TU Braunschweig
Jan Ehrhardt, Universität zu Lübeck
Sandy Engelhardt, Universitätsklinik Heidelberg
Ralf Floca, DKFZ Heidelberg
Nils Forkert, University of Calgary, Canada
Jürgen Frikel, OTH Regensburg
Horst Hahn, Fraunhofer MEVIS, Bremen
Heinz Handels, Universität zu Lübeck
Tobias Heimann, Siemens Healthcare, Erlangen
Mattias Heinrich, Universität zu Lübeck
Anja Hennemuth, Charité-Universitätsmedizin Berlin
Alexander Horsch, The Arctic University of Norway, Tromsø, Norwegen
Dagmar Kainmüller, MDC Berlin
Ron Kikinis, Harvard Medical School, Boston, USA
Dagmar Krefting, Universität Göttingen
Andreas Maier, Universität Erlangen
Klaus Maier-Hein, DKFZ Heidelberg
Lena Maier-Hein, DKFZ Heidelberg
Andre Mastmeyer, Hochschule Aalen
Dorit Merhof, RWTH Aachen
Jan Modersitzki, Fraunhofer MEVIS, Lübeck
Heinrich Müller, TU Dortmund
Nassir Navab, TU München
Marco Nolden, DKFZ Heidelberg
Christoph Palm, OTH Regensburg
Bernhard Preim, Universität Magdeburg
Srefanie Remmele, HAW Landshut
Petra Ritter, BIH Berlin
Karl Rohr, Universität Heidelberg
Eva Rothgang, OTH Amberg-Weiden
Sylvia Saalfeld, Universität Magdeburg
Dennis Säring, FH Wedel
Ingrid Scholl, FH Aachen
Stefanie Speidel, HZDR (NCT Dresden)
Thomas Tolxdorff, Charité-Universitätsmedizin Berlin
Klaus Tönnies, Universität Magdeburg
Gudrun Wagenknecht, Forschungszentrum Jülich
René Werner, UKE Hamburg
Thomas Wittenberg, Fraunhofer IIS, Erlangen
Ivo Wolf, Hochschule Mannheim

Sponsoren und Unterstützer des Workshops BVM 2021

Wir bedanken uns für die Unterstützung durch die Regensburger Forschungsein-
richtungen:

- Regensburg Center for Artificial Intelligence (RCAI)
- Regensburg Center of Biomedical Engineering (RCBE)
- Regensburg Center of Health Sciences and Technology (RCHST)

Darüber hinaus freuen wir uns sehr über die langjährige kontinuierliche Unterstützung mancher Firmen sowie auch über das neue Engagement anderer. Die
BVM wäre ohne diese finanzielle Unterstützung in ihrer erfolgreichen Konzeption
nicht durchführbar.

Platin-Sponsoren

Canon Medical Systems GmbH, Hellersbergstr. 4, 41460 Neuss
Continental Engineering Services GmbH, Breitlacherstr. 94, 60489 Frankfurt
DEKOM Engineering GmbH, Hoheluft-Chaussee 108, 20253 Hamburg
Moysis & Partner IT Managementberatung, Adolfstr. 15, 65343 Eltville

Gold-Sponsoren

arxes-tolina GmbH, Piesporter Str. 37, 13088 Berlin
Dell Technologies GmbH, Raffineriestr. 28, 06112 Halle (Saale)
Fotofinder Systems GmbH, Industriestr. 12, 84364 Bad Birnbach
ID GmbH & Co KGaA, Platz vor dem Neuen Tor 2, 10115 Berlin
numares AG, Am BioPark 9, 93053 Regensburg

Silber-Sponsoren

BioPark Regensburg GmbH, Am BioPark 13 (BioPark III), 93053 Regensburg
Haption GmbH, Dennewartstr. 25, 52068 Aachen
NEXUS/CHILI GmbH, Friedrich-Ebert-Str. 2, 69221 Dossenheim
Olympus Deutschland GmbH, Amsinckstr. 63, 20097 Hamburg

Bronze-Sponsoren

1000shapes GmbH, Hamerlingweg 5, 14167 Berlin
AKTORmed GmbH, Borsigstr. 13, 93092 Barbing
Springer Vieweg Verlag, Abraham-Lincoln-Str. 46, 65189 Wiesbaden

Preisträger der BVM 2020 in Berlin

Beste wissenschaftliche Arbeiten

1. **Leonie Henschel**
   (Forschungsgruppe Bildanalyse (Reuter), Deutsches Zentrum für Neurode-
   generative Erkrankungen (DZNE), Bonn)
   Henschel L, Reuter M:
   Parameter Space CNN for Cortical Surface Segmentation.

1. **Alexander Preuhs**
   (Lehrstuhl für Mustererkennung, Friedrich-Alexander-Universität Erlangen-
   Nürnberg)
   Preuhs A, Manhart M, Roser P, Stimpel B, Syben C, Psychogios M, Kowar-
   schik M, Maier A:
   Deep Autofocus with Cone-Beam CT Consistency Constraint.

3. **Felix Denzinger**
   (Lehrstuhl für Mustererkennung, Friedrich-Alexander-Universität Erlangen-
   Nürnberg)
   Denzinger F, Wels M, Breininger K, Reidelshöfer A, Eckert J, Sühling M,
   Schmermund A, Maier A:
   *Deep Learning Algorithms for Coronary Artery Plaque Characterisation from
   CCTA Scans.*

Bester Vortrag

Marc Aubreville
(Lehrstuhl für Mustererkennung, Friedrich-Alexander-Universität Erlangen-
Nürnberg)
Aubreville M, Bertram CA, Jabari S, Marzahl C, Klopfleisch R, Maier A:
*Inter-Species, Inter-Tissue Domain Adaptation for Mitotic Figure Assessment:
Learning New Tricks from Old Dogs.*

Bestes Poster

Sonja Jäckle
(Fraunhofer-Institut für Digitale Medizin MEVIS, Lübeck)
Jäckle S, García-Vázquez V, Haxthausen F, Eixmann T, Sieren MM, Schulz-
Hildebrandt H, Hüttmann G, Ernst F, Kleemann M, Pätz T:
3D Catheter Guidance Including Shape Sensing for Endovascular Navigation.

Vorwort

Die Tagung *Bildverarbeitung für die Medizin (BVM 2021)* wird seit weit mehr als 20 Jahren an wechselnden Orten Deutschlands veranstaltet. Inhaltlich fokussiert sich die BVM dabei auf die computergestützte Analyse medizinischer Bilddaten mit vielfältigen Anwendungsbieten, z.B. im Bereich der Bildgebung, der Diagnostik, der Operationsplanung, der computerunterstützten Intervention und der Visualisierung.

In dieser Zeit hat es bemerkenswerte methodische Weiterentwicklungen und Umbrüche gegeben, an denen die BVM-Community intensiv mitgearbeitet hat. Hervorzuheben ist das Gebiet des Maschinellen Lernens, das gerade für Aufgaben der Klassifikation und Segmentierung, aber zunehmend auch in der Bildregistrierung zu signifikanten Verbesserungen geführt hat. In der Folge dominieren inzwischen Arbeiten im Zusammenhang mit *Deep Learning* die BVM. Auch diese Entwicklungen haben dazu beigetragen, dass die Medizinische Bildverarbeitung an der Schnittstelle zwischen Informatik und Medizin als eine der Schlüsseltechnologien zur Digitalisierung des Gesundheitswesens etabliert ist.

Zentraler Aspekt der BVM ist neben der Darstellung aktueller Forschungsergebnisse schwerpunktmäßig aus der vielfältigen deutschlandweiten BVM-Community insbesondere die Förderung des wissenschaftlichen Nachwuchses. Die Tagung dient vor allem Doktorand*innen und Postdoktorand*innen, aber auch Studierenden mit hervorragenden Bachelor- und Masterarbeiten als Plattform, um ihre Arbeiten zu präsentieren, dabei in den fachlichen Diskurs mit der Community zu treten und Netzwerke mit Fachkolleg*innen zu knüpfen. Trotz der vielen Tagungen und Kongresse, die auch für die Medizinische Bildverarbeitung relevant sind, hat die BVM deshalb nichts von Ihrer Bedeutung und Anziehungskraft eingebüßt und ihren festen Platz im jährlichen Tagungsrhythmus behalten.

Aufbauend auf diesem Fundament gibt es in diesem Jahr einige Neuerungen und Veränderungen. So wird die BVM 2021 erstmalig an der Ostbayerischen Technischen Hochschule Regensburg (OTH Regensburg) ausgerichtet. Regensburg ist nach Aachen, Berlin, Erlangen, Freiburg, Hamburg, Heidelberg, Leipzig, Lübeck und München nicht nur ein neuer Veranstaltungsort. Mit der OTH Regensburg wird die Tagung erstmalig nicht durch eine Universität, eine Universitätsklinik oder ein Helmholtz-Forschungszentrum organisiert, sondern durch eine Hochschule für Angewandte Wissenschaften (HAW). Damit wird auch der Weiterentwicklung der Forschungslandschaft in Deutschland Rechnung getragen, wo HAWs zunehmend neben ihrem Fokus auf der Lehre auch in der angewandten Forschung einen wichtigen Beitrag leisten. Diese Entwicklung spiegelt sich auch in den eingereichten Beiträgen zur BVM in den letzten Jahren.

Die OTH Regensburg ist eine sehr forschungsstarke Hochschule mit der größten Informatikfakultät aller HAWs in Bayern. Gerade in den für die BVM relevanten Bereichen gibt es einschlägige Studiengänge: Bachelorstudiengang und Masterschwerpunkt Medizinische Informatik und ein seit Oktober 2020 neu eingeführter Bachelorstudiengang Künstliche Intelligenz und Data Science. Die Tagungsleitung für die BVM 2021 übernimmt Prof. Dr. rer. nat. Christoph Palm,

Leiter des Labors Regensburg Medical Image Computing (ReMIC), der seit 2017 dem BVM-Komitee angehört und seitdem die Neugestaltung der BVM-Webseite sowie den BVM-Newsletter verantwortet. Während die lokale Organisation in Regensburg liegt, konnte darüber hinaus in bewährter Weise auf die weitere überregionale Organisation durch Fachkollegen des BVM-Komitees aus Berlin, Braunschweig, Erlangen, Heidelberg und Lübeck zurückgegriffen werden.

Neben dem neuen Veranstaltungsort bedingt die Corona-Pandemie eine weitere maßgebliche Veränderung. Nachdem die Präsenzveranstaltung der BVM 2020 in Berlin nur Tage vor dem Start abgesagt werden musste, wird auch in diesem Jahr keine „normale" BVM wie in den letzten Jahren möglich sein. Derzeit werden zwei Varianten parallel geplant: Bei einer *hybriden Variante* sind nur Vortragende, Sessionchairs und Industrievertreter*innen vor Ort in Regensburg, der Großteil der Teilnehmenden wird virtuell dazu geschaltet. Über Live-Streaming der Vorträge mit virtueller Fragemöglichkeit und hybride Postersessions soll eine Verzahnung stattfinden. Bei einer *rein virtuellen BVM* sind alle Teilnehmenden im virtuellen Raum, so dass dafür Möglichkeiten der Interaktion und Kommunikation geschaffen werden müssen. Die Tatsache, dass zum Zeitpunkt der Verfassung dieses Vorworts die Entscheidung für eine der beiden Varianten noch nicht gefallen ist, zeigt, dass es sich die Veranstalter in Regensburg nicht leicht gemacht haben und in jedem Fall, egal zu welcher Veranstaltungsform es am Ende kommen wird, eine für alle bereichernde Tagung organisieren werden.

Inhaltlich kann auch bei der BVM 2021 ein attraktives und hochklassiges Programm geboten werden. Erfreulicherweise stieg die Zahl der Einreichungen deutlich. So konnten aus 97 Einreichungen über ein anonymisiertes Reviewing-Verfahren mit jeweils drei Reviews 26 Vorträge, 51 Poster und 5 Softwaredemonstrationen angenommen werden. Die drei besten Arbeiten werden mit BVM-Preisen ausgezeichnet, die von einem eigenen Komitee vergeben werden. Alle Beiträge werden auch in diesem Jahr wieder im Springer Verlag in der Reihe Informatik aktuell zu einem Tagungsband zusammengefasst, der zur BVM erscheint.

Das Programm wird durch drei eingeladene Vorträge ergänzt:

- **Prof. Dr. Marleen de Bruijne** vom Erasmus MC, Rotterdam, Niederlande und der University of Copenhagen, Dänemark:
  Learning from Imperfect Data: Weak Labels, Shifting Domains, and Small Datasets in Medical Imaging
- **Prof. Dr. Alexandre Xavier Falcão** von der University of Campinas, Brasilien:
  Interactive Design of Convolutional Neural Networks for Medical Image Analysis
- **Prof. Dr. Helmut Messmann** vom Universitätsklinikum Augsburg:
  Artificial Intelligence in Endoscopy

Außerdem werden im Vorfeld der BVM vier Tutorials angeboten:

- Deep Design Patterns (FAU Erlangen-Nürnberg)
- Advanced Deep Learning (DKFZ Heidelberg)

- Deep Learning in Medical Image Registration (Universität zu Lübeck)
- Of Bones and Muscles – Musculoskeletal Human Body Modelling (OTH Regensburg)

Das Programm und alle weiteren Informationen finden sich unter:

https://www.bvm-workshop.org

Zum Schluss möchten wir allen danken, die sich bei der umfangreichen Vorbereitung und Organisation des Workshops engagiert haben: der Gastreferentin und den Gastreferenten, den Autor*innen der Beiträge, den Referent*innen der Tutorien, den Sponsoren, dem Programmkomitee, den Fachgesellschaften und den Mitgliedern des BVM-Komitees. Ein besonderer Dank gilt dem lokalen Organisationsteam aus Regensburg: Simone Böttger, Dr. Alexander Leis, Leonard Klausmann, Robert Mendel, Prof. Dr. Christoph Palm, David Rauber, Sümeyye Yildiran und allen weiteren Mitarbeiter*innen des Labors Regensburg Medical Image Computing der OTH Regensburg.

Wir wünschen allen Teilnehmer*innen spannende Vorträge, anregende Gespräche über die Poster bzw. Softwaredemonstrationen, mit den industriellen Sponsoren sowie untereinander. Lassen Sie sich auf die neuen Formate ein und nutzen Sie die vielen Möglichkeiten der aktiven Mitgestaltung.

Januar 2021

Christoph Palm (Regensburg)
Thomas M. Deserno (Braunschweig)
Heinz Handels (Lübeck)
Andreas Maier (Erlangen)
Klaus Maier-Hein (Heidelberg)
Thomas Tolxdorff (Berlin)

Inhaltsverzeichnis

Die fortlaufende Nummer am linken Seitenrand entspricht den Beitragsnummern, wie sie im endgültigen Programm des Workshops zu finden sind. Dabei steht V für Vortrag, P für Poster und S für Softwaredemonstration.

Session 2: Navigation / Guidance / Visualization

Postersession / Software Demonstration I

Session 3: Data Sets / Challenges

Postersession / Software Demonstration II

Session 4: Visible Light

Session 5: Segmentation and Regression

Postersession / Software Demonstration III

Session 6: Imaging and Image Reconstruction

Session 7: Autoencoder

Learning from Imperfect Data
Weak Labels, Shifting Domains, and Small Datasets in Medical Imaging

Marleen de Bruijne[1,2]

[1]Erasmus MC, Rotterdam, The Netherlands
[2]University of Copenhagen, Denmark
marleen.de.bruijne@gmail.com

Machine learning approaches, and especially deep neural networks, have had tremendous success in medical imaging in the past few years. Machine learning-based image reconstruction techniques are used to acquire high-resolution images at a much faster pace than before. Automated, quantitative image analysis with convolutional neural networks is as accurate as the assessment of an expert observer. Imaging biomarkers extracted via machine learning improve diagnosis, prognosis, and treatment decisions, and the first autonomous AI systems have been approved for diagnostic use and for patient triage in emergency radiology settings.

Machine learning however requires training datasets that are representative of the target data to analyze, cover the range of variation that will be observed in the target data, and are carefully labelled, often with time-consuming manual annotation strategies that require input from clinical experts. This hampers the adoption of machine learning in many medical image analysis tasks. In this talk, various approaches are discussed to make machine learning techniques work in practical situations, where training data is limited, data is highly heterogeneous, annotations are difficult to obtain or may be wrong, and training data may not be representative. Possible solutions include semi-supervised and weakly labeled learning, domain adaptation, and crowd-sourcing of visual analysis.

The potential of direct, machine learning-based diagnostics and prognostics is also discussed. Currently, most quantitative imaging biomarkers used for diagnosis and prognosis are factors that are already well-known to indicate disease. With such image quantification designed by experts–and AI models trained to mimic these experts–simplifications are made and the focus is on a small number of easily quantifiable image aspects. Machine learning enables a new, more data-driven approach. Image characteristics related to disease outcome can be learned directly from databases that combine medical imaging data with patient outcomes (e.g., the clinical diagnosis, therapy outcome, or future disease progression). This fully exploits the rich information present in medical imaging data and does not require time-consuming and error-prone manual annotations. This can result in stronger, more predictive imaging biomarkers, which is emphasized on applications in neuro-, pulmonary, and vascular imaging.

© Der/die Autor(en), exklusiv lizenziert durch
Springer Fachmedien Wiesbaden GmbH, ein Teil von Springer Nature 2021
C. Palm et al. (Hrsg.), *Bildverarbeitung für die Medizin 2021*,
Informatik aktuell, https://doi.org/10.1007/978-3-658-33198-6_1

Interactive Design of Convolutional Neural Networks for Medical Image Analysis

Alexandre Xavier Falcão

Institute of Computing, University of Campinas, Brazil
afalcao@ic.unicamp.br

Convolutional neural networks (CNNs) have played a role in image analysis with several well-succeeded applications involving object detection, segmentation, and identification. The design of a CNN model traditionally relies on the pre-annotation of a large dataset, the choice of the model's architecture, and the tunning of the training hyperparameters. These models are sought as "black-boxes", implying that one cannot explain their decisions. Explainable artificial intelligence (XAI) has appeared to address the problem and avoid the wrong interpretation of the results. However, the importance of user and designer participation in the machine learning loop has called little attention yet.

In medical image computing, data annotation is costly, often scarce, and depends on an expert in the application domain (the user). The choice of the model's architecture and the training hyperparameter tunning rely on the network designer (an expert in AI). The user absence in the machine learning loop leaves essential questions with no answer (e.g., what are the most relevant samples for annotation?), while the lack of interactive methodologies to learn filters and model's architecture limits the designer to the interpretation of the model. The user and designer should then actively participate in the data annotation and training processes, both assisted by the machine, to increase human understanding and control, reduce human effort, and improve interpretation of the results.

This lecture addresses part of the above problems by presenting an interactive methodology for the design of CNN filters from markers in medical images, and a semi-automatic data annotation method guided by feature projection. The user starts the training process by selecting a few images per class and drawing strokes (markers) in regions that discriminate the classes. The designer defines an initial network architecture, and the filters of the CNN are automatically computed with no need for backpropagation. The user and designer may decide about the most suitable filters based on data visualization. The image features extracted by the CNN are projected in 2D for semi-automatic data annotation. The user analyzes the 2D projection, annotates the most challenging samples, while a semi-supervised classifier propagates the labels to the remaining ones. The annotated dataset can then be used to revisit the design of the CNN model, as illustrated for applications of medical image computing.

Artificial Intelligence in Endoscopy

Helmut Messmann

III. Medizinische Klinik, Universitätsklinikum Augsburg
helmut.messmann@uk-augsburg.de

Artificial intelligence (AI) will revolutionize our daily life and will have tremendous impact on health care. Especially the influence in disciplines where imaging plays an important role seems to be substantial. Radiology, pathology and endoscopy will benefit from these developments. So far diagnosis of diseases by using images is based on the experience of the physician (radiologist, pathologist, endoscopist) and highly subjective with low inter- and intra-observer agreement.

Meanwhile AI has become routine in some parts of endoscopy such as screening colonoscopy. The quality of screening endoscopy depends on the number of detected polyps, which is called adenoma detection rate (ADR). Usually an ADR of at least 20% (women) or 25% (men) is recommended. Different techniques such as (virtual) chromo-endoscopy, caps on the distal end of the endoscope or optimizing withdrawal time have shown to increase ADR. By using AI first randomized trials could show a significant increase of ADR, mainly for small polyps (< 5mm). However, it is questionable whether these small polyps have any clinical impact. Besides detection the differentiation of polyps is of major impact. First prototypes showed the possibility to differentiate adenoma from non-adenoma polyps which is of clinical relevance.

Meanwhile similar efforts are made for gastric cancer or esophageal cancer. Our group was the first worldwide to show that AI can differentiate normal Barrett mucosa from dysplastic mucosa, which is a precursor of cancer. Meanwhile we are able to detect cancer real time during endoscopy.

Besides detection and differentiation of polyps and cancer the invasion depth of a cancer is of clinical importance. Usually endoscopic ultrasound is used for staging early cancers to predict whether endoscopic treatment or surgery is necessary. AI seems to have the potential to diagnose the invasion depth of early tumors and so guiding the optimal therapy.

In addition AI can control the endoscopist during his procedure to avoid incomplete visual observation of the Gi-tract.

Learning-based Patch-wise Metal Segmentation with Consistency Check

Tristan M. Gottschalk[1,2,3], Andreas Maier[1,3,4], Florian Kordon[1,2,3],
Björn W. Kreher[2]

[1]Pattern Recognition Lab, Universität Erlangen-Nürnberg (FAU), Erlangen
[2]Siemens Healthcare GmbH, Forchheim
[3]Erlangen Graduate School in Advanced Optical Technologies (SAOT), Universität Erlangen-Nürnberg (FAU), Erlangen
[4]Machine Intelligence, Universität Erlangen-Nürnberg (FAU), Erlangen
Tristan.Gottschalk@fau.de

Abstract. Metal implants that are inserted into the patient's body during trauma interventions cause heavy artifacts in 3D X-ray acquisitions. Metal Artifact Reduction (MAR) methods, whose first step is always a segmentation of the present metal objects, try to remove these artifacts. Thereby, the segmentation is a crucial task which has strong influence on the MAR's outcome. This study proposes and evaluates a learning-based patch-wise segmentation network and a newly proposed Consistency Check as post-processing step. The combination of the learned segmentation and Consistency Check reaches a high segmentation performance with an average IoU score of 0.924 on the test set. Furthermore, the Consistency Check proves the ability to significantly reduce false positive segmentations whilst simultaneously ensuring consistent segmentations.

1 Introduction

Trauma interventions regularly require an intraoperative evaluation of the correct positioning of inserted metallic implants. This oftentimes not only includes a 2D- but also a 3D-X-ray scan performed by a mobile C-arm. Due to heavy image artifacts caused by the inserted implants the surgeon is in need of a well functioning metal artifact reduction method (MAR). Thereby, the overall ability of the particular MAR method to reduce the artifacts heavily depends on the quality of the so-called metal segmentation [1]. Experiments show that missed metal parts in the segmentation lead to still present streak artifacts in the reconstructions even after the MAR, whereas falsely segmented anatomical structures lead to a blurred or even vanished representation. Such segmentation can be done in the 2D projections as well as in the corresponding 3D reconstructed volume. Whereas classic MAR methods like normalized and frequency split metal artifact reduction method (NMAR,FSMAR) [2, 3] use advanced threshold-based metal segmentation methods in 3D, recent segmentation methods has shown the high potential of deep learning based models like e.g. shown by Ronneberger et al. [4]. Despite these advancements, recent MAR methods oftentimes still use thresholding methods in 3D for metal segmentation in the volume [5, 6] although this method has clear disadvantages. Firstly, the present artifacts in the 3D volume (caused by the metal itself) strongly aggravates the segmentation task and makes a clean thresholding difficult and secondly, metal which lies outside the field of view (FOV) of the reconstructed volume can not be segmented at all. Thus, the unsegmented metal parts will not be processed by the MAR and consequently still cause heavy artifacts in the volume. In contrast, segmentation methods on the 2D projection images have the possibility to find all present metal and thus should be preferred.

In order to tackle the mentioned problems, we investigate the difference in performance of 2D projection-based networks, the first using a patch-wise segmentation which is trained and tested for two patch-sizes and using a sliding window with stitching and the second performing segmentation on the complete projection image at once. Furthermore, a segmentation Consistency Check (CC) is introduced as a post processing step, which robustly removes falsely segmented structures, whilst ensuring consistent segmentation masks.

2 Materials and methods

2.1 Network architectures

Due to the proven performance of the U-Net architecture in segmenting medical images [4], the proposed networks are inspired by it. Thereby, the non-patched architecture version which has an input image size of 976×976 pixels, consists of seven contracting blocks and seven expanding blocks with skip-connections in between. Starting with 8 feature maps in its first layer, the network has 1024 feature maps at its bottleneck, each with a size of 8×8 pixels. The expanding path of the network is designed that it expands the processed image to its initial size. In accordance with that, its patch-based counterpart has input image sizes of 128×128 and 256×256 pixels and the same-/doubled-sized bottleneck. Thus, it consists of only 4 contracting and 4 expanding blocks.

2.2 Data

To train the networks, we acquired suitable X-ray projection images by performing two consecutive 3D short-scans, the first with and the second without metal implants. These scans were collected during two cadaver studies of human knees, using a Siemens Cios Spin system and following an acquisition protocol similar to [7]. During both studies, in total 32 corresponding 3D scans were acquired, each consisting of 400 projection images, covering a variety of metal implants, that were placed on the skin or directly on and inside the bone. The corresponding ground truth (GT) labels for the metal segmentation task can be

6   Gottschalk et al.

generated by subtraction. Thus, we are able to train our networks using real acquired X-ray projections which should provide a good generalization to clinical knee data. The data set was split into 22 3D scans for training, 8 for testing and 2 for validation.

2.3 Experiment protocol

As a preprocessing step, the acquired RAW data was converted into line integral data. This was done by using Lambert-Beer Law [8], where the measured intensities were normalized with the initially emitted intensity and then the logarithm was applied. Both networks were trained from scratch using the same data split, the same cross-entropy based loss function, a decaying learning rate (start: $1e^{-6}$) and an online augmentation scheme with randomized left-right flips, rotations, contrast and brightness scaling and different amount of added Poisson noise to mimic varying image acquisition qualities. For training of the patch-based segmentation networks, a randomized cropping with sizes of 128 or 256, resp. is added to the online augmentation scheme. All networks were trained until convergence. In cases of patch-wise segmentation, a sliding window (step size 32 or 64 resp.) with stitching was implemented, where the values of the overlapping windows are summed up in order to segment the complete projection.

2.4 Consistency check

By exploiting the underlying consistency conditions of 3D reconstructions, we propose a segmentation Consistency Check which is able to reduce false positive segmentations and simultaneously accounts for consistency of the mask among the stack of segmentations and which consists of three steps. The first step is a back-projection of the complete stack of binarized segmentation masks into a 3D volume. In contrast to the initial diagnostic volume which has in our case 512^3 voxels (voxel size of 0.31 mm), the size of this volume is chosen larger and in a way that the reconstruction of the binarized masks includes all metal parts present. This leads to a volume size of 920^3 voxels with again a voxel size of 0.31 mm. Due to the fact that we back-project binary masks, each voxel of the corresponding volume can be understood as a "visitor counter" which provides information about how many of the 2D metal masks actually contributed to each specific voxel. By normalizing each voxel value with the maximal amount of possible "visitors", we account for the reduced amount of rays outside the FOV of the volume. Consequently, the voxel values lie in the range of 0 and 1, where a voxel with a value of 0 corresponds to no contribution and a voxel with a value of 1 corresponds to a contribution from all 2D metal masks. Thus, each voxel value provides information about how consistently the corresponding metal part was segmented across the projections. Consequently, applying a threshold of e.g. 0.95 in order to create a binary 3D metal mask in the reconstruction, is equivalent to only including the parts into the 3D mask that were segmented in at least 95% of the projections. Thus, by performing the final forward projection, a

Table 1. Results for the AUC of the three different segmentation networks.The results are calculated over the complete test data set.

Patch Size	Avg.	Min	Max
No patching	0.967	0.952	0.990
256x256	0.972	0.960	0.984
128x128	0.983	0.973	0.994

Table 2. Average results of the 128 patch-sized network for IoU, Dice Score, Precision and Recall for different thresholds for mask binarization in combination with or without the proposed CC.

Thres.	CC	Avg. IoU	Avg. Dice	Avg. Precision	Avg. Recall
5	no	0.783±0.107	0.855+0.095	0.598±0.200	0.995±0.023
5	yes	0.924±0.032	0.959±0.024	0.873±0.039	0.975±0.038
30	no	0.913±0.034	0.952±0.026	0.850±0.052	0.978±0.041
30	yes	0.917±0.042	0.954±0.029	0.917±0.031	0.908±0.073
55	no	0.913±0.040	0.952±0.029	0.895±0.042	0.925±0.076
55	yes	0.832±0.084	0.954±0.060	0.954±0.027	0.707±0.171

stack of 2D metal masks that only include consistently segmented parts, is provided. Consequently, the inconsistent false positive segmentations are removed. Thereby, the classification into consistent or inconsistent parts is defined by the chosen threshold.

3 Results

By having a look at Tab. 1, it can be observed that all three networks perform on a high level. Whereas the patch-based segmentation using the patch-size of 128 results in the largest AUC, the increased patch-size of 256 results in a slightly decreased AUC. Using the network segmenting on the complete projection, generates the lowest AUC.

In Tab. 2 the results for the combination of three different thresholds (5, 30, 55) for the binarization of the patch-wise network's output with and without the proposed CC are illustrated. It can be seen that using the thresholds 30 and 55 for binarization without CC result in overall high metric scores, whereas using a threshold of 5 results in significant lower scores for all metrics, expect the avg. recall. The shown images b) to d) of Fig. 1 support the quantitative results. It can be seen that the mask in image b) contains a higher amount of falsely segmented structures. However, especially at the bottom edge, the metal implant is still segmented, whereas those parts are missing in images c) and d). Having a look at the configurations applying the proposed CC, it can be observed that the evaluation metrics are significantly increased when being combined with the lowest threshold of 5. This combination reaches the highest avg. IoU and Dice score among all tested configurations (Tab. 2). Whereas the scores marginally increase for the threshold 30 with CC, decreasing scores can be investigated for threshold 55 with CC. The observed effects are also visible in images f) to h) in Fig. 1.

4 Discussion

By investigating the AUC values for the three evaluated network setups, it becomes clear that all setups perform on a high level with mean AUC values of almost reaching 1. Having a closer look shows that patching in general seems to be beneficial and that a reduction of the patch-size further increases the performance. However, in future work, the influence of more patch-sizes should be investigated. Based on these results the subsequent tests of the proposed CC were evaluated using the best-performing network with a patch size of 128.

When neglecting the CC at first, it can be investigated that using thresholds 30 and 55 result in an supposedly high performance with respect to the quantitative results (Tab. 2), whereas using the threshold 5 leads to a poor performance. This effect is due to the high amount of falsely segmented structures as can be seen in Fig. 1 image b). However, despite the high metric scores and rather convenient looking mask for threshold 30 and 55, neither the quantitative nor the qualitative evaluation provide distinct information about how consistent the respective segmentations are. Due to the fact that consistency among the complete stack of segmented masks of a 3D scan is crucial for the quality of the corresponding reconstruction, this information is important. Inconsistencies in the segmented metal masks will lead to streaking artifacts in the volume. Having a look at the results after applying the proposed CC, it can be observed that the performance of the threshold 5 is significantly boosted with respect to the quantitative results, whereas the performance of the threshold 30 only marginally

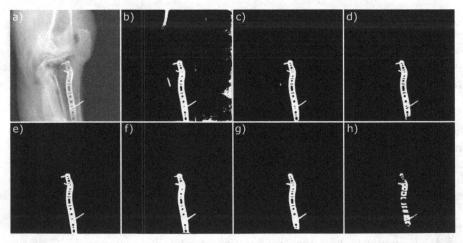

Fig. 1. a) and e) show the 2D projection and GT mask, whereas b),c) and d) correspond to the binary result masks for the thresholds 5, 30 and 55 using the 128 patch-sized network. Images f) to h) show the masks after being processed by the proposed CC.

increases and the performance for the threshold of 55 even decreases. The distinct increase for the threshold of 5 can be explained by the complete removal of false positive segmentations. The same holds for threshold 30. However, a more interesting result can be drawn from image h) in Fig. 1. Applying the CC reveals and simultaneously fixes the problem that the initial segmentation using a threshold of 55 was inconsistent which results in removed metal parts. Despite the correspondingly decreased segmentation metrics, we are confident that the newly reached consistency within the mask will result in less artifacts in the corresponding volume. However this hypothesis needs to be further investigated. Concluding the discussion about the proposed Consistency Check, it can be stated that CC is able to remove falsely positive segmented structures whilst simultaneously enforcing consistency of the segmentation. Both should be beneficial for subsequent MAR methods. Based on the fact that the proposed patch-wise segmentation networks were trained using real X-ray scans, we are confident that the method generalizes well to clinical cases. Nonetheless, this should be further investigated in future work.

Acknowledgement. The authors gratefully acknowledge funding of the Erlangen Graduate School in Advanced Optical Technologies (SAOT) by the Bavarian State Ministry for Science and Art. Furthermore, the authors like to thank the Rimasys GmbH for their extensive support during the cadaver studies.

Disclaimer. The methods and information presented here are based on research and are not commercially available.

References

1. Stille M, Kratz B, Müller J, et al. Influence of metal segmentation on the quality of metal artifact reduction methods. In: Medical Imaging 2013: Physics of Medical Imaging. vol. 8668. International Society for Optics and Photonics. SPIE; 2013. p. 902 – 907.
2. Meyer E, Raupach R, Lell M, et al. Normalized metal artifact reduction (NMAR) in computed tomography. Med Phys. 2010;37(10):5482–5493.
3. Meyer E, Raupach R, Lell M, et al. Frequency split metal artifact reduction (FS-MAR) in computed tomography. Med Phys. 2012;39(4):1904–1916.
4. Ronneberger O, Fischer P, Brox T; Springer. U-net: Convolutional networks for biomedical image segmentation. Proc MICCAI. 2015; p. 234–241.
5. Yu L, Zhang Z, Li X, et al. Deep sinogram completion with image prior for metal artifact reduction in CT images. IEEE Trans Med Imaging. 2020; p. 1–1.
6. Peng C, Li B, Li M, et al. An irregular metal trace inpainting network for X-ray CT metal artifact reduction. Med Phys. 2020;47(9):4087–4100. Available from: https://aapm.onlinelibrary.wiley.com/doi/abs/10.1002/mp.14295.
7. Gottschalk TM, Kreher BW, Kunze H, et al. Deep learning based metal inpainting in the projection domain: Initial results. In: Proc MLMIR. Springer; 2019. p. 125–136.
8. Maier A, Steidl S, Christlein V, et al. Medical imaging systems: An introductory guide. vol. 11111. Springer; 2018.

Localization of the Locus Coeruleus in MRI via Coordinate Regression

Max Dünnwald[1,2], Matthew J. Betts[3,4,6], Emrah Düzel[3,4,5],
Steffen Oeltze-Jafra[1,6]

[1]Department of Neurology, Otto von Guericke University Magdeburg (OVGU)
[2]Faculty of Computer Science, OVGU
[3]German Center for Neurodegenerative Diseases (DZNE), Magdeburg
[4]Institute of Cognitive Neurology and Dementia Research, OVGU
[5]Institute of Cognitive Neuroscience, University College London
[6]Center for Behavioral Brain Sciences (CBBS), OVGU
`max.duennwald@med.ovgu.de`

Abstract. The locus coeruleus (LC) is a small nucleus in the brain stem. It is gaining increasing interest of the neuroscientific community due to its potentially important role in the pathogenesis of several neurodegenerative diseases such as Alzheimer's disease. In this study, an existing LC segmentation approach has been improved by adding a preceding LC localization to reduce false positive segments. For the localization, we propose a network that can be trained using coordinate regression and allows insights into its function via attention maps.

1 Introduction

The locus coeruleus (LC) is a small brain structure in the upper dorsolateral pontine tegmentum of the brainstem. It is involved in several important functions, such as memory, learning, attention, arousal and pain modulation [1]. The LC currently attracts increasing interest, since it may also play an important role in the pathogenesis of neurodegenerative diseases [1]. It has been found, that so-called neuromelanin sensitive Magnetic Resonance Imaging (MRI) allows the in-vivo visualization of the LC. Further investigations require a delineation of the LC for which manual segmentation methods have primarily been applied to date [2]. One of the few exceptions employed a Convolutional Neural Network for this task, namely an adapted version of the 3D-Unet [3], and was published recently [4].

LC segmentation is a challenging task that results in relatively low inter-rater agreements, which are characterized by a Dice Similarity Coefficient (DSC) in the range of 0.499 to 0.64 [5, 6], depending on the used acquisition and segmentation protocols as well as the experience of the rater. A reason for this is the substantial uncertainty in the measurements, which is mostly caused by the small size of the LC, requiring an appropriate resolution. Higher resolutions however, yield worse

© Der/die Autor(en), exklusiv lizenziert durch
Springer Fachmedien Wiesbaden GmbH, ein Teil von Springer Nature 2021
C. Palm et al. (Hrsg.), *Bildverarbeitung für die Medizin 2021*,
Informatik aktuell, https://doi.org/10.1007/978-3-658-33198-6_5

signal to noise ratios (SNRs) jeopardizing the relatively weak signal. Nonetheless, reasonable compromises can be found and the resulting hyperintense regions (or properties of them) were shown to correspond to LC properties obtained in post-mortem studies, such as anatomical position and dimensions, LC cell density [7] and age-related effects of neuromelanin aggregation [1].

In this work, we propose a pipeline for LC segmentation (Fig. 1) that outperforms the approach in [4]. Instead of a false positives removal requiring careful parameterization, we apply an initial localization network, that was trained to regress the coordinates of LCs centers of mass (COMs) to obtain a single relevant patch containing the LC. This patch is then, processed by the 3D-Unet of [4]. This pipeline is more efficient, as the number of inferences is substantially lower, since the application is no longer done in a sliding window manner, while reducing false positive segments outside of the relevant region. For the localization network, we propose a combination of 3D-Unet and a differentiable spatial to numerical transform (DSNT) [8]. This architecture offers two major advantages: it allows insights into the networks function via attention maps as well as the processing of input volumes of arbitrary shape.

2   Materials and methods

2.1   Data

This work utilizes the same data set as in [9] and [4]. It contains T_1-weighted FLASH 3T MRI whole-brain acquisitions of 82 healthy subjects, of which 25 are younger (22-30 years old; 13 male, 12 female) and 57 are older adults (61-80 years; 19 male, 38 female). The LCs were manually segmented by two expert raters, however, for this study, we made use of the masks of just one of the raters. Prior to delineation, the data was upsampled from an isotropic voxel size of 0.75mm^3 to 0.375mm^3 by means of a sinc filter. Additionally, a bias field correction was applied. For more details on the data set, see [9].

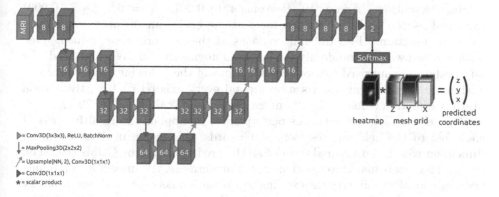

Fig. 1. Schematic illustration of CoRe-Unet, which directly predicts the coordinates of a voxel in the input volume. The white numbers denote the number of features.

2.2   Network architecture

Our network is based on the version of 3D-Unet [3] described in [4]. However, a major adaption was applied. The Unet is followed by a DSNT [8] that has been adapted to work with 3D data. It applies a softmax function, such that the sum over the Unet's output's spatial dimensions (a heatmap) equals 1 and, afterwards, calculates the scalar product between the result and a mesh grid of equal size, which encodes the coordinates of each of the volumes voxels. This adaption enables the model to directly predict coordinates and has three prime advantages. It's prediction is independent of the size and shape of the input volume, which is especially useful if both whole-brain as well as slab acquisitions shall be processed without any further adaptation. Furthermore, this model can be trained directly via a regression loss of the coordinates. And finally, the heatmap that can be obtained allows insight into the network's behaviour. In contrast to [8], no further regularization steps were performed on the heatmap. To take account of GPU memory limitations, the number of features of the Unet was reduced. We will refer to the network as coordinate regression Unet or CoRe-Unet for short. The CoRe-Unet is illustrated in Fig. 1.

2.3   Evaluation scheme

The following scheme was used for the evaluation of the networks performance. First, a test set of 23 randomly selected subjects was held out. On the remaining 59 subjects, a 5-fold crossvalidation was performed. Hence, they were subdivided into 5 sets and during 5 trainings each subset was used as the validation set once, while the rest formed the training set for the respective training iteration. Every training lasted 500 epochs and converged without exception, while the final weights were chosen based on the validation set loss performance.

The network was trained with the data of the original isotropic resolution of 0.375mm^3. As the ground truth, we determined the COMs of the LCs based on the manual segmentations and propagated their coordinates into the lower, original resolution. Adam [10] (learning rate 0.001, $\beta_1 = 0.9$, $\beta_2 = 0.999$) was used as the optimization scheme and the euclidean distance was chosen as a loss function. Two different versions of the network were trained. One with and one without randomly applied data augmentation. When applied, the augmentation comprised random combinations of the following transformations within the specified ranges: rotation around every axis (-15°, 15°), translation in every direction (-image_size/2, image_size/2) and scaling (-20%, 20%).

For determining the networks performance, we applied the resulting nets of each fold to the held-out test set. Afterwards, the euclidean distance and a dimension-wise mean squared error of all the predictions to the COMs (based on the manual raters mask) were calculated. Furthermore, the impact of combining the CoRe localization with the existing segmentation network of [4] was assed by computing and comparing the resulting DSC ($DSC = \frac{2TP}{2TP+FP+FN}$) and False Discovery Rates ($FDR = \frac{FP}{FP+TP}$) for three cases: First, applying the 3D-Unet

Table 1. Errors measured in euclidean distance of the respective networks predicted coordinates and the COM of the manually created LC masks. Every cell contains the values for left and right LC in Millimeters (mm) and voxels (vx).

	no augmentation	with augmentation
mean	2.97mm (3.96vx), 3.13mm (4.18vx)	1.34mm (1.79vx), 1.23mm (1.64vx)
std	1.56mm (2.08vx), 1.52 (2.02vx)	0.86mm (1.15vx), 0.67mm (0.89vx)

[4] in a sliding window fashion without any post-processing, apart from a tresholding with a value of 0.5 (labeled "no post-processing" - NPP). Second, the same with the post-processing steps suggested by [4] (labeled "post-processing" - PP), which requires setting several parameters that had been determined empirically. Third, using the CoRe localizer for pre-processing, i.e. passing only one patch, generated with the localizers predicted coordinates as the center (labeled "localizer pre-processing" - LPP), to the 3D-Unet without any further post-processing. The median and maximum contrast ratios (CRs) between LC and a reference region in the pons represent popular LC biomarkers [2]. To gain insights into how the addition of the localizer affects them, they were determined for the aforementioned three variants as well and the intra-class coefficients (ICCs) (confidence 0.95) were calculated for each fold to compare them to the CRs determined using the manual masks.

3 Results

The errors measured as euclidean distances, which are reported in Table 1, indicate better performance for the network that was trained with augmentation (AUG), as its errors are often less than half than those of the version, that was trained without augmentation (NoAUG). For AUG, we determined the mean squared errors of each dimension and found that in axial direction

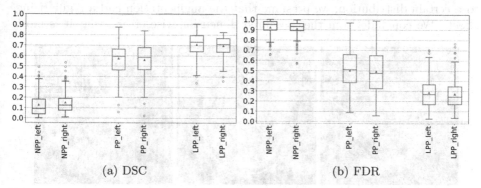

(a) DSC   (b) FDR

Fig. 2. Boxplots of DSCs and FDRs calculated for different scenarios: NPP: applied the segmentation net from [4] without its post-processing step; PP: same as NPP, but with the post-processing; LPP: using the proposed localizer (CoRe-Unet + AUG) to extract a patch that is passed to the net of [4]. "_left" and "_right" encode the respective LC.

(left LC: 2.27mm ±2.99mm, right LC: 1.68mm ±1.85mm), the errors are substantially larger than in both sagittal (left LC: 0.13mm ±0.16mm, right LC:
0.12mm ±0.17mm) and coronal (left LC: 0.14mm ±0.18mm, right LC: 0.15mm
±0.18mm) direction. This trend was not observed in NoAUG.

Furthermore, the boxplots in Figure 2 show, that the scenario including the
CoRe-Unet as a pre-processing step to determine the relevant patch first (LPP),
yielded preferable segmentation performance of the subsequent 3D-Unet in terms
of both reported metrics as compared to the other tested options (NPP, PP [4]).
This trend continues when assessing the ICCs of the CRs. The average ICC
of NPP was close to zero (for median CRs: 0.06, for maximum CRs: 0.01).
PP slightly improved to averages of 0.37 and 0.16 for median and maximum
CRs respectively. LPP obtained average ICCs of 0.89 (median CRs) and 0.66
(maximum CRs).

4   Discussion

The calculation of the errors and their standard deviations reported in Table 1
indicated, that using augmentation during the training increases the performance
of the network. Although the statistical significance of the performance difference
remains to be determined, further investigation of possible reasons for this was
carried out. We examined the heatmaps that are produced as a byproduct and
that allow insight into the attention of the network. A clear trend, which is
illustrated in Figure 3 by an example could be found. While the heatmaps of
AUG have focussed on the actual position of LC, the NoAUG version merely
highlighted structures that, when the scalar product is calculated, result in a
coordinate roughly in the center of the pons. The latter is undesirable behaviour
that indicates that the network did not learn to localize the LC itself, but relied
on correlating, more prominent structures. Similar to the additional weighted
term in the loss function proposed by [8] that forces similarity of the heatmap
to a certain distribution, we presume that the augmentation had a regularizing
effect. We conclude from the measured dimension-wise errors, that it is most

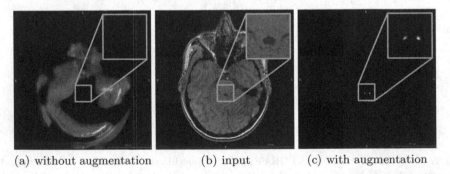

(a) without augmentation   (b) input   (c) with augmentation

Fig. 3. An exemplary slice of a testset sample (b) and the corresponding heatmaps of
the network once trained without augmentation (a) and once with augmentation (c).
The heatmaps for left and right LC have been added for better visualization.

challenging for the network to determine the rostrocaudal extent of the LC. The experiments wrt. the different LC segmentation pipeline versions (NPP, PP, LPP) suggest that the option utilizing the CoRe localizer performs preferable to the others. We found quite substantial differences between the results of our PP option and the values reported in [4], which we assume have their origin in the different evaluation scheme applied in this study.

The results of this work suggest that including a CoRe-Unet localizer as a pre-processing step in the established LC segmentation pipeline can improve the performance. This improvement is mostly achieved by reducing false positive regions outside the relevant vicinity of the LC. Visual inspection of the heatmaps found that the method shows potential for generating segmentation masks. In this case, instead of laborously delineating a complete mask, it would be sufficient to merely select single points per LC as the ground truth for training. Therefore, we will investigate this approach as a weakly supervised segmentation method in future work.

Acknowledgement. This work received funding from the federal state of Saxony-Anhalt, Germany (Project I 88).

References

1. Betts MJ, Kirilina E, Otaduy MCG, et al. Locus coeruleus imaging as a biomarker for noradrenergic dysfunction in neurodegenerative diseases. Brain. 2019;142(9):2558–2571.
2. Liu KY, Marijatta F, Hämmerer D, et al. Magnetic resonance imaging of the human locus coeruleus: a systematic review. Neuroscience & Biobehavioral Reviews. 2017;83:325–355.
3. Çiçek O, Abdulkadir A, Lienkamp SS, et al. 3D U-Net: learning dense volumetric segmentation from sparse annotation. Med Image Comput Comput Assist Interv – MICCAI 2016. 2016; p. 424–432.
4. Dünnwald M, Betts MJ, Sciarra A, et al. Automated segmentation of the locus coeruleus from neuromelanin-sensitive 3T MRI using deep convolutional neural networks. Bildverarbeitung für die Medizin 2020. 2020; p. 61–66.
5. Ariz M, Abad RC, Castellanos G, et al. Dynamic atlas-based segmentation and quantification of euromelanin-rich brainstem structures in parkinson disease. IEEE Trans Med Imaging. 2019;38(3):813–823.
6. Tona KD, Keuken MC, de Rover M, et al. In vivo visualization of the locus coeruleus in humans: quantifying the test–retest reliability. Brain Struct Funct. 2017;222(9):4203–4217.
7. Keren NI, Lozar CT, Harris KC, et al. In vivo mapping of the human locus coeruleus. NeuroImage. 2009;47(4):1261–1267.
8. Nibali A, He Z, Morgan S, et al. Numerical coordinate regression with convolutional neural networks. arXiv:180107372 [cs]. 2018;.
9. Betts MJ, Cardenas-Blanco A, Kanowski M, et al. In vivo MRI assessment of the human locus coeruleus along its rostrocaudal extent in young and older adults. NeuroImage. 2017;163:150–159.
10. Kingma DP, Ba J. Adam: a method for stochastic optimization. arXiv:14126980 [cs]. 2017;.

Semantically Guided 3D Abdominal Image Registration with Deep Pyramid Feature Learning

Mona Schumacher[1,2], Daniela Frey[3], In Young Ha[1], Ragnar Bade[2],
Andreas Genz[2], Mattias Heinrich[1]

[1]Institute of Medical Informatics, University of Lübeck
[2]MeVis Medical Solutions AG, Bremen
[3]University of Applied Sciences, Lübeck
Mona.Schumacher@mevis.de

Abstract. Deformable image registration of images with large deformations is still a challenging task. Currently available deep learning methods exceed classical non-learning-based methods primarily in terms of lower computational time. However, these convolutional networks face difficulties when applied to scans with large deformations. We present a semantically guided registration network with deep pyramid feature learning that enables large deformations by transferring features from the images to be registered to the registration networks. Both network parts have U-Net architectures. The networks are trained end-to-end and evaluated with two datasets, both containing contrast enhanced liver CT images and ground truth liver segmentations. We compared our method against one classical and two deep learning methods. Our experimental validation shows that our proposed method enables large deformation and achieves the highest Dice score and the smallest surface distance of the liver in contrast to other deep learning methods.

1 Introduction

Medical imaging techniques are important for diagnosis and treatment planning. In order to be able to ensure a detailed analysis of the structures to be examined, different images with complementary information are acquired and the information of these images have to be combined in order to be able to make a valid decision. One important example is the registration of contrast enhanced liver CT images. The organs in the abdomen are, due to their soft tissue structures, flexible and can be deformed by the (respiratory) movement of the patient, which makes a mapping of the liver and vascular systems necessary, e.g., to plan a liver surgery.

To address this issue, most classical image registration algorithms iteratively optimise a similarity metric in order to spatially align images, which leads to long computation times [1].

© Der/die Autor(en), exklusiv lizenziert durch
Springer Fachmedien Wiesbaden GmbH, ein Teil von Springer Nature 2021
C. Palm et al. (Hrsg.), *Bildverarbeitung für die Medizin 2021*,
Informatik aktuell, https://doi.org/10.1007/978-3-658-33198-6_6

Convolutional neural networks overcome the drawback of a long processing time since the iterative optimization takes place during training and not during inference [2, 3]. Most of the currently available approaches show a good performance on regions with small deformations, e.g. brain images, but have difficulties registering images with large deformations.

The aim of this work is to overcome the drawback using learning-based networks and enable large deformations. Since it is rather difficult to create ground truth data for a registration, most methods are unsupervised. One example is VoxelMorph that was introduced by Balakrishnan et al. in 2018 [2]. It is based on the intensity values in the image and can use mutual information as similarity metric to maximize the image correspondence. Besides approaches that learn in an unsupervised manner, there are also methods that use other expert information as guidance. Ha et al. in 2020 [3] focus on the 2D registration of segmentations as regions of interest and combine a U-Net segmentation and a registration network that are jointly optimized. In 2D optical flow learning, the concept of feature pyramids proposed in the PWC-Net has led to huge advances [4]. Our work combines and extends the ideas of Sun et al. and Ha et al. First, we adapted the networks to enable 3D registrations. Additionally, we overcome the drawback of the registration network, which outputs a coarse deformation field. Instead we use a U-Net architecture that additionally has a decoder path and outputs a larger deformation field. To further guide the registration, we transfer the information of each resolution of the decoder path of the semantic network to the corresponding resolution of the encoder path of registration network with skip connections.

2 Material and method

Our method consists of two parts (Fig. 1): a feature extraction and a registration part. The first part extracts the semantic features by generating a liver segmentation of the fixed and the moving image with two U-Nets that have shared weights. The deformation field is estimated in the second part by two registration networks that have U-Net architecture, hence an encoder and a decoder path. The input of the first registration network are the concatenated outputs of the fixed and moving feature extraction networks. In the downsampling path, the feature maps of the feature extraction networks are concatenated to the corresponding resolution. The output of the first registration network is an initial deformation field. The input of the second registration network are the outputs of the feature extraction networks that are warped with the initial deformation field. The feature maps of the upsampling path of the feature extraction network are also warped with the initial deformation field and are concatenated to the corresponding resolution level in the encoder path. The resulting deformation field of the second registration network is added to the initial deformation field. This sequential generation of the final deformation field enables us to align large deformations.

2.1   Semantic feature extraction

To extract semantic features in the images to be registered, two U-Nets with shared weights are used to generate liver probabilities of the fixed and the moving image. The U-Net contains three downsampling steps with convolutions with a kernel size of $3 \times 3 \times 3$, stride of 2 and a padding of 1, followed by 3D instance normalization and leaky ReLU with a slope of 0.1. The decoder part is structured parallel to the encoder part but contains only two upsampling steps. Additionally, the network contains skip connections from the encoder path to the decoder path. The output corresponds to the halved resolution of the input images. The semantic loss is a weighted cross-entropy with weights computed by the square root of the inverse class frequency for each label.

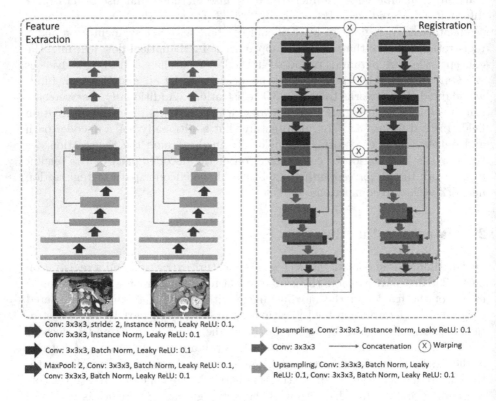

Fig. 1. Pipeline of semantically guided registration. The feature extraction part consists of two U-Nets with shared weights that extract the features of the moving and the fixed image. These features are transferred to the second part, the registration, which consists of two U-Nets connected in series. The first U-Net creates an initial deformation field, which is finalized by the second U-Net. All added elements (compared to the original architecture) are marked orange.

2.2 Registration networks

The deformation field is estimated by two registration networks with the same architecture. It comprises three downsampling and upsampling steps. In contrast, the original approach consists of four downsampling steps without upsampling. The downsampling steps contain convolutions with a kernel size of $3 \times 3 \times 3$, stride of 2 and padding of 1, followed by 3D batch normalization and leaky ReLU with a parameter of 0.1. The decoder part is structured parallel to the encoder part. The deformation and regularization loss is calculated as described in [3].

2.3 Image data

To train, validate and test our approach, and to compare it to other registration techniques, two contrast enhanced liver CT datasets are used.

The first dataset consists of 170 images: 85 images of the venous phase and 85 images of the late-venous phase. For all of these images, ground truth labels of the liver are available. The data has been manually segmented and reviewed by three experienced radiologic technicians. The CT scans and the corresponding segmentations are resampled to a voxel size of $0.9 \times 0.9 \times 1.3$ mm^3 and an initial affine registration is applied. Around the center of the segmented liver, the image is cropped to $304 \times 240 \times 144$ voxels and zero padded if necessary. The segmentations of the liver of the corresponding phases are processed in the same way. 43 images of each of the two phases are assigned to the training data set, 42 image of each phase to the test data set.

The second dataset is a publicly available dataset from the Learn2Reg MICCAI Registration Challenge 2020[1] that consists of 30 abdominal CT scans of different patients of the portal venous phase. The dataset includes ground segmentations of 13 organs, in particular also of the liver. In contrast to the first dataset, the initial average liver Dice score is much lower so that even larger deformations are required. The images are already preprocessed to the same voxelsize of $2.0 \times 2.0 \times 2.0$ mm^3, a spatial dimension of $192 \times 160 \times 256$ voxels and affine registered. For the following experiments only the liver segmentation is taken into account. 20 images are included in the training process, while 10 are used as test dataset.

3 Results

All networks are trained across patients to ensure a sufficient number of image pairs and obtain a good generalization. During training, two random images are chosen as fixed and moving images so that the choice of phases is randomized. We have performed an ablation study for the proposed pipeline. First, we adapted the original approach of Ha et al. [3] to a 3D approach and trained it with the two datasets. The resulting deformation field is of the size $9 \times 7 \times 4$ voxels for our dataset and $6 \times 5 \times 8$ for the Learn2Reg dataset. The deformation field

---

[1] https://learn2reg.grand-challenge.org/Datasets/Task 3

Table 1. Results of deformable registration with our test dataset (upper part) and the Learn2Reg test dataset (lower part). Average Dice Scores, mean of the Average Surface Distance (ASD), 95% Hausdorff Distance (HD95), lowest 30% of the Dice coefficients (Dice30), standard deviation of the Jacobian determinant, and the percentage of negative elements of the Jacobian are presented.

Method	Dice	ASD	HD95	Dice30	JacStd	JacDet<0
Affine	0.71 ± 0.12	11.74 ± 5.68	34.79 ± 17.56	0.58 ± 0.09	-	-
deeds	0.82 ± 0.11	7.73 ± 5.54	29.23 ± 20.44	0.70 ± 0.08	0.42	0.0
VoxelMorph	0.74 ± 0.11	10.56 ± 5.42	33.20 ± 17.25	0.63 ± 0.09	0.36	0.15
Ha et al.	0.87 ± 0.11	4.61 ± 2.02	16.24 ± 9.77	0.83 ± 0.04	0.77	4.62
Ours	0.90 ± 0.03	4.07 ± 2.30	15.76 ± 10.75	0.87 ± 0.02	1.55	6.22
Ours+Skip	0.91 ± 0.03	3.90 ± 2.06	15.36 ± 10.21	0.87 ± 0.02	1.30	6.12
Affine	0.62 ± 0.10	15.39 ± 4.60	49.27 ± 13.21	0.51 ± 0.06	-	-
deeds	0.83 ± 0.06	7.72 ± 4.03	35.54 ± 17.45	0.77 ± 0.06	0.49	3.78
VoxelMorph	0.68 ± 0.08	12.88 ± 3.99	45.04 ± 12.85	0.59 ± 0.05	0.35	0.38
Ha et al.	0.72 ± 0.07	10.86 ± 3.46	35.73 ± 11.77	0.65 ± 0.04	0.25	0.19
Ours	0.77 ± 0.08	9.16 ± 3.80	33.22 ± 14.61	0.67 ± 0.04	0.46	2.01
Ours+Skip	0.79 ± 0.07	8.56 ± 3.48	31.78 ± 13.80	0.71 ± 0.04	0.46	1.75

is upsampled to the cropped image size. The networks are trained end-to-end with an Adam optimizer with a learning rate of 0.01. A number of 300 epochs is carried out for the datasets.

Next, we adapted the registration networks, whereas the learning parameters remain as in the first experiment. First, the decoding path is added. Additionally, the number of downsampling steps is reduced to three. The downsampling path therefore results in a larger feature map of dimension $19 \times 15 \times 9$ for our dataset and $12 \times 10 \times 16$ for the Learn2Reg dataset. The final deformation field has the size of the input feature map. Second, further skip connections are introduced to additionally guide the registration network with semantic features (Fig. 1).

In addition, we compared our method to the classical registration algorithm deeds [1] and the deep learning registration approach VoxelMorph [2]. We adapted VoxelMorph from an atlas-based registration to an image to image registration and trained it with our image data. The mutual information loss is weighted with $\lambda = 2.0$. Due to the limited GPU memory, 20 is chosen as the number of intensity bins and a total number of 100 epochs is trained.

We used the average Dice score and the lowest 30% of the liver segmentations as metric for evaluation. Additionally, the average surface distance, the 95% Hausdorff distance, the standard deviation of the Jacobian determinant and the percentage of negative elements of the Jacobian are used as evaluation metrics.

The results for all methods for both datasets are listed in Table 1. An example slice of both networks for all methods are displayed in Fig. 2. Deeds took on average six times longer than the deep learning approaches, with all deep learning approaches taking less than 10 seconds.

Fig. 2. Exemplary registration results. The images show corresponding slices of the 3D volumes (top: our dataset, bottom: Learn2Reg dataset) with the liver segmentation as red overlay. From left to right: fixed image, moving image, deeds, VoxelMorph, Ours.

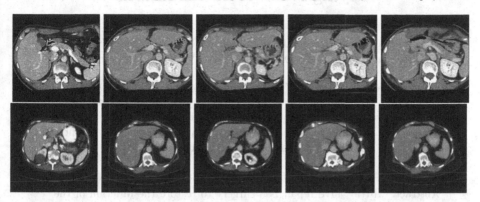

4   Discussion and conclusion

Considering inter-patient registration of the first dataset, our semantically guided registration network outperforms the remaining approaches with Dice score of 0.91 and an average surface distance of 3.90 which corresponds to an improvement of at least +4% and -0.71 voxels, respectively.

In case of the second dataset, our semantically guided registration network also outperforms the other deep learning-based methods by at least +7% for the Dice score and -2.3 voxels for the average surface distance. However, the classical method deeds is the best method for this dataset and has a higher Dice score (+4%) and a smaller surface distance (-0.84 voxels) than our method.

The different results for the two datasets can be explained trough the small number of training images for the second dataset. In general, learning-based methods are strongly dependent of the amount and quality of the dataset which leads to a good generalization of the model.

Overall, our presented approach can overcome the problems of most deep learning-based methods that have difficulties to register large deformations.

References

1. Heinrich MP, Jenkinson M, Brady M, et al. MRF-based deformable registration and ventilation estimation of lung CT. IEEE Trans Med Imaging. 2013;32(7):1239–1248.
2. Balakrishnan G, Zhao A, Sabuncu MR, et al. Voxelmorph: a learning framework for deformable medical image registration. IEEE Trans Med Imaging. 2019;38(8):1788–1800.
3. Ha IY, Wilms M, Heinrich M. Semantically guided large deformation estimation with deep networks. Sensors. 2020;20(5):1392.
4. Sun D, Yang X, Liu MY, et al. PWC-Net: CNNs for optical flow using pyramid, warping, and cost volume. Proc IEEE CVPR. 2018; p. 8934–8943.

Heatmap-based 2D Landmark Detection with a Varying Number of Landmarks

Antonia Stern[1], Lalith Sharan[1], Gabriele Romano[2], Sven Koehler[1], Matthias Karck[2], Raffaele De Simone[2], Ivo Wolf[3], Sandy Engelhardt[1]

[1]Group Artificial Intelligence in Cardiovasular Medicine (AICM), Department of Internal Medicine III, Heidelberg University Hospital, Heidelberg
[2]Department of Cardiac Surgery, Heidelberg University Hospital, Heidelberg
[3]Faculty of Computer Science, University of Applied Sciences, Mannheim
sandy.engelhardt@med.uni-heidelberg.de

Abstract. Mitral valve repair is a surgery to restore the function of the mitral valve. To achieve this, a prosthetic ring is sewed onto the mitral annulus. Analyzing the sutures, which are punctured through the annulus for ring implantation, can be useful in surgical skill assessment, for quantitative surgery and for positioning a virtual prosthetic ring model in the scene via augmented reality. This work presents a neural network approach which detects the sutures in endoscopic images of mitral valve repair and therefore solves a landmark detection problem with varying amount of landmarks, as opposed to most other existing deep learning-based landmark detection approaches. The neural network is trained separately on two data collections from different domains with the same architecture and hyperparameter settings. The datasets consist of more than $1,300$ stereo frame pairs each, with a total over $60,000$ annotated landmarks. The proposed heatmap-based neural network achieves a mean positive predictive value (PPV) of $66.68 \pm 4.67\%$ and a mean true positive rate (TPR) of $24.45 \pm 5.06\%$ on the intraoperative test dataset and a mean PPV of $81.50 \pm 5.77\%$ and a mean TPR of $61.60 \pm 6.11\%$ on a dataset recorded during surgical simulation. The best detection results are achieved when the camera is positioned above the mitral valve with good illumination. A detection from a sideward view is also possible if the mitral valve is well perceptible.

1 Introduction

Mitral valve reconstruction is a complicated surgery, where the surgeon implants a prosthetic ring to the tissue by placing approx. 12 to 15 sutures on the mitral annulus [1]. Analysing how sutures are placed (e.g., their pattern and distances) can help in improving the quality and consistency of the procedure. This could be useful in surgery itself and in preoperative simulation for trainees [2]. Besides that, the position of the sutures may be utilized to reconstruct the 3D position of the mitral annulus in a stereo-setting and a virtual ring model can be superimposed onto the endoscopic video stream prior to ring implantation [3, 4].

Springer Fachmedien Wiesbaden GmbH, ein Teil von Springer Nature 2021
C. Palm et al. (Hrsg.), *Bildverarbeitung für die Medizin 2021*,
Informatik aktuell, https://doi.org/10.1007/978-3-658-33198-6_7

Several deep learning-based methods exist for landmark detection in computer-vision and medical applications. In general, they can be classified into heatmap approaches [5, 6], coordinate regression and patch-based [7] approaches. Gilbert et al. [5] used a U-Net-like architecture to detect anatomical landmarks by predicting one heatmap per landmark. The input label heatmaps contain 2D Gaussians centred at the annotated point location. In contrast to that, coordinate regression approaches directly output the coordinates instead of heatmaps, which is less computationally expensive as no upsampling is necessary. Usually, these approaches consist of a sequence of convolutional layers along with a fully connected layer or a 1×1-convolution. Another common approach is to detect landmarks in global and local patches with the help of displacement vectors [7].

State-of-the-art literature on deep learning-based landmark detection focuses mainly on detecting a predefined number of keypoints. In medical applications, landmarks are often used to define a fixed number of anatomical points. These approaches output one heatmap for each landmark or use a vector representation of fixed length with the length corresponding to the number of keypoints. However, these methods cannot be applied to a setting with an arbitrary number of keypoints. Furthermore, in our scenario, unlike in most other works, the landmarks can lie in close proximity to each other, which makes the application of patch-based approaches difficult.

The work presented in this paper uses a network architecture that is able to deal with a varying number of landmarks, since, in principle, a varying number of sutures can be placed. This work uses a U-Net based architecture with a *single* foreground heatmap as output. Thresholding this heatmap allows us to detect a non-predefined number of points in endoscopic images, which represent the positions where the sutures enter the tissue.

2   Materials and methods

2.1   Network architecture

This work uses a U-Net-based [8] architecture with a depth of 4. After each 3×3-convolution, batch normalisation is applied. The padded 3×3-convolutional layers use the *ELU* activation function. The final layer is a 1×1-convolutional layer with a *sigmoid* activation function. The first convolutional layer has 16 filter maps, while the bottleneck layer has 256 filter maps. The number of filters is doubled/halved after every maxpooling/upsampling in the downsampling/upsampling path. The dropout rate is set to values between 0.3 and 0.5 with the lowest dropout rate in the first downsampling/last upsampling block. Unlike the original U-Net [8], our architecture applies zero-padding in the convolutional layers. Therefore, the input size has to be divisible by 4^{depth}, which equals 16 in this work. The loss function is of the form $MSE - SDC$, where MSE is the mean squared error function and SDC, the Sørensen dice coefficient.

To preserve the aspect ratio of the images, a width of 512 pixels and a height of 288 pixels was chosen as the input size. The input images are RGB-images with 3 channels. The two-channel output masks contain one channel for the suture landmarks and one for the background. This design is more efficient than heatmaps approaches, which use one channel for each landmark. The predicted output heatmap is converted into a binary mask by thresholding. Then, the centre of mass for each region is determined as point of interest.

2.2 Dataset

Two instances of the same neural network approach proposed in this work were trained separately on two different data sub-collections (Tab. 1, A.1 and B) consisting of endoscopic images of mitral valve repair. One data collection contains very heterogeneous *intraoperative* images extracted from videos which were recorded during surgery (different view angles, light intensities, number of sutures, surgical instruments, prosthesis etc.). Different amounts of frames were annotated from these datasets, therefore an additional hold-out test set was created from surgeries with significantly less frames (A.2). The other *simulation* data collection was extracted from videos of operations performed on an artificial mitral valve replica made of silicone, which was first introduced in [2] and used in surgical training applications.

The endoscopic videos were recorded from an Image S1 stereo camera (Karl Storz SE & Co. KG, Tuttlingen, Germany) in full HD resolution or larger at 25 fps. Frames were saved in top-down format (left image top, right image bottom). Relevant scenes were identified before extracting the frames from the videos and afterwards every 120*th* frame was extracted. In scenes with rapid changes, every 10*th* frame was extracted and in scenes with only few changes, every 240*th* frame was extracted. These characteristics were identified manually.

This work uses the two subimages of the stereo recording as separate input images to the network, thus the final number of frames for training and testing is twice as large as given in Tab. 1. The intraoperative dataset used for training consists of 2654 frames, which were extracted from 5 surgeries (mean 530,8 $\pm$ 213,6 frames per surgery). An additional balanced intraoperative test dataset was annotated, containing 200 frames extracted from 4 surgeries (mean 100 $\pm$ 0 frames per surgery). The simulator datasets consists of 2708 frames extracted from 10 simulated surgeries (mean 270,7 $\pm$ 77,7 frames per surgery).

The frames were manually annotated with the tool *labelme* [9]. During annotation, corresponding suture points in the left and right image of the stereo pair are joined with a line. If a suture point is only visible in one of the subimages it is marked as a point. The ground truth heatmaps were then created by placing 2D Gaussians at the position of the landmarks. For a down-scaled input size of 512×288, a variance σ of 1 was used.

During training the images are randomly augmented with a probability of 80% using tensorflow functions: rotation of $\pm 60°$, pixel shifting in a range of $\pm 10\%$, mask pixel shifting in a range of $\pm 1\%$, shearing in a range of ± 0.1, brightness in a range of ± 0.2, contrast in a range from 0.3 to 0.5, random saturation in a range from 0.5 to 2.0 and hue in a range of ± 0.1. Additionally the images were flipped horizontally and vertically with a probability of 50%.

Table 1. Three sub-collections from two different domains were used. Note that we treat left and right stereo frame independently in our work, therefore training frames are doubled. The additional intraop test set has significantly lower number of labeled frames, hence we decided to not include it directly in the cross validation (CV).

Domain	Usage	# stereo frame	# suture endpoints	# surgeries
A.1 intraop	5-fold CV (train, test)	1,327	26,937	5
A.2 intraop	test	200	4,305	4
B simulator	5-fold CV (train, test)	1,354	33,893	10

2.3 Evaluation

During method development, which involved hyperparameter tuning, training and validation was performed on dataset A.1. The best neural network had a total of $2.1M$ trainable parameters. The initial learning rate was set to 10^{-3} with a decay factor of 0.1. After fixing these parameters, final evaluation was conducted on A.1, A.2 and B, involving two 5-fold cross validations (CV) on different splits of dataset A.1 and B. Furthermore, an additional disjoint test set was used (A.2) to further assess method generalizability. To prevent data leakage, dataset splitting was always carried out on the level of the surgeries. The results are given for the epoch ≤ 200 with the lowest value of the validation loss. In total, 10 different models were trained, one for each fold of each application (intraop and simulation).

A suture point detection is considered successful if the centres of mass of ground truth and prediction are less than 6 pixels apart. On an image of size 512×288, this radius roughly corresponds to the thickness of a suture when it enters the tissue. If a point in the produced mask or the ground truth mask is assigned multiple times, only the matched pair with the least distance is kept. Every matched point from the produced mask is considered a true positive (TP). Predicted points that could not be matched to any ground truth point are defined as false positives (FP) and all ground truth points without a corresponding point in the produced mask are false negatives (FN). To evaluate the precision (positive predictive value, PPV) and sensitivity (true positive rate, TPR) are used. Precision and sensitivity are defined as $PPV = TP/(TP + FP)$ and $TPR = TP/(TP + FN)$. The values of PPV and TPR are displayed over a threshold from 0.05 to 1.0 to show the influence of thresholding the heatmap on the detection rate.

3 Results

Some visual examples are provided in Fig. 1(a) and Fig.1(b). In intraoperative images, green sutures are better recognized than white ones because they can be better distinguished from the background. During surgery (not during simulation), white sutures often appear red because they are soaked with blood which makes it even harder to distinguish them from the background.

The model achieved a mean PPV of $67.99 \pm 7.69\%$ and a mean TPR of $29.03 \pm 7.74\%$ on the intraoperative dataset (A.1) for a threshold of $t = 0.8$ during testing on the respective hold-out folds (Fig. 2(a)). All models from the CV were also applied to the separate test set (A.2) and comparable results were obtained with a mean PPV of $66.68 \pm 4.67\%$ and a mean TPR of $24.45 \pm 5.06\%$ (Fig. 2(b)), meaning that it generalizes beyond the surgeries where hyperparameter tuning was performed on. When training the model on the simulator dataset (B) with the same settings, a mean PPV of $81.50 \pm 5.77\%$ and a mean TPR of $61.60 \pm 6.11\%$ is achieved during CV (Fig. 2(c)). As can be seen in the plots, the estimated TPR and PPV are not sensitive with regard to the chosen threshold. Performance differences between the folds are expressed by the bars in Fig. 2.

4 Discussion

The developed approach is able to detect a varying number of landmarks, which represent the position of sutures stitched through the mitral annulus. Evaluation on a large dataset of two domains revealed that the neural networks detects sutures in most of the scenes, but had difficulties in cases where the mitral annulus is partly occluded by the prosthetic ring, the surgical tools or tissue (Fig. 1(a) 4th image). Reflections or embossings on tools has also led to an increase in FPs (Fig. 1(b) 3rd image). The best detection results were achieved when the camera

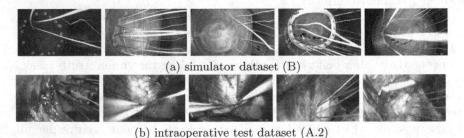

(a) simulator dataset (B)

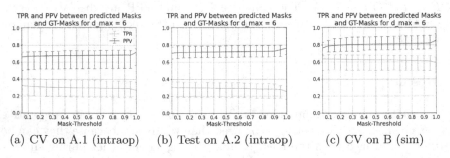

(b) intraoperative test dataset (A.2)

Fig. 1. Example predictions on the two domains. Green circles represent true positives (TP), red circles show false positives (FP) and orange circles show false negatives (FN).

(a) CV on A.1 (intraop)   (b) Test on A.2 (intraop)   (c) CV on B (sim)

Fig. 2. The mean PPV and TPR of all folds with variable mask threshold. The bars show the value of the fold with the lowest and highest value respectively.

was positioned above the mitral valve with good illumination. Comparing both domains, the network performance was better on the simulation domain, where the camera angle is often more favorable and the silicone appearance is more homogeneous in comparison to intraoperative scenes with various tissue textures and blood. However, the performance differences could be also explained by the higher numbers of simulated surgery instances used during training in the simulator domain.

In this work, two neural networks were trained separately on two datasets from different domains with the same architecture and hyperparameter settings. Future work includes incorporating image-to-image translation by generative adversarial networks [10] to adapt between the domains and to allow for joint landmark detection in both domains.

Acknowledgement. The research was supported by the German Research Foundation DFG Project 398787259, DE 2131/2-1 and EN 1197/2-1 and by Informatics for Life funded by the Klaus Tschira Foundation.

References

1. Carpentier A, Adams D, Filsoufi F. Carpentier's reconstructive valve surgery. Saunders; 2010.
2. Engelhardt S, Sauerzapf S, Preim B, et al. Flexible and comprehensive patient-specific mitral valve silicone models with chordae tendinae made from 3D-printable molds. Int J Comput Assist Radiol Surg. 2019;14(7):1177–1186.
3. Engelhardt S, De Simone R, Zimmermann N, et al. Augmented reality-enhanced endoscopic images for annuloplasty ring sizing. In: Augmented Environments for Computer-Assisted Interventions. Springer International Publishing; 2014. p. 128–137.
4. Engelhardt S, Kolb S, De Simone R, et al. Endoscopic feature tracking for augmented-reality assisted prosthesis selection in mitral valve repair. In: Proc SPIE, Medical Imaging: Image-Guided Procedures, Robotic Interventions, and Modeling. vol. 9786; 2016. p. 402–408.
5. Gilbert A, Holden M, Eikvil L, et al. Automated left ventricle dimension measurement in 2D cardiac ultrasound via an anatomically meaningful CNN approach. In: Smart Ultrasound Imaging and Perinatal, Preterm and Paediatric Image Analysis. Springer International Publishing; 2019. p. 29–37.
6. Jin H, Liao S, Shao L. Pixel-in-pixel net: towards efficient facial landmark detection in the wild. arXiv:200303771v1 [csCV]. 2020;.
7. Noothout JMH, De Vos BD, Wolterink JM, et al. Deep learning-based regression and classification for automatic landmark localization in medical images. IEEE Trans on Med Imag. 2020; p. 1–1.
8. Ronneberger O, Fischer P, Brox T. U-Net: convolutional networks for biomedical image segmentation. Proc MICCAI. 2015;9351:234–241.
9. Wada K. labelme: image polygonal annotation with python; 2016. https://github.com/wkentaro/labelme.
10. Engelhardt S, Simone RD, Full PM, et al. Improving surgical training phantoms by hyperrealism: deep unpaired image-to-image translation from real surgeries. Proc MICCAI. 2018; p. 747–755.

Ultrasound-based Navigation of Scaphoid Fracture Surgery

Peter Broessner[0], Benjamin Hohlmann[0], Klaus Radermacher

[0]Both authors contributed equally
Chair of Medical Engineering, RWTH Aachen
hohlmann@hia.rwth-aachen.de

Abstract. For minimally-invasive surgery of the scaphoid, navigation based on ultrasound images instead of fluoroscopy reduces costs and prevents exposure to ionizing radiation. We present a machine learning based two-stage approach that tackles the tasks of image segmentation and point cloud registration individually. For this, Deeplabv3+ as well as the PRNet architecture were trained on two newly generated datasets. An evaluation on in-vitro data results in an average surface distance error of 1.1 mm and a mean rotational deviation of $6.2°$ with a processing time of 9 seconds. We conclude that near real-time navigation is feasible.

1 Introduction

Of all carpal bones, the scaphoid is the most frequently fractured one, accounting for about 60% of all fractures [1]. For diagnosis of fractures a comprehensive exam including bi-planar radiography as well as computed tomography (CT) and possibly magnetic resonance imaging (MRI) and ultrasound (US) is standard. Given this rich image based pre-operative information, the decision upon conservative treatment using a cast, or operative treatment is based on the stability of the fracture. Fractures of the proximal third as well as displaced fractures indicate an operative treatment. Stable or non-displaced cases may also be treated operatively to fasten the recovery [1].

Surgery can be performed in an open as well as minimally-invasive fashion. While strongly dislocated cases require an open surgery, minimally-invasive surgery (MIS) is recommended whenever possible due to minimized operative trauma, preservation of carpal ligaments and faster recovery. During surgery, the bone fragments are united using an osteosynthesis screw. The exact placement of this screw is crucial for surgical success. In MIS, placement and validation, which takes place under continuous fluoroscopy, is a challenging task due to the limited spatial perception of the three-dimensional position in the two-dimensional projected radiographs. Furthermore, the patient and surgeon are exposed to ionizing radiation. Therefore, this work investigates ultrasound as a cheap and readily available alternative to fluoroscopy. Yet, ultrasound is limited in terms of signal-to-noise ratio as well as occlusion.

Intra-operative registration of ultrasound images to pre-operatively acquired models is a common concept in navigated surgery. For surgery of the scaphoid, which poses a hard problem due to the small size of the bone, several authors proposed concepts and validated them in in-vitro, ex-vivo as well as in-vivo studies. The earliest procedure, proposed by Beek et al., involves a semi-automatic heuristic, requiring the user to set seed points. Subsequently, the pre-operative plan is manually aligned to the intra-operative ultrasound image and the position is refined using the iterative closest point algorithm (ICP). While the method proofed viable regarding realization of the surgical plan, it requires manual interaction with reported times of 5-10 minutes [2]. Following a breakthrough of ultrasound segmentation techniques, Anas et al. improved the procedure by incorporating phase symmetry pre-processing as well as statistical shape and pose models into the segmentation process [3]. They enhance the symmetric high intensity interfaces, like the bone surface, in the ultrasound image by computing the phase symmetry. To distinguish bone from soft-tissue interfaces, the bone's shadow is incorporated as an additional feature. After that, a statistical shape and pose model of all carpal bones is manually aligned to the ultrasound image. The alignment is optimized in an Expectation Maximization framework using Gaussian Mixture Models. This algorithm reduces the manual interaction while at the same time improving the registration accuracy. They evaluated their technique in in-vitro [3], ex-vivo [4] and in-vivo [3] studies and achieved a processing time of about 90 seconds.

In recent years, the computer vision community achieved great advances in automatic semantic segmentation of the bone surface in in-vivo ultrasound images. Pandey et al. reviewed 56 articles on this specific task [5]. Most of the publications included fully automatic methods with a clear tendency to machine learning based approaches in the recent past.

Given the success of Convolutional Neural Networks (CNN) on images the concept was transferred to point sets. Wang et al. used a graph based approach for convolution-like computations [6]. Their Dynamic Graph CNN (DGCNN) is the backbone used in the Partial Registration Network (PRNet), a machine learning based architecture for partial point set registration [7].

In this work, we present the first fully automatic as well as near-real time capable algorithm for ultrasound based navigation of scaphoid fracture surgery. We further proof its feasibility in an in-vitro study. We propose a two-stage architecture, tackling the problems of segmentation and registration individually. As machine learning based segmentation is a well studied problem, we focus on evaluating the registration.

2 Materials and methods

In order to allow a navigated fixation of scaphoid fractures, a preoperative virtual object, including the surgical plan, has to be intra-operatively registered to the therapeutical object. For this purpose, the aforementioned two-stage approach is proposed (Fig. 1): in a first step, a tracked 3D US probe is used for the acquisition of slice images, which are subsequently segmented by a neural network. The pixels labeled as scaphoid surface are then skeletonized and uniformly sampled to obtain a surface point set (depicted in red). In a second step, the point set of the source model (depicted in blue) is registered to this sampled point set, again using a neural network.

2.1 Architectures

For the task of semantic segmentation, the DeepLabv3+ [8] architecture is selected. It is characterized by an encoder-decoder structure with atrous separable convolution for spatial pyramid pooling. In combination with a MobileNetv2 [9] backbone it offers a compromise between performance on the one hand and a reduced number of trainable parameters on the other hand, which is favorable given the rather small size of the training data set.

The subsequent task of registration is quite challenging: Points sampled from a partial surface have to be registered to points representing the complete surface, without real point correspondences and disturbed by errors of segmentation. The task is further complicated by the fact that the use of shared architectures for feature extraction requires the point sets to be of equal size, which in our case leads to different spatial resolutions. To meet these challenges, the PRNet architecture in combination with a DGCNN backbone seems most promising and is employed in the course of this work. The DGCNN utilizes a convolution-like learning of filters on dynamically updated k-nearest neighbors for the extraction of local and global point features; in PRNet, these feature vectors are co-contextualized by a Transformer, which in combination addresses the difficulty of partial-to-full registration. Furthermore, PRNet aims at establishing non-bijective correspondences with variable sharpness by using gumbel softmax, which addresses the lack of real correspondences and the difficulty of different spatial resolutions.

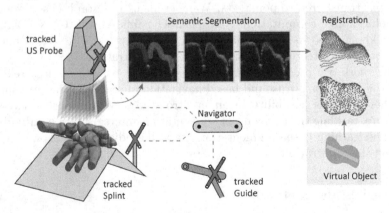

Fig. 1. Intra-operative procedure for the registration of therapeutical object and virtual object: the US image slices acquired by a 3D US probe are fed into a segmentation network. The resulting masks are thinned and sampled to a partial point set, which is registered to the point set obtained from CT.

2.2 Datasets

In order to train models for the tasks of semantic segmentation and registration, two datasets are created. The first dataset is created for semantic segmentation of carpal bones in US images. It is based on four printed carpal phantoms, two male and two female, and consists of automatically annotated US phantom images. For the automated annotation, tracked phantoms are placed in a water basin, where a tracked 3D US probe is then used for the acquisition of 22 volume images per phantom, with 81 image slices each. By transforming the respective carpal model to these US volume images of the carpal phantom, a surface annotation is generated. Since neighboring slice images are very similar, only every third slice is included, resulting in a total of 2376 annotated US images. These are split according to the underlying wrist phantom for the creation of similar composed and hence comparable datasets. With four wrist phantoms available, images are split in 1782 images (three phantoms) for training and 594 images (one phantom) for validation and testing.

The second dataset is created for the training of point-based scaphoid registration. It is based on 105 scaphoid models provided by Moore et al. [10], which were generated from CT images of both male and female patients. From these 105 models, a statistical shape model (SSM) is derived in order to obtain a greater variety of data. The resulting dataset consists of pairs of aligned point sets with equal sizes of 1024 points. For each of these pairs of point sets, the first set is derived from the SSM with variances in the range of ±2 standard deviations (SD), while the second is generated by synthetic sampling of the first set, which imitates US imaging. The dataset contains about 74,000 pairs of data, divided into about 41,000 pairs for training and about 16,500 pairs for validation and testing respectively. Fig. 1 examplarily shows a pair of point sets from the created dataset in the registration section.

2.3 Training

For training of the segmentation model, weights pretrained on the PASCAL VOC dataset are used as initialization. Using Adam for optimization and a set of hyperparameters derived from grid search, the final segmentation model is obtained by early stopping after 156 epochs based on results on the combined validation/test set.

For training of the registration model, ground truth (GT) has to be generated from the aligned pairs of point sets by applying a random transform to the sampled point set. This random transform consists of a rotation around each axis uniformly sampled from $[0°, 45°]$, and a translation uniformly sampled from $[-25\%, 25\%]$ of object size. Again, Adam is employed for optimization, with hyperparameters determined by grid search; the final registration model is obtained by early stopping after 14 epochs based on results on the validation set.

Table 1. Rotational and translational registration errors on point sets derived from segmentation GT and segmentation results, with mean and SD respectively.

	Derived from GT		Derived from Segmentation	
	MAE(R) / °	MAE(t) / mm	MAE(R) / °	MAE(t) / mm
Initial	23.17 ± 7.14	3.29 ± 1.09	22.02 ± 7.35	3.72 ± 1.34
ICP	24.68 ± 14.05	2.23 ± 1.42	22.77 ± 13.62	2.88 ± 1.82
PRNet	5.29 ± 3.79	0.92 ± 0.47	10.22 ± 7.37	1.73 ± 1.16
PRNet+ICP	1.42 ± 3.94	0.13 ± 0.25	6.20 ± 8.80	0.72 ± 1.50

2.4 Testing

Test results for registration are reported for two different test scenarios, which are based on the segmentation validation/test dataset: registration results on point sets derived from GT, in comparison to results of registration on point sets derived from segmentation results. For each of the two test scenarios, initial errors are compared to registration results of ICP and PRNet. Moreover, results of a combination of PRNet and ICP are included, with ICP starting from the estimated transformation of PRNet. Results of registration are measured by means of mean absolute error (MAE) between GT and predicted transformation, decomposed into a rotational error MAE(R) and a translational error MAE(t). Furthermore, the surface distance error (SDE) is computed as a point to surface distance. All experiments are repeated 10 times, results are reported as mean and SD.

3   Results

Test results for registration can be seen in Tab. 1, with results on point sets derived from GT in the left column, and results of registration on point sets derived from segmentation results in the right column. The SDE after registration of GT is 0.49 mm ±0.02 mm and after registration of predicted segmentations is 1.10 mm ±0.86 mm. Computation times for the whole process add up to 9.09 s ±0.89 s, of which the major part is attributed by segmentation with 7.70 s ±0.75 s, while only 0.21 s ±0.03 s are needed for registration.

4   Discussion

The proposed two-stage approach removes the need for manual interaction while simultaneously reducing the processing time to 9 seconds. This is an at least tenfold improvement over previous methods [2, 3, 4]. Our evaluation results in an axis deviation of 6.2° MAE and 1.1 mm SDE, which is roughly equal to 5° absolute deviation and 1-1.2 mm SDE reported by Anas et al [3]. In an ex-vivo evaluation of their method, Anas et al. successfully performed 10 out of 13 screw placements [4]. Thus, for clinical application, the overall error needs to be reduced further. Additionally, given the limitation to non-displaced fractures, only few patients could receive an ultrasound-based treatment, yet. Extending the application to displaced fractures requires an evaluation of bone fragment registration as well as visibility. An obvious limitation of this work is the evaluation on in-vitro data, which is a comparably simple task. Finally, the absence of an independent test set limits the significance of the segmentation evaluation of this study.

As shown in Tab. 1, scaphoid registration poses a difficult task, as the gold standard algorithm ICP is not able to converge to the global minimum solution. Combining it with a machine learning based global prior registration however, our approach achieves significant improvements. The segmentation on the other hand is not yet sufficiently fast and precise, as can be concluded from the high errors when processing segmented point sets. Future work will therefore focus on improving the first stage: A preceding classifier may reduce the number of false positive segmentations. Lightweight architectures designed for real-time segmentation could speed up the computation. Additionally, the pipeline needs to be adapted to and evaluated on in-vivo data.

Acknowledgement. We would like to thank Moore et al. for providing carpal and scaphoid models.

References

1. Mehling IM, Sauerbier M. Skaphoidfrakturen und Skaphoidpseudarthrosen. Z Orthop Unfall. 2013;151(6):639–660.
2. Beek M, Abolmaesumi P, Luenam S, et al. Validation of a new surgical procedure for percutaneous scaphoid fixation using intra-operative ultrasound. Med Image Anal. 2008;12(2):152–162.
3. Abu Anas EM, Seitel A, Rasoulian A, et al. Bone enhancement in ultrasound using local spectrum variations for guiding percutaneous scaphoid fracture fixation procedures. Int J Comput Dent. 2015;10(6):959–969.
4. Anas EMA, Seitel A, Rasoulian A, et al. Registration of a statistical model to intraoperative ultrasound for scaphoid screw fixation. Int J Comput Assist Radiol Surg. 2016;11(6):957–965.
5. Pandey PU, Quader N, Guy P, et al. Ultrasound bone segmentation: a scoping review of techniques and validation practices. Ultrasound Med Biol. 2020;46(4).
6. Wang Y, Sun Y, Liu Z, et al. Dynamic graph CNN for learning on point clouds. ACM Trans Graph. 2019;38(5):1–12.
7. Wang Y, Solomon JM. PRNet: self-supervised learning for partial-to-partial registration. In: Wallach H, editor. Adv Neural Inf Process Syst 32. Curran Associates, Inc.; 2019. p. 8814–8826.
8. Chen LC, Zhu Y, Papandreou G, et al. Encoder-decoder with atrous separable convolution for semantic image segmentation. In: Proceedings of the European conference on computer vision (ECCV); 2018. p. 801–818.
9. Sandler M, Howard A, Zhu M, et al. Mobilenetv2: inverted residuals and linear bottlenecks. In: Proc IEEE Comput Soc Conf Comput Vis Pattern Recognit; 2018. p. 4510–4520.
10. Moore DC, Crisco JJ, Trafton TG, et al. A digital database of wrist bone anatomy and carpal kinematics. J Biomech. 2007;40(11):2537–2542.

Abstract: 3D Guidance Including Shape Sensing of a Stentgraft System

Sonja Jäckle[1], Verónica García-Vázquez[2], Tim Eixmann[3], Florian Matysiak[4],
Felix von Haxthausen[2], Malte Sieren[5], Hinnerk Schulz-Hildebrandt[3,6,7],
Gereon Hüttmann[3,6,7], Floris Ernst[2], Markus Kleemann[4], Torben Pätz[8]

[1]Fraunhofer MEVIS, Institute for Digital Medicine, Lübeck, Germany
[2]Institute for Robotics and Cognitive Systems, Universität zu Lübeck, Germany
[3]Institute of Biomedical Optics, Universität zu Lübeck, Germany
[4]Department of Surgery, UKSH, Lübeck, Germany
[5]Department for Radiology and Nuclear Medicine, UKSH, Lübeck, Germany
[6]Medical Laser Center Lübeck GmbH, Lübeck, Germany
[7]German Center for Lung Research (DZL), Großhansdorf, Germany
[8]Fraunhofer MEVIS, Institute for Digital Medicine, Bremen, Germany
sonja.jaeckle@mevis.fraunhofer.de

During endovascular aneurysm repair (EVAR) procedures, medical instruments are guided with two-dimensional (2D) fluoroscopy and conventional digital subtraction angiography. However, this guidance requires X-ray exposure and contrast agent administration, and the depth information is missing. To overcome these drawbacks, a three-dimensional (3D) guidance approach based on tracking systems is introduced and evaluated [1]. A multicore fiber with fiber Bragg gratings for shape sensing and three electromagnetic (EM) sensors for measuring the position and orientation were integrated into a stentgraft system. A model for obtaining the located shape of the first 38 cm of the stentgraft system with two EM sensors is introduced and compared with a method based on three EM sensors. Both methods were evaluated with a phantom containing a 3D printed vessel made of silicone and agar-agar simulating the surrounding tissue. The evaluation of the guidance methods resulted in average errors from 1.35 to 2.43 mm and maximum errors from 3.04 to 6.30 mm using three EM sensors, and average errors from 1.57 to 2.64 mm and maximum errors from 2.79 to 6.27 mm using two EM sensors. The results showed that an accurate guidance with two and three EM sensors is possible and that two EM sensors are already sufficient. Thus, the introduced 3D guidance method is promising for navigation in EVAR procedures. Future work will focus on developing a method with less EM sensors and a detailed latency evaluation of the guidance method.

References

1. Jäckle S, García-Vázquez V, Eixmann T, et al. Three-dimensional guidance including shape sensing of a stentgraft system for endovascular aneurysm repair. Int J Comput Assist Radiol Surg. 2020;15(6):1033–1042.

Abstract: Move Over There

One-click Deformation Correction for Image Fusion during Endovascular Aortic Repair

Katharina Breininger[1], Marcus Pfister[2], Markus Kowarschik[2], Andreas Maier[1]

[1]Pattern Recognition Lab, Friedrich-Alexander-Universität Erlangen-Nürnberg (FAU), Erlangen, Germany
[2]Siemens Healthcare GmbH, Forchheim, Germany
katharina.breininger@fau.de

Endovascular aortic repair (EVAR) is an X-ray guided procedure for treating aortic aneurysms with the goal to prevent rupture. During this minimally invasive intervention, stent grafts are inserted into the vasculature to support the diseased vessel wall. By overlaying information from preoperative 3-D imaging onto the intraoperative images, radiation exposure, contrast agent volume, and procedure time can be reduced. However, the reliability of this fusion can deteriorate during the course of the procedure because the interventional instruments deform the vasculature. In [1], we propose an approach that models the deformation caused by stiff wires by integrating minimal user action into the otherwise fully automatic deformation correction method. Based on a single click on a relevant vascular landmark in a 2-D fluoroscopic image, we derive a projective constraint that is used in an as-rigid-as-possible deformation modeling approach. This allows to deform the preoperative information of the aortic and iliac vessels in 3-D to match the intraoperative situation with clinically relevant accuracy. The proposed approach recovers the position of the right and the left iliac bifurcation up to a mean 3-D error of 1.9 mm, with an error of 0.5 mm orthogonal to the viewing direction, and an error of 1.7 mm in depth, compared to 11.6, 7.8 and 7.9 mm before deformation correction. With a mean computation time of 6 s, the approach can be integrated smoothly into existing clinical workflows for EVAR.

References

1. Breininger K, Pfister M, Kowarschik M, et al. Move over there: one-click deformation correction for image fusion during endovascular aortic repair. Proc MICCAI. 2020; p. 713–723.

Interactive Visualization of Cerebral Blood Flow for Arteriovenous Malformation Embolisation

Ulrike Sprengel[1], Patrick Saalfeld[1], Sarah Mittenentzwei[1], Moritz Drittel[1],
Belal Neyazi[2], Philipp Berg[3,4], Bernhard Preim[1], Sylvia Saalfeld[1,4]

[1]Department for Simulation and Graphics, University of Magdeburg, Germany
[2]University Hospital Magdeburg, Department of Neurosurgery, Germany
[3]Laboratory of Fluid Dynamics and Technical Flows, University of Magdeburg, Germany
[4]Research Campus STIMULATE, University of Magdeburg, Germany
sylvia.saalfeld@ovgu.de

Abstract. Arteriovenous malformations in the brain are abnormal connections between cerebral arteries and veins without the capillary system. They might rupture with fatal consequences. Their treatment is highly patient-specific and includes careful analysis of the vessels' configuration. We present an application that visualizes the blood flow after different combinations of blockages of feeder arteries. In order to convey a detailed representation of flow in all regions of the vascular structure, we utilized the visual effect graph of the Unity game engine that allows displaying several million particles simultanously. We conducted an informal evaluation with a clinical expert. He rated our application as beneficial in addition to the tools used in clinical practice, since the interactive blockage of arteries provides valuable feedback regarding the influence of the blood flow of the remaining arteries.

1 Introduction

Arteriovenous malformations (AVMs) are vascular malformations in which the blood feeding arteries are directly fused with the veins without an intermediate capillary bed. Their center is called *nidus* and consists of interwoven vessel channels. The channels leading to the nidus arteries are called *feeders*, which are important for treatment since they are supplying the AVM. Cerebral AVMs may rupture and can lead to neurological disorders and epileptic seizures with even fatal consequences [1]. The treatment often comprises a combination of embolization, irradiation or surgical removal.

We describe an application to support a patient-specific planning of cerebral AVM treatment focusing on embolization of the AVM's feeder arteries. In clinical practice, embolization is performed with the aid of a sclerosing agent to close the arteries. Since in general a nidus has several feeders, the order in which these feeder arteries are embolized is highly relevant. For example, the occlusion of one artery can alter the blood flow in the other arteries such that a rupture may be induced [2]. With our application, which represents the different sequence of embolization steps, the treating physician may get additional information about the best possible sequence. For neuroradiology, advances in imaging and computer technology have led to the development of different simulation application including sophisticated virtual reality simulators with haptic feedback, but an intuitive visualization of interactive blood flow in AVM is still missing [3].

In this work, we employ the *Visual Effect Graph* (VFX Graph) of the game engine Unity that is used to display special effects with millions of particles. We use the VFX Graph to create an effective and intuitive blood flow visualization.

2 Materials and methods

2.1 Medical image dataset

For the blood flow visualization, a patient-specific dataset was used (Fig. 1). A cerebral AVM was segmented from a 3D rotational subtraction dataset and the feeder arteries were identified with the treating neurosurgeon. Next, to focus on the relevant vascular sections, we edit the model such that only the feeders and a smaller part of the nidus are contained for the sake of feasibility. In the following, we focus on the three feeding arteries.

2.2 Embolization and blood flow simulation

The aim of our AVM blood flow visualization was an intuitive presentation that is easy to understand for medical experts. To ensure a visual representation capable of rendering millions of particles depicting flow patterns even in small regions, we chose the cross-platform game engine Unity (Unity Technologies, Unity v2019.1.3f1, https://unity.com/) together with Unity's VFX Graph. Since the VFX Graph relies heavily on the GPU, an adequate processing of the dataset is required, which is depicted in Fig. 2 and will be described in the following.

2.2.1 Simulation of embolization. First, we replicated the embolization of the feeder artery, imitating the clinical procedure [1]. A sclerosant consisting of small, often spherical particles, is injected at the root of the artery to prevent

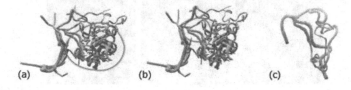

(a)   (b)   (c)

Fig. 1. Depiction of the medical dataset: segmentation of the 3D rotational subtraction data with highlighted nidus (a) and highlighted feeder arteries (b). The model is reduced to focus on these arteries (c).

disturbances in the blood flow. To analyze if the blood flow simulation can be influenced by a different surface, we tested the simulation with two embolization techniques (Fig. 3). First, we inserted small spheres in the 3D model and second, we cut the feeder arteries such that a gap is created. The 3D models were created with Blender 2.9 (Blender Foundation, Amsterdam, the Netherlands). To enable the selection of the feeders, we prepared all combinations of closed or unaltered feeders, i.e., based on three feeder arteries, we created 2^3 models.

2.2.2 Blood flow simulation. STAR-CCM+ 15.04 (Siemens PLM Software Inc., Plano, TX, USA) was chosen for the blood flow simulation. Based on parameters from the literature [4, 5], we set the following attributes: a constant inflow velocity of 0.1 m/s, zero-pressure boundary conditions at all outlets, rigid vessel walls, constant density (1055 kg/m^3) and viscosity (0.004 Pa ∗ s) values. Hence, steady-state conditions and a laminar flow was assumed. We conducted simulations of both closure techniques (Fig. 3) yielding no difference regarding the flow behavior. Therefore, we used the plain cuts. Simulation results of each configuration were stored as binary-encoded *.case files.

2.2.3 Usage of Unity's VFX graph. To use the VFX graph a *VF* file containing a binary 3D texture is required. For this purpose, the binary-encoded *.case files

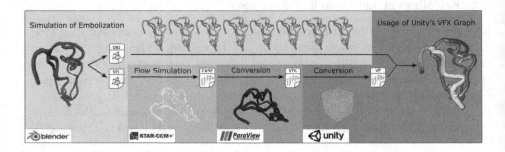

Fig. 2. Depiction of our pipeline containing the workflow from 3D editing, over the flow simulation to the usage of the VFX Graph.

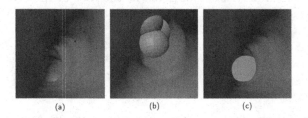

Fig. 3. Depiction of the embolization techniques: (a) unaltered artery, (b) closed artery with spherical particles, (c) closed artery based on cutting.

were converted into ASCII-coded VTK files using ParaView (Kitware Inc., New York, USA, https://www.paraview.org/). To convert from VTK to VF files, we mapped the given points on a Cartesian grid using the information provided on the VF file documentation [6]. The step size can be adjusted to influence the spatial resolution. We empirically chose a step size of 0.2 mm.

3 Results

3.1 Interactive blood flow application

Our application was implemented in Unity (Unity Technologies, San Francisco, USA)(Fig. 4). The user can navigate with the keyboard (translate, rotate and scale). In the user interface, she or he can switch between the eight models and adjust the blood flow and the opacity. For the surface visualization of the model, we adapted a ghosted view technique to reveal the underlying particles [7].

The VFX graph has four components: spawn, initialize, update and output. Parameters decide how many particles spawn and simultaneously exist, how long a particle survives and the size of the particles. Furthermore, different blend modes (*alpha/ additive*) and visualization types (*particle quads/particle strips*) can be chosen (Fig. 5). The particles with additive blending offer a better depth perception because the color values of particles lying on top of each other add up. The user can also choose a color scale to represent the velocity.

To display all 2 million particles using particle quads 259.39 MB memory are needed while the particle strips need only 137.32 MB. Both CPU and GPU are mostly running between 100 and 200 FPS. These values were taken on a PC running Windows 10 x64, with a 3.60GHz AMD Ryzen 5 3600 6-core processor and 16 GB of RAM (1600 MHz) using the AMD Radeon RX 480 graphics card.

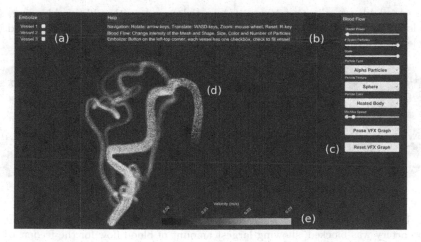

Fig. 4. Depiction of the GUI. On top are the menus for (a) switching between models, (b) usage instructions and (c) adjustable parameters for the visualization. In the center, (d) the surface model and particles as well as (e) the color bar are presented.

3.2   Evaluation

We evaluated our application via a demonstration session with a neurosurgeon, who is familiar with cerebral AVM treatment. Although he focuses on neurosurgical treatment, he is familiar with embolization therapy as well and interested in the virtual blocking of the different feeder arteries. We used the think-aloud method [8], where the user is encouraged to comment and to provide feedback.

The neurosurgeon liked the visualization especially the possibility to close or open each feeder artery individually. The rainbow-color scale with additive blending was chosen (Fig. 6), but he stated that there is no strong advantage or disadvantage between the scales. Additive blending could better highlight areas with increased blood flow, since the overlaying of multiple particles yields to brighter areas. During evaluation, the visualization of the unaltered arteries indicated that the largest amount of blood flow w.r.t. velocity and particles can be seen in the centered artery, and the artery at the bottom shows the smallest amount. Thus, he would recommend to close first the artery at the bottom, then the artery at top and the artery in the center at last. The neurosurgeon appreciated the visualization of the AVM after the selected blockages and the combination of the eight configurations. For clinical usage, he requested

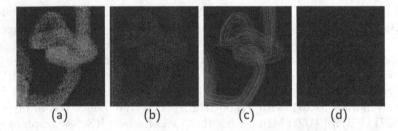

(a)   (b)   (c)   (d)

Fig. 5. Available visualization types: (a) particle quads with additive blending, (b) particle quads with alpha blending, (c) particle strips with additive blending and (d) particle strips with alpha blending.

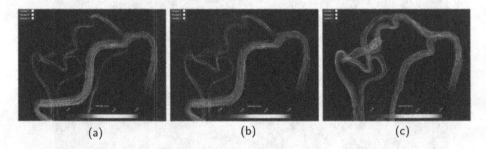

(a)   (b)   (c)

Fig. 6. Blood flow visualization with the rainbow-color scale and additive blending. In (a), no artery was blocked, showing largest amount of blood flow for the feeder artery in the center. In (b), the bottom vessel was closed, yielding little changes to the other arteries. In (c) the vessel at the center was closed that inflicts large amounts of blood flow change in the remaining arteries.

more quantitative information, including wall shear stress as well as volume of the blood flow velocity in the parent vessels compared to the feeder arteries as presented for the characterization of intracranial aneurysm blood flow [9]. He emphasized that a patient-specific planning solely based on the application is not sufficient, but it would be a useful addition for the planning based on pre-surgical datasets, anamnesis and patient's treatment history.

4 Discussion and outlook

We presented an interactive blood flow visualization of cerebral AVMs. For a representation that allows the visualization of flow patterns even in small regions, we decided to use the game engine Unity including its VFX graph that exploits the graphics hardware to simultaneously render millions of particles. By creating all combinations of feeder artery blockage, the application allows for interactively closing the arteries. A clinical evaluation partner rated it as supportive but in addition to the existing clinical practice. Future work should include quantitative blood flow information and should be tested with multiple and more complex malformations. Also the cutout of the vessels should be larger to enable an evaluation of the blood flow within the veins.

Acknowledgements. This work was supported by the Federal Ministry of Education and Research within the Research Campus *STIMULATE* (grant number 13GW0095A).

References

1. Spetzler RF, Martin NA, Carter LP, et al. Surgical management of large AVM's by staged embolization and operative excision. J Neurosurg. 1987;67(1):17–28.
2. Wu EM, El Ahmadieh TY, McDougall CM, et al. Embolization of brain arteriovenous malformations with intent to cure: a systematic review. J Neurosurg. 2019;132(2):388–399.
3. Rehder R, Abd-El-Barr M, Hooten K, et al. The role of simulation in neurosurgery. Childs Nerv Syst. 2016;32(1):43–54.
4. Ballyk C, Steinman P, Ethier D. Simulation of non-Newtonian blood flow in an end-to-side anastomosis. Biorheology. 1994;31(5):565–586.
5. Sousa L, Castro C, Conce C, et al. Blood flow simulation and vascular reconstruction. J Biomech. 2012;45(15):2549–2555.
6. Iché T. VectorFieldFile data format; 2020. https://github.com/peeweek/ VectorFieldFile.
7. Behrendt B, Berg P, Beuing O, et al. Explorative blood flow visualization using dynamic line filtering based on surface features. Comput Graph Forum. 2018;37(3):183–194.
8. Van Someren M, Barnard Y, Sandberg J. The think aloud method: a practical approach to modelling cognitive. London: AcademicPress. 1994;.
9. Cebral JR, Mut F, Weir J, et al. Quantitative characterization of the hemodynamic environment in ruptured and unruptured brain aneurysms. AJNR Am J Neuroradiol. 2011;32(1):145–151.

Rotation Invariance for Unsupervised Cell Representation Learning

Analysis of The Impact of Enforcing Rotation Invariance or Equivariance on Representation for Cell Classification

Philipp Gräbel[1], Ina Laube[1], Martina Crysandt[2], Reinhild Herwartz[2],
Melanie Baumann[2], Barbara M. Klinkhammer[3], Peter Boor[3],
Tim H. Brümmendorf[2], Dorit Merhof[1]

[1]Institute of Imaging and Computer Vision, RWTH Aachen University, Germany
[2]Department of Hematology, Oncology, Hemostaseology and Stem Cell
Transplantation, University Hospital RWTH Aachen University, Germany
[3]Institute of Pathology, University Hospital RWTH Aachen University, Germany
graebel@lfb.rwth-aachen.de

Abstract. While providing powerful solutions for many problems, deep neural networks require large amounts of training data. In medical image computing, this is a severe limitation, as the required expertise makes annotation efforts often infeasible. This also applies to the automated analysis of hematopoietic cells in bone marrow whole slide images. In this work, we propose approaches to restrict a neural network towards learning of rotation invariant or equivariant representation. Even though the proposed methods achieve this goal, it does not increase classification scores on unsupervisedly learned representations.

1 Introduction

Analysis of hematopoietic cells in bone marrow samples is a critical step for diagnosis of many hematological diseases, e.g. leukemia. Currently, medical experts have to manually perform the tedious task of identifying and counting a large number of cells in bone marrow slides. An automated analysis, particularly the classification of various cell types, is a challenging problem but could potentially improve throughput as well as objectivity.

While supervised learning of deep neural networks was shown to be a promising approach [1], it requires a large number of manually created expert annotations. Since this is a time-consuming task, it is infeasible to rely solely on fully supervised methods. Cell detection, however, is comparatively simple [2]. Furthermore, manual validation of automated detection results can be performed by non-experts in short time. Consequently, there is an abundance of patches centered around an individual cell (of unknown type) that can be used for unsupervised representation learning.

© Der/die Autor(en), exklusiv lizenziert durch
Springer Fachmedien Wiesbaden GmbH, ein Teil von Springer Nature 2021
C. Palm et al. (Hrsg.), *Bildverarbeitung für die Medizin 2021*,
Informatik aktuell, https://doi.org/10.1007/978-3-658-33198-6_12

In this work, we focus on auto-encoders [3], which allow extracting a representation of an image in the bottleneck by minimizing a reconstruction loss. As cells occur in arbitrary orientation, a network often learns different representations for the same cell type – even when using rotation augmentations. Finding rotation invariant representations is not straight-forward as the auto-encoder requires orientation information to reconstruct an image. As the classification of cell types is inherently rotation invariant it would be desirable to have rotation invariant representations as well.

A typical solution is data augmentation [4]: training a network with arbitrarily rotated images to force it to learn valid representations for each angle. However, the network still learns multiple representations even for the same image. Intrinsically rotation invariant operations in the network architecture therefore offer a more suitable solution. The HNet [5] uses harmonic convolutions instead of classical convolutional layers to make each operation rotation invariant or equivariant (depending on the chosen rotation order). Even in theory, however, a rotation invariant network cannot be used for reconstruction with the orientation information missing in the representation. Additionally, the proposed HNet is shallow and not suitable for the complex data of hematopoietic cells.

We thus propose the following approach (Fig. 1): A spatial transformer network (STN) [6] is used to normalize the images in rotation direction by minimizing the Kullback Leibler (KL) Divergence [7] between two rotated versions of the same image. A rotation invariant network architecture finds a rotation invariant representation of these normalized images. All methods are further evaluated with respect to the suitability of learned representations for supervised cell classification.

2   Materials and methods

2.1   Image data

The dataset consists of several Whole Slide Images (WSI) of human bone marrow, acquired with a $63\times$ magnifying lens and automated immersion oiling. Each sample is pre-processed with Pappenheim staining to highlight hematologically relevant structures. In this work, we utilize patches of size $256 \times 256\,\mathrm{px}^2$ centered around an individual cell. The cell positions are determined automatically

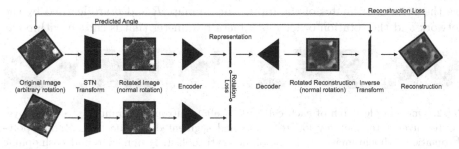

Fig. 1. Overall pipeline.

using U-Net [8] and Watershed [9] and subsequently manually validated and, if necessary, corrected. Hematological experts assigned each patch a cell type corresponding to the cell in the center, which might be surrounded by other cells as well. This results in a dataset of 6 085 samples of ten different cell types, as shown in Fig. 2.

A larger unlabelled dataset is employed to learn representations in an unsupervised fashion. This dataset contains approx. 11,000 patches centered around a cell of unknown cell type each from different images than the fully labelled dataset. It should further be noted that the influence of surrounding cells on image reconstruction tasks is reduced through decreasing the influence of pixels on the loss based on their distance to the center. This is a necessary prerequisite as surrounding cells are neither generally relevant for the classification of the cell nor rotation invariant per se.

2.2 Rotation loss

We apply a rotation loss by sending two arbitrarily rotated versions of an image through the network and comparing the output representations. As the representation of a Variational Auto Encoder [10] is described by a Gaussian distribution with mean μ and variance σ^2, we can compute the similarity between representations using the Kullback Leibler (KL) divergence [7] d_{KL}. We use the symmetric KL divergence of the two representations as an additional loss term, which penalizes representations that differ from the representations of rotated versions of the same image

2.3 Harmonic convolutions

Using spherical harmonics in convolutional layers, a specific rotation order can be enforced as shown in the HNet [5]. In our work, we use the proposed definitions for invariance and equivariance: a mapping is rotation equivariant if and only if each rotation in the image domain can be associated with a unique transformation in the feature domain. For invariance, the transformation needs to be the identity function.

In HNet, rotation equivariance is achieved by restricting the filters of convolutional layers to be of the form $W_m(r, \theta, R, \beta) = R(r)e^{i(m\theta + \beta)}$, where (r, θ) are the polar coordinates of the input feature map, R and β are learned by the network and the rotation order r is a meta parameter that is chosen within the

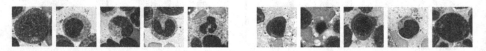

Fig. 2. One sample patch of each cell type. Left (neutrophilic granulocytes): promyelocyte, myelocyte, metamyelocyte, band and segmented granulocyte. Right: polychromatic, orthochromatic and basophilic erythroblast, lymphocyte and eosinophilic granulocyte.

architecture design. Rotational invariance requires rotation order $r = 0$, while equivariance only requires the existence of a unique rotation order. In this paper, rotation order $r = 2$ is chosen for rotation equivariant networks.

Since the originally proposed network is comparatively shallow, we introduce a ResNet-like architecture that is deeper and has residual connections [11]. In order to keep the rotation order consistent, we enforce that the rotation order of sub-networks skipped by a residual connection is zero. We further apply Harmonic Batch Normalization. As it is not possible to use a stride larger than one or maximum pooling with equivariant convolutions, we employ average pooling for downsampling.

2.4 Experimental setup

For the evaluation, several VAEs are trained unsupervisedly using reconstruction losses to learn a useful representation of hematopoietic cells. To this end, the dataset with unlabeled cell patches is employed in six-fold cross-validation. Training is performed using the Adam optimizer until an early stop criterion based on a separated validation set is reached. First of all, the reconstruction quality is evaluated in terms of SSIM between original and reconstructed images of the test sets. Secondly, the network is used to extract representations (feature vectors) of the dataset with labelled cell patches. These vectors are used as input to a shallow classification network, which is evaluated in terms of F1-score in five-fold cross-validation.

Each VAE has a Spatial Transform Subnetwork and utilizes the weight rotation loss wL_{rot} with the weight $w \in [0.2, 0.5, 0.9]$. The network is either a classical VAE (denoted as *only-STN*), a VAE with harmonic layers of rotation order zero (*inv-HNet*) or a VAE with harmonic layers of rotation order two (*equ-HNET*). As a baseline, we us a normal VAE without additional efforts to establish rotation invariant representations.

3   Results

Fig. 3 shows the KL Divergence between representations of test images in different rotations. Fig. 4 shows reconstruction results for three sample images. All methods yield representations that fulfill the desired condition: being invariant with respect to rotation of input images. As expected, this effect is stronger with larger weights for the rotation loss. Visual inspection of the reconstructions suggests that the network achieves rotation invariance or equivariance mostly through reconstructing a rotation symmetric image.

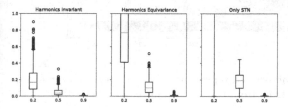

Fig. 3. Results in terms of KL Divergence between the representations of different rotations of test images. For each of the networks types, three different rotation loss weight factors are tested.

Fig. 4. From left to right: original image, baseline reconstruction, reconstructions from only STN, equivariant HNet and invariant HNet (with rotation loss weight $w = 0.5$ each). Note that effects at the patch border are due to the surrounding cell suppression.

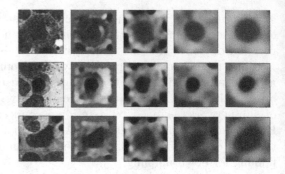

Fig. 5 shows the corresponding classification results on labelled cell images. It can be seen that the representations from networks trained with rotation invariance methods have generally lower or similar scores compared to the baseline. For most methods, a higher rotation loss weight yields a lower classification score.

4   Discussion

The qualitative results suggest that the presented methods to obtain rotation invariant or equivariant representations mostly achieve this by learning rotation symmetric reconstructions. While this lowers the reconstruction accuracy slightly, it has a larger impact on classification accuracy with learned representations. Enforcing rotation invariant harmonic convolutions (rotation order zero) is most detrimental to the F1-score, while harmonic networks with rotation order two perform slightly better. The trend generally shows that the learned embeddings are less descriptive with respect to the classification of cell types with higher focus on rotation invariance or equivariance. With low rotation loss weight and no harmonic convolutions, similar results compared to the baseline can be reached while having a more rotation independent model.

It remains to be evaluated whether the restriction to a rotation invariant representation is a beneficial constraint in semi-supervised learning approaches.

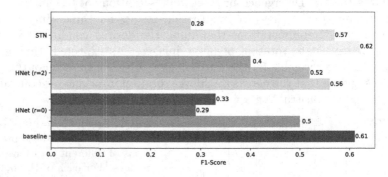

Fig. 5. Classification results using the learned representations. Lighter colors indicate lower values for the rotation loss weight (from top to bottom: 0.2, 0.5 and 0.9).

As it has been shown that domain-dependent suitable constraints improve semi-supervised strategies, it could be a valuable approach in these settings. Furthermore, losses that penalize purely rotation symmetric reconstructions for non-symmetric images might increase the usefulness of the presented methods. Further research should include the amount of labelled data as well as additional augmentations.

Acknowledgement. This study was supported by the following grants: DFG: SFB/TRR57, SFB/TRR219, BO3755/6-1, STE 2802/1-1, BMBF: STOP-FSGS-01GM1901A, BMWi: EMPAIA project to PB.

References

1. Gräbel P, Crysandt M, Herwartz R, et al. Evaluating out-of-the-box methods for the classification of hematopoietic cells in images of stained bone marrow. 1st MICCAI Workshop COMPAY. 2018;.
2. Gräbel P, Özcan Özkan, Crysandt M, et al. Circular anchors for the detection of hematopoietic cells using retinaNet. IEEE ISBI. 2020;.
3. Kramer MA. Nonlinear principal component analysis using autoassociative neural networks. AIChE J. 1991 02;37:233–243.
4. Krizhevsky A, Sutskever I, Hinton GE. ImageNet classification with deep convolutional neural networks. Adv Neural Inf Process Syst 25. 2012; p. 1097–1105. Available from: http://papers.nips.cc/paper/4824-imagenet-classification-with-deep-convolutional-neural-networks.pdf.
5. Worrall DE, Garbin SJ, Turmukhambetov D, et al. Harmonic networks: deep translation and rotation equivariance. CoRR. 2016;abs/1612.04642. Available from: http://arxiv.org/abs/1612.04642.
6. Jaderberg M, Simonyan K, Zisserman A, et al. Spatial transformer networks. Adv Neural Inf Process Syst 28. 2015; p. 2017–2025. Available from: http://papers.nips.cc/paper/5854-spatial-transformer-networks.pdf.
7. Kullback S, Leibler RA. On information and sufficiency. Ann Math Statist. 1951 03;22(1):79–86. Available from: https://doi.org/10.1214/aoms/1177729694.
8. Ronneberger O, Fischer P, Brox T. U-Net: convolutional networks for biomedical image segmentation. CoRR. 2015;abs/1505.04597. Available from: http://arxiv.org/abs/1505.04597.
9. Beucher S, Meyer F. The morphological approach to segmentation: the watershed transformation. Opt Eng-New York-Marcel Dekker Inc. 1992;34:433–433.
10. Kingma D, Welling M. Auto-encoding variational bayes. ICLR. 2013 12;.
11. He K, Zhang X, Ren S, et al. Deep residual learning for image recognition. CoRR. 2015;abs/1512.03385. Available from: http://arxiv.org/abs/1512.03385.

Abstract: Deep Learning-based Quantification of Pulmonary Hemosiderophages in Cytology Slides

Christian Marzahl[1,2], Marc Aubreville[1], Christof A. Bertram[3], Jason Stayt[4],
Anne Katherine Jasensky[5], Florian Bartenschlager[3], Marco Fragoso[3],
Ann K. Barton[6], Svenja Elsemann[7], Samir Jabari[8], Jens Krauth[2],
Prathmesh Madhu[1], Jörn Voigt[2], Jenny Hill[4], Robert Klopfleisch[3],
Andreas Maier[1]

[1]Pattern Recognition Lab, Department of Computer Science,
Friedrich-Alexander-Universität Erlangen-Nürnberg (FAU), Germany
[2]R & D Projects, EUROIMMUN Medizinische Labordiagnostika AG
[3]Institute of Veterinary Pathology, Freie Universität Berlin, Germany
[4]VetPath Laboratory Services, Ascot,Western Australia
[5]Laboklin GmbH und Co. KG, Bad Kissingen, Germany
[6]Equine Clinic, Freie Universität Berlin, Berlin, Germany
[7]Department of Neurosurgery, Universitätsklinikum Erlangen, Erlangen, Germany
[8]Institute of Neuropathology, Universitätsklinikum Erlangen, Erlangen, Germany
c.marzahl@euroimmun.de

Exercise-induced pulmonary hemorrhage (EIPH) is a common condition in sport horses with negative impact on performance. Cytology of bronchoalveolar lavage fluid by use of a scoring system is considered the most sensitive diagnostic method. Manual grading of macrophages, depending on the degree of cytoplasmic hemosiderin content, on whole slide images (WSI) is however monotonous and time-consuming. We evaluated state-of-the-art deep learning-based methods for macrophage classification and compared them against the performance of nine cytology experts. Additionally, we evaluated object detection methods on a novel data set of 17 completely annotated cytology WSI containing 78,047 hemosiderophages [1]. Our deep learning-based approach reached a concordance of 0.85, partially exceeding human expert concordance (0.68 to 0.86, mean of 0.73, SD of 0.04). Our object detection approach has a mean average precision of 0.66 over the five classes from the whole slide gigapixel images. To mitigate the high inter- and intra-rater variability, we propose our automated object detection pipeline, enabling accurate and reproducible EIPH scoring in WSI.

References

1. Marzahl C, Aubreville M, Bertram CA, et al. Deep learning-based quantification of pulmonary hemosiderophages in cytology slides. Sci Rep. 2020;10(1):1–10.

© Der/die Autor(en), exklusiv lizenziert durch
Springer Fachmedien Wiesbaden GmbH, ein Teil von Springer Nature 2021
C. Palm et al. (Hrsg.), *Bildverarbeitung für die Medizin 2021*,
Informatik aktuell, https://doi.org/10.1007/978-3-658-33198-6_13

Learning the Inverse Weighted Radon Transform

Philipp Roser[0], Lina Felsner[0], Andreas Maier, Christian Riess

[0]Both authors contributed equally
Pattern Recognition Lab, FAU Erlangen-Nürnberg
lina.felsner@fau.de

Abstract. X-ray phase-contrast imaging enhances soft-tissue contrast. The measured differential phase signal strength in a Talbot-Lau interferometer is dependent on the object's position within the setup. For large objects, this affects the tomographic reconstruction and leads to artifacts and perturbed phase values. In this paper, we propose a pipeline to learn a filter and additional weights to invert the weighted forward projection. We train and validate the method with a synthetic dataset. We tested our pipeline on the Shepp-Logan phantom, and found that our method suppresses the artifacts and the reconstructed image slices are close to the actual phase values quantitatively and qualitatively. In an ablation study we showed the superiority of our fully optimized pipeline.

1 Introduction

Medical applications could benefit from the high soft-tissue contrast of X-ray phase contrast imaging techniques [2]. Especially, the Talbot-Lau interferometer (TLI) is a promising setup to acquire phase contrast images in a medical context, due to the comparably low overall system requirements and the high robustness of the setup [1]. The TLI setup contains three gratings that are placed between the source and detector (Fig. 1).

Engelhard et al. reported a correlation between the object magnification and the measured signal strength of the differential phase image in the TLI [3].

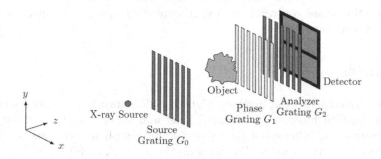

Fig. 1. Schematic setup of a Talbot-Lau interferometer. From [1].

© Der/die Autor(en), exklusiv lizenziert durch
Springer Fachmedien Wiesbaden GmbH, ein Teil von Springer Nature 2021
C. Palm et al. (Hrsg.), *Bildverarbeitung für die Medizin 2021*,
Informatik aktuell, https://doi.org/10.1007/978-3-658-33198-6_14

Donath et al. confirmed these findings, and clarified that the measured phase value depends on the position of the object relative to the phase grating G1 [4]. More concretely, the interferometer's angular sensitivity is given as

$$S = \frac{1}{2\pi} \frac{\Delta\varphi}{\alpha} \tag{1}$$

where $\Delta\varphi$ is the measured intensity oscillation of the phase scan (normalized to 2π) and α is the refraction angle caused by the object.

The position-dependent sensitivity plays a critical role in the tomographic reconstruction of large objects. The differential phase contrast at tomographic angle θ and detector position t is [5]

$$\varphi(\theta, t) = \frac{\partial}{\partial t} \int_{-\infty}^{\infty} S(r)\delta(t, r)\mathrm{d}r \tag{2}$$

where $\delta(t, r)$ encodes the objects phase values, and integration is along the ray direction r, which depends on the tomographic angle θ. In general, the position-dependent sensitivity changes the forward projection process, such that it is not possible to use conventional filtered backprojection (FBP) algorithms. Chabior et al. [5] first discussed the changing contrast formation in tomographic imaging. One particular effect is that a parallel-beam geometry requires a circular trajectory of 2π instead of π, and Chabior et al. show that a trajectory over π leads to severe reconstruction artifacts. This shows that the reconstruction task changes such that the standard analytic inversion is not possible. Furthermore, Felsner et al. showed that the task can also not be exactly solved if it is split into a standard general-purpose reconstruction and another part that is specific to the differential phase [6]. In view of this challenge to find a direct solution, we propose as an alternative a data-driven approach to differential phase reconstruction. One particularity of our approach is that we propose a specialized neural network architecture that integrates domain knowledge to remain true to the physical model [7]. For standard CT, this has been used to learn redundancy weights [8] or dedicated reconstruction filters [9]. In this work, we learn a tailored reconstruction filter, normalization weights, and voxel weights for differential phase-contrast, and experimentally show that it provides highly accurate reconstructions.

2   Methods

This work investigates the inverse weighted radon transform, more specifically its reconstruction filter and additional pixel and voxel weights. Although the TLI measures the differential phase signal, for simplicity we consider in this work direct refraction angles. We describe the network architecture in Sec. 2.1, introduce our training and test data in Sec. 2.2, and describe the experimental setup in Sec. 2.3.

2.1 Inverse weighted radon transform

Our approach is similar to previous works, where either redundancy weights [8] or filter kernels [9] are estimated in a data-driven fashion. To this end, we model the reconstruction task with a neural network (NN), where each step in the pipeline is interpreted as a layer. A schematic sketch of the pipeline can be found in Fig. 2.

The input of the NN is a sinogram that contains line integrals of weighted phase values. The first layer corresponds to the reconstruction filter H, which is carried out in the Fourier domain. Then, a layer of pixel-wise multiplicative normalization weighting W_N is added. The next layer represents the (analytical) row-wise parallel backprojection. Afterwards, a voxel-wise multiplicative weighting layer W_V accounts for the position of the phase values in the volume. The final step comprises averaging of the row-wise backprojections and masking of the reconstructed volume. The filter and the weighting layers (as highlighted in Fig. 2) can be optimized.

2.2 Data

For training, we used 1000 synthesized two-dimensional phantoms of 400×400 voxels. Each phantom is a superposition of up to six randomly scaled and sized distributions of binary blobs [10]. Figure 3 shows several examples. Based on the phantoms, we computed an ideal sinogram $P \in \mathbb{R}^{m \times n}$ without voxel weights, and a sinogram $\tilde{P} \in \mathbb{R}^{m \times n}$ with voxel weights $w_{i,j} \in [0.1, 0.9]$, with $m = 400$ projections comprising $n = 400$ pixels acquired over π. We use the weighted sinogram $\tilde{P}$ as input to our method and the FBP of the ideal sinogram P as target for optimizing the model parameters. For validation, we used 20 % of the training data. To evaluate our method's performance on unseen data, we selected the Shepp-Logan phantom [11].

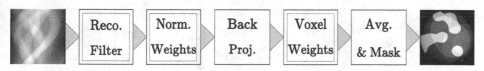

Fig. 2. Proposed Pipeline. The highlighted blocks contain parameters that can be trained in data-driven fashion.

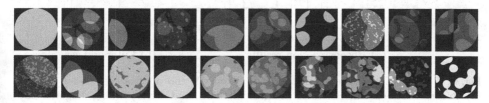

Fig. 3. Exemplary synthetic blobs phantoms used for training our model.

2.3 Experiments

We initialized the reconstruction filter with the Ram-Lak filter [12], which is the optimal filter for the conventional reconstruction problem. The normalizing weights were initialized with ones and the voxel weights were initialized homogeneously to the average of the weight interval, i.e., $\bar{w} = 0.5$ on our data. Overall, we performed three experiments. First, as a baseline, we used the the pipeline with the initialized weights for reconstruction. This correspond to an offset corrected FBP reconstruction [5]. Second, in our method, the filter and weights of the baseline were optimized on the training data (Sec. 2.2). Third, to provide an ablation, we also separately trained for (i) a projection-wise reconstruction filter, (ii) a global reconstruction filter, (iii) the normalizing weights, and (iv) the voxel weights. Where applicable, we optimized the free parameters with respect to the mean absolute error (MAE) using stochastic gradient descent with adaptive moments [13] with 10^{-4} learning rate. In addition to the MAE, we investigate the structural similarity index (SSIM) concerning our test dataset within a centered ciruclar region of interest (ROI).

3 Results

The reconstruction of the Shepp-Logan phantom is shown for the average-corrected baseline and our proposed method in top row of Fig. 4(a). The difference images to the ideal reconstruction are shown below. We found that

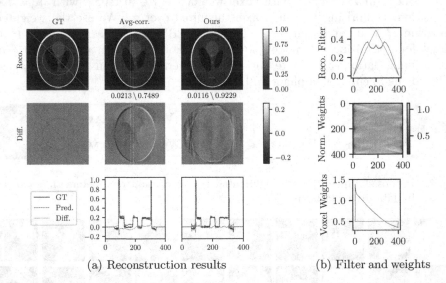

(a) Reconstruction results   (b) Filter and weights

Fig. 4. Results of the baseline method (Avg. corr.) and our trained model (Ours): (a) Reconstructions, differences to the ground truth, and corresponding diagonal line profiles. MAE and SSIM (<MAE> \ <SSIM>) refer to the circular ROI. (b) Averaged reconstruction filter (top), the learned normalization weights (mid), and voxel weights (bottom) of our trained model (blue) and the baseline/initialization (orange).

our proposed method remarkably reduces the error in the ROI compared to the average-corrected reconstruction. This can be seen from the line plots in Fig. 4(a), as well as from the quantitative values. The MAE is almost reduced by half, and the SSIM is increased by over 20 %. Figure 4(b) (top) shows the learned reconstruction filter averaged over all projection angles in blue. The comparison to the Ram-Lak (orange) shows that especially the high-frequency components get reduced in favor of low to medium frequencies. Figure 4(b) (mid) shows the normalization weights that were applied in the projection domain. Although we found that the sinogram is nearly point-symmetric, it is interesting to note that the weights along one projection are *not* symmetric. Figure 4(b) (bottom) shows the voxel weights along (each) ray, plotted from the source to the detector. As expected, we observed a strong dependence of voxel weights on the position along the ray.

The results of the ablation study are shown in Fig. 5. For all the configurations, we show from top to bottom reconstruction, difference image, and line plot. Overall, we found that the pipeline with different single layers does not improve the reconstruction. The MAE and SSIM are close to MAE and SSIM for the average-corrected reconstruction (Fig. 4(a)). Especially the offset of the left air cavity is prominent in the line plots, and only reduced with our proposed pipeline.

4   Discussion and outlook

In a proof-of-concept study, we showed that optimizing reconstruction parameters in a data-driven manner has the potential to improve generally ill-posed reconstruction problems. We improved average error rates and SSIM values by large margins without utilizing costly iterative approaches. Still, our approach preserves the interpretability of the conventional reconstruction pipeline

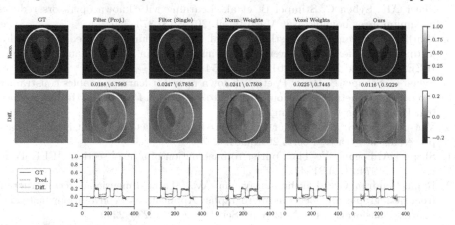

Fig. 5.   Ablation study for the proposed pipeline. Reconstructions, differences to the ground truth, and corresponding diagonal line profiles. The MAE and SSIM (<MAE> \ <SSIM>) are given for the circular ROI.

and somewhat ensuring data integrity. However, there are certain limitations that need to be addressed. First, this study is performed on simulated data. Second, especially close to the border of the reconstructed volume, our method introduced considerable artifacts, whose origin and severity need to be further investigated. Furthermore, we investigated direct phase measurements instead of differential phase, which shall be investigated in the future. In addition, we want to point out promising directions for future studies. We believe the combination of a bilateral or guided filter, or additional regularization with our method is desirable. Using a backprojection filtering approach instead of the FBP-like pipeline aims in the same direction. Also, the learned filter and weights can give insight of a theoretically/physically sound analytical solution.

References

1. Maier A, Steidl S, Christlein V, et al. Medical imaging systems: An introductory guide. vol. 11111. Springer; 2018.
2. Pfeiffer F, Weitkamp T, Bunk O, et al. Phase retrieval and differential phase-contrast imaging with low-brilliance X-ray sources. Nat Phys. 2006;2(4):258–261.
3. Engelhardt M, Baumann J, Schuster M, et al. High-resolution differential phase contrast imaging using a magnifying projection geometry with a microfocus X-ray source. Appl Phys Lett. 2007;90(22):224101.
4. Donath T, Chabior M, Pfeiffer F, et al. Inverse geometry for grating-based X-ray phase-contrast imaging. J Appl Phys. 2009;106(5):054703.
5. Chabior M, Schuster M, Schroer C, et al. Grating-based phase-contrast computed tomography of thick samples. Nucl Instrum Methods Phys Res A. 2012;693:138–142.
6. Felsner L, Würfl T, Syben C, et al. Reconstruction of voxels with position- and angle-dependent weightings. In: The 6th Int. Conf. on Image Formation in X-Ray Computed Tomography; 2020. p. 502 – 505.
7. Maier AK, Syben C, Stimpel B, et al. Learning with known operators reduces maximum error bounds. Nat Mach Intell. 2019;1(8):373–380.
8. Würfl T, Hoffmann M, Christlein V, et al. Deep learning computed tomography: learning projection-domain weights from image domain in limited angle problems. IEEE Trans Med Imaging. 2018;37(6):1454–1463.
9. Syben C, Stimpel B, Roser P, et al. Known operator learning enables constrained projection geometry conversion: Parallel to cone-beam for hybrid MR/X-ray imaging. IEEE Trans Med Imaging. 2020;.
10. Van der Walt S, Schönberger JL, Nunez-Iglesias J, et al. Scikit-image: image processing in python. PeerJ. 2014;2:e453.
11. Shepp LA, Logan BF. The Fourier reconstruction of a head section. IEEE Trans Nucl Sci. 1974;21(3):21–43.
12. Ramachandran GN, Lakshminarayanan AV. Three-dimensional reconstruction from radiographs and electron micrographs: Application of convolutions instead of Fourier transforms. Proc Natl Acad Sci. 1971;68(9):2236–2240.
13. Kingma DP, Ba J. Adam: a method for stochastic optimization. In: Bengio Y, LeCun Y, editors. 3rd Int. Conf. on Learning Representations; 2015. p. 1–15.

Table Motion Detection in Interventional Coronary Angiography

Junaid R. Rajput[1,2], Karthik Shetty[1,2], Andreas Maier[1], Martin Berger[2]

[1]Pattern Recognition Lab, FAU Erlangen-Nürnberg
[2]Siemens Healthcare GmbH, Forchheim, Germany
junaid.rajput@fau.de

Abstract. The most common method for detecting coronary artery stenosis is interventional coronary angiography (ICA). However, 2D angiography has limitations because it displays complex 3D structures of arteries as 2D X-ray projections. To overcome these limitations, 3D models or tomographic images of the arterial tree can be reconstructed from 2D projections. The 3D modeling process of the arterial tree requires accurate acquisition geometry since in many ICA acquisitions the patient table is translated to cover the entire area of interest, the original calibrated geometry is no longer valid for the 3D reconstruction process. This study presents methods for identifying the frames acquired during table translation in an angiographic scene. Spatio-temporal methods based on deep learning were used to identify translated frames. Three different architectures – 3D convolutional neural network (CNN), bi-directional convolutional long short term memory (CONVLSTM), and fusion of bi-directional CONVLSTM and 3D CNN – were trained and tested. The combination of CONVLSTM and 3D CNN surpasses the other two methods and achieves a macro f1-score (mean f1-scores of two classes) of 93%.

1 Introduction

X-ray based interventional coronary angiography (ICA) is the most widely used technique to detect coronary diseases, which is still considered the gold standard for diagnosis and treatment. The 2D X-ray image of the 3D vessel structure lacks depth information, resulting in projection artifacts such as vessel overlap and foreshortening. These inherent limitations of ICA can be overcome by reconstructing a 3D representation of the arterial tree that allows 3D quantitative coronary analysis (QCA) [1]. This can be done either by creating a symbolic 3D model of the coronary tree or by reconstructing a tomographic volume [2].

The symbolic 3D image of the coronary tree can be reconstructed from at least two projection images of the arterial tree obtained at least 30° apart for an identical cardiac phase with minimum vessel overlap [3]. This requires prior information about the acquisition geometry, e.g., the distance between source and image, the pixel spacing of the detector, and the distance between source and isocenter. The translation of the patient table which regularly occurs in ICA acquisitions to cover the entire arterial tree in projection images, disrupts the original imaging geometry. Hence, that initial calibrated geometry does not remain valid for reconstruction. An example of a right coronary artery (RCA) acquisition with typical table translation is illustrated in Fig. 1. In prior work, an additional translation vector based on the known distance of table displacement was integrated into the optimization of correspondence matching in projection images [4]. In another study, the translation vector was integrated into physical space instead of in projections [5]. However, these methods require prior information about the table displacement and manual selection of centerline correspondences of two projection images.

Spatio-temporal neural networks can detect and distinguish movements in a 3D scene, and they have outperformed traditional machine learning algorithms [6]. This work attempts to use these spatio-temporal networks to identify the frames in ICA acquisitions that are recorded during the table translation. This information allows to accurately determine when exactly in an acquisition the table has been moved, i.e., which frames are deviating from the known acquisition geometry. Based on that, a subset of frames from different view angles, which still correspond to the given acquisition geometries, can be selected automatically.

2 Materials and methods

2.1 Datasets and annotation

The datasets used for all experiments consisted of angiographic scenes from three different clinical sites. All scenes were acquired at 15 frames per second (FPS), with varying scene length, image size, and pixel spacing using Siemens Artis imaging devices (Siemens Healthineers, Erlangen, Germany). All required information, e.g., the corresponding electrocardiogram (ECG), the orientation of the scene, and the image data were stored as DICOM files. A total of 158 scenes from 28 patients were manually annotated, frames were labeled as translated frames (moving) if the rib or spine changed position compared to the previous frame, otherwise frames were termed static. Tab. 1 provides a detailed overview of the datasets.

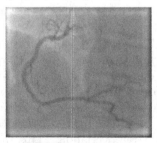 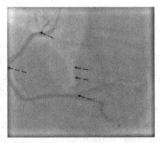
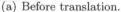

(a) Before translation.   (b) After translation.

Fig. 1. Impact of table translation on angiographic scene.

Table 1. Detailed overview of the angiographic scenes.

Site	Number of scenes	Table movement	Left coronary artery (LCA)	Right coronary artery (RCA)	Frames per second	Pixel spacing
Training and validation sets						
Site 1	104	94	74	30	15	0.18 mm
Site 2	2	2	1	1	15	0.16 mm
Site 3	2	2	0	2	15	0.4 mm
Test set						
Site 1	24	23	10	14	15	0.18 mm
Site 2	25	17	19	6	15	0.16 mm
Site 3	1	1	0	1	15	0.4 mm

2.2 Preprocessing

The angiographic scenes were of varying lengths, with a number of 12 to 182
frames. Fig. 2 depicts the overview of the preprocessing pipeline. The scenes
were divided into temporal blocks so that each block of the scene has 32 frames –
for the training, blocks of 32 frames were extracted from the angiographic scenes
without any overlap. If the scene length was not a multiple of 32, temporally
symmetrically mirrored frames were added to fill the blocks, e.g. the second block
of the scene with 40 frames consists of [33, 34, ..., 40, 39, 38, ..., 17, 16] frames
– then each frame of these temporal blocks was resized to 512×512, afterwards
contrast was enhanced using adaptive histogram equalization, and in the final
step the frames were downsampled to 128×128 using minimum pooling. The
application of minimum pooling was to highlight high-density structures (ribs
and spine) in the angiography scene. During the training, the first frame of each
block was marked as static. During the evaluation, the scene was split up so
that the following block starts with the last frame of the previous block, i.e. if
the scene has 63 frames, then block 1 and 2 have frames 1 - 32 and 32 - 63
respectively, the prediction of frame number 32 comes from block 1.

2.3 Network architectures

Three different spatio-temporal networks were designed and trained. Fig. 2
shows the overview of network architectures. Network 1 consisted of a 3D convolutional neural network (CNN), 3D CNN captures the spatial and temporal

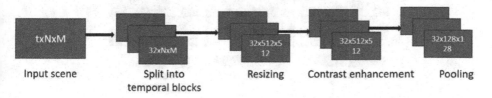

Fig. 2. Overview of the preprocessing pipeline for angiographic input scenes.

information among adjacent frames of the scene [7]. Network 2 consisted of bi-directional convolutional long short term memory (CONVLSTM) layers. This layer contains a convolution operation within the LSTM cell, allowing it to learn spatial information and long-term dependencies between frames of the scene [8]. Network 3 (3D CNN-CONVLSTM) contained both 3D CNN and the CONVL-STM layers. The bi-directional CONVLSTM layer stacked on top of the 3D CNN layer in the fusion network enables the learning of longer temporal information with much less complexity compared to the CONVLSTM network.

3 Results

All three networks were trained with the binary cross-entropy loss and the Adam optimizer. The class imbalance was addressed by adding multiple copies of temporal blocks that consisted only of moving frames from the respective training and validation sets. Tab. 2 gives an overview of the performance of network architectures for the test set. The 3D CNN-CONVLSTM network outperformed the other two networks and was able to successfully predict the moving frames based on the rigid structures of the angiography. It achieved a macro f1-score of 93% on the complete test set, the macro f1-score was 93%, 92%, 95% for Site 1, Site 2, and Site 3. Macro f1-score was 94% and 92% for RCA and LCA scenes, respectively. The results for Site 2 and RCA show that the trained model generalized well, as they were severely underrepresented in the training data. Increasing the depth of CONVLSTM and 3D CNN architectures leads to overfitting and further degrades their performance.

Fig. 4a shows the binary classification and the ground truth labels for an example scene. The angiographic scene was resliced along a vertical line in temporal direction (right Fig. 4b), highlighting a part that focuses on a selected vertebra. The superimposition of a selected vertebra and the classification results in Fig. 4a confirm that the 3D CNN-CONVLSTM architecture can accurately distinguish between static and moving frames. Furthermore, the overlaid ECG signal shows that there is a sufficient number of cardiac cycles before table translation, hence, these frames still correspond to a correctly known acquisition geometry and could be used directly for further processing, e.g., 3D QCA.

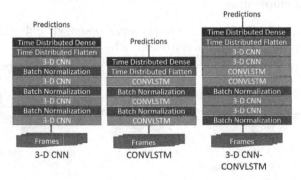

Fig. 3. Overview of network architectures.

Table 2. Overview of the performance of network architectures.

Frames	Precision	Recall	F1-score	# frames	Macro F1-score
3D CNN					
Moving	0.74	0.64	0.69	969	0.8
Static	0.89	0.92	0.91	2968	
CONVLSTM					
Moving	0.85	0.71	0.78	969	0.86
Static	0.91	0.96	0.93	2968	
3D CNN-CONVLSTM					
Moving	0.91	0.87	0.89	969	0.93
Static	0.96	0.97	0.97	2968	

Misclassifications were mainly due to the difference between the leading edge (static to moving) and the trailing edge (moving to static) of the predictions and the ground truth, shown as black arrows pointing up and down in Fig. 4a. This provides a quantitative measure for temporal accuracy. Fig. 5 shows the distributions of these temporal errors. Both the leading and trailing edges have almost similar temporal accuracy with a mean deviation of 1.37 and 1.61 frames, respectively. An Overlay of all data points on the box plots shows that the maximum error was 5 frames for both the leading and trailing edge.

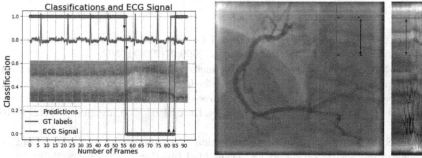

(a) Classification result superimposed on the temporal movement of a disc. (b) Temporal movement along a vertical line within an angiographic scene.

Fig. 4. Output of the 3D CNN-CONVLSTM network for an example scene.

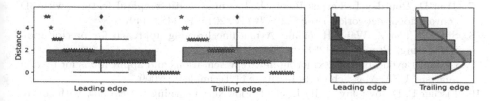

Fig. 5. Distance between the leading and trailing edges of ground truth and predictions.

4 Discussion

The 3D CNN-CONVLSTM network successfully distinguishes table motion in the angiographic scene from heart and respiratory movements as it encodes longer temporal information. The CONVLSTM network also works reasonably well, but it usually incorrectly classified static frames as moving when there was a sudden change in successive frames, usually at the beginning of the contrast flow. The 3D CNN network only worked well when there was no significant diaphragm motion and the effects of heart movement and heart shadow were minimal. The results show that the trained model can robustly classify table motion frames since all three clinical sites and RCA and LCA scenes yield similar f1-scores. The temporal error of the leading and trailing edge was less than 2 frames on average. This uncertainty can easily be taken into account when selecting suitable frames by adding an appropriate safety margin to the classification results. Currently, this study is limited to angiographic acquisitions with a framerate of 15 FPS. In future work, angiographic scenes will be up- or downsampled to a common framerate using motion interpolation techniques [9]. Furthermore, we aim to incorporate the information of the table motion predictor from this study to an extended network trained to estimate the optical flow [10]. This information could then be used to further reduce the effects of table motion when modeling the arterial tree.

References

1. Pantos I, Efstathopoulos EP, Katritsis DG. Two and three-dimensional quantitative coronary angiography. Cardiol Clin. 2009;27(3):491–502.
2. Çimen S, Gooya A, Grass M, et al. Reconstruction of coronary arteries from x-ray angiography. Med Image Anal. 2016;32:46–68.
3. Chen SJ, Hoffmann KR, Carroll JD. Three-dimensional reconstruction of coronary arterial tree based on biplane angiograms. Proc SPIE Med Imaging. 1996;2710:103–114.
4. Chen SJ, Carroll JD. 3-D reconstruction of coronary arterial tree to optimize angiographic visualization. IEEE Trans Med Imaging. 2000;19:308–336.
5. Yang J, Wang Y, Liu Y, et al. Novel approach for 3D reconstruction of coronary arteries from two uncalibrated angiographic images. IEEE Trans Med Imaging. 2009;18:1563–1572.
6. Xiao X, Xu D, Wan W. Video recognition from handcrafted method to deep learning method. Proc ICALIP. 2016; p. 646–651.
7. Tran D, Bourdev L, Fergus R, et al. Learning spatiotemporal features with 3D convolutional networks. Proc IEEE ICCV. 2015; p. 4489–4497.
8. Shi X, Chen Z, Wang H, et al. A machine learning approach for precipitation nowcasting. Proc NIPS. 2015; p. 802–810.
9. Ce Liu. Beyond pixels: Exploring new representations and applications for motion analysis. USA: Massachusetts Institute of Technology; 2009.
10. Fischer P, Dosovitskiy A, Ilg E, et al. FlowNet: Learning optical flow with convolutional networks. Proc IEEE ICCV. 2015; p. 2758–2766.

Semi-permeable Filters for Interior Region of Interest Dose Reduction in X-ray Microscopy

Yixing Huang[0,1], Leonid Mill[0,1], Robert Stoll[1], Lasse Kling[2,4], Oliver Aust[3], Fabian Wagner[1], Anika Grüneboom[3], Georg Schett[3], Silke Christiansen[2,4,5], Andreas Maier[1]

[0]Both authors contributed equally
[1]Pattern Recognition Lab, Friedrich-Alexander-University Erlangen-Nuremberg
[2]Korrelative Mikroskopie und Materialdaten, Fraunhofer-Institut für Keramische Technologien und Systeme IKTS, Forchheim
[3]Institute of clinical Immunology, University Hospital Erlangen
[4]Institut für Nanotechnologie und korrelative Mikroskopie, Forchheim
[5]Physics Department, Freie Universität Berlin, Berlin
yixing.yh.huang@fau.de

Abstract. In osteoporosis research, the number and size of lacunae in cortical bone tissue are important characteristics of osteoporosis development. In order to reconstruct lacunae well in X-ray microscopy while protecting bone marrow from high-dose damage in in-vivo experiments, semi-permeable X-ray filters are proposed for dose reduction. Compared with an opaque filter, image quality with a semi-permeable filter is improved remarkably. For image reconstruction, both iterative reconstruction with reweighted total variation (wTV) and FDK reconstruction from penalized weighted least-square (PWLS) processed projections can reconstruct lacunae when the transmission rate of the filter is as small as 5%. However, PWLS is superior in computation efficiency.

1 Introduction

In today's aging society, there has been a dramatic increase in the occurrence of osteoporosis and related diseases. Osteoporosis is a "progressive systemic skeletal disease characterized by low bone mass and microarchitectural deterioration of bone tissue, with a consequent increase in bone fragility and susceptibility to fracture", as described by WHO. To investigate the development of osteoporosis and its corresponding treatment, the microanalysis of bone tissue is necessary. In this work, tibial bones from aging mouse models are used, which in general have very fine structures. A mouse tibial bone mainly contains exterior cortical bone tissue and interior bone marrow. The number and size of lacunae in the cortical bone tissue are important characteristics of osteoporosis development. Therefore, the bone tissue region is of interest for osteoporosis research. The bone marrow consists of hematopoietic cells, marrow adipose tissue and supportive stromal cells, which is vital for the health of mice.

© Der/die Autor(en), exklusiv lizenziert durch
Springer Fachmedien Wiesbaden GmbH, ein Teil von Springer Nature 2021
C. Palm et al. (Hrsg.), *Bildverarbeitung für die Medizin 2021*,
Informatik aktuell, https://doi.org/10.1007/978-3-658-33198-6_16

With modern X-ray microscopy (XRM) systems, high resolution images are reconstructed with a voxel size up to 500 nm, which allows the investigation of bone structures in nano-scale in a nondestructive manner [1]. However, such a high resolution reconstruction requires around 2000 projections with acquisition time up to several hours. The large amount of X-ray dose will damage bone marrow [2] and thereby affects the natural osteoporosis development in in-vivo experiments. Therefore, we aim to avoid the high dose exposure to bone marrow while preserving the good image quality of exterior cortical bone tissue.

For dose reduction, collimators are widely used in computed tomography (CT) for region-of-intrest (ROI) imaging. They are typically placed to block exterior X-ray exposure for interior tomography [3]. However, in our application, since the exterior region is of interest, blocking the X-rays for the central bone marrow area leads to insufficient measured data for the exterior area as well, which is an exterior tomography problem [4]. Image reconstruction for exterior tomography is very challenging because of data truncation and missing data. Therefore, semi-permeable collimators, commonly called X-ray filters [5], are proposed for our application. In this work, the image quality using filters of different transmission rates and different reconstruction algorithms is investigated[1].

2 Materials and methods

2.1 Filter design

The attenuation of X-rays in a filter follows the Beer-Lambert Law

$$I_c = I_0 e^{-\eta} \tag{1}$$

where I_0 is the intensity of the incident X-ray without filtration and I_c is the X-ray after filtration. η is the filter attenuation determined by the X-ray energy E, the filter material type (defining the mass attenuation coefficient $\mu_m(E)$ and the density ρ), and the filter thickness l

$$\eta = \mu_m(E) \cdot l \cdot \rho \tag{2}$$

The mass attenuation coefficient μ_m and the density ρ for different materials are available in the NIST Standard Reference Database 126 We further denote the filter transmission rate by $\alpha = I_c/I_0 = e^{-\eta}$. In order to design a filter with a transmission rate α, the filter thickness needs to be $l = -\ln(\alpha)/(\rho \cdot \mu_m)$. For example, with a photon energy of 40 KeV, aluminum has $\mu_m = 0.5685 \text{ cm}^2/\text{g}$ and $\rho = 2.70 \text{ g/cm}^3$. Thus, an aluminum filter with a transmission rate of 5% requires a thickness of around 2.0 cm.

In a cone-beam XRM system, we denote the source-to-isocenter distance by D_1 and the filter length by L_0. The filter is placed between the X-ray source and the isocenter with distance D_c to the source. During a 360° scan, a circular

---

[1] https://www.nist.gov/pml/x-ray-mass-attenuation-coefficients

area with a diameter of $L = L_0 * D_1/D_c$ is affected by the filter. In practice, the filter length or position can be adjusted according to a preliminary scan using two orthogonal views to align the affected area close to the bone marrow area.

If an opaque filter is applied, i.e. $\alpha = 0$, it changes the angular coverage of X-rays at different locations. Particularly, a point with a distance of d $(d > L)$ to the isocenter has an angular range of $\theta = \pi - 2\arctan(L/d)$ for X-ray coverage, as displayed in Fig. 1(a). The closer the points are to the affected area $(d \rightarrow L)$, the smaller θ is. Therefore, it is very challenging to reconstruct them.

However, with a semi-permeable filter, i.e. $0 < \alpha < 1$, the point still has a full X-ray coverage, but with fewer X-ray photons passing through it (Fig. 1(b)). Due to the reduced number of photons, the X-ray projections contain more quantum (Poisson) noise. According to the Beer-Lambert Law, the detected intensity for the filtered region is as follows

$$I(u, v, \beta) = I_c \cdot e^{-p(u,v,\beta)} = \alpha \cdot I_0 \cdot e^{-p(u,v,\beta)} \tag{3}$$

where $I(u, v, \beta)$ is the ideal number of X-ray photons at detector pixel (u, v) given the rotation angle β, and $p(u, v, \beta)$ is the total attenuation of the imaged object along the path from the X-ray source at angle β to the detector pixel (u, v). However, due to quantum noise, the actual detected photon number follows a Poisson distribution

$$I_{\text{Poi}} = \mathcal{P}(I(u, v, \beta)) \tag{4}$$

where $\mathcal{P}(\lambda)$ is a Poisson random variable with a mean parameter λ.

2.2 Image reconstruction

In this work, we investigate three algorithms for image reconstruction from filtered data: conventional FDK, iterative reconstruction with reweighted total variation (wTV) regularization [6], and FDK with penalized weighted least-squares (PWLS) [7].

The objective function for wTV with a semi-permeable filter is

$$\min \|f\|_{\text{wTV}}, \text{ subject to } \|A_c f - p_c\| < e_c, \text{ and } \|A_n f - p_n\| < e_n \tag{5}$$

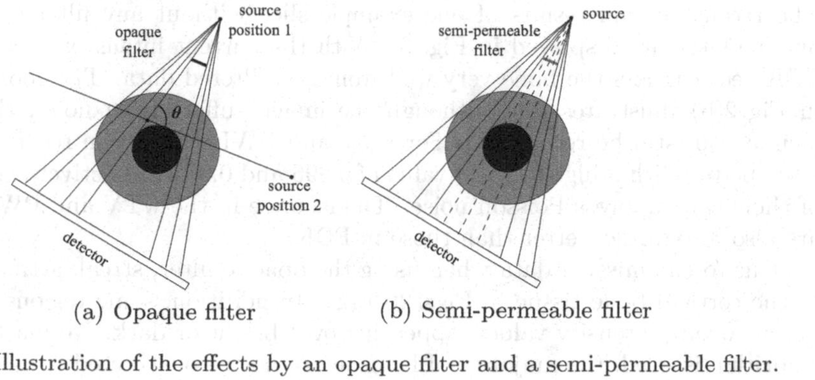

(a) Opaque filter   (b) Semi-permeable filter

Fig. 1. Illustration of the effects by an opaque filter and a semi-permeable filter.

where $||f||_{\text{wTV}}$ is the wTV term defined in [6], p_c and p_n are the filtered and non-filtered projection vectors respectively, A_c and A_n are their corresponding system matrices respectively, and e_c and e_n are two error tolerance parameters to account for different levels of noise. For image reconstruction with an opaque filter, the data fidelity term $||A_c f - p_c|| < e_c$ is omitted. The above objective function is optimized by alternating simultaneous algebraic reconstruction technique (SART) and the gradient descent of the wTV term [6].

The PWLS objective function in the projection space can be described as [7]

$$\min(\hat{p} - p)^\top \Lambda^{-1}(\hat{p} - p) + \frac{1}{2} \sum_i \sum_{m \in \mathcal{N}_i} (\hat{p}_i - \hat{p}_m)^2 \tag{6}$$

where p is the measured projection vector, $\hat{p}$ is the denoised projection vector, i and m are projection pixel index, and $\mathcal{N}_i$ is the four-nearest neighbor of the i-th pixel. The iterative algorithm in [7] is applied to solve the above objective function. Afterwards, FDK is applied for image reconstruction.

2.3 Experimental setup

We investigate the effect of different filters using a mouse tibial bone in a simulation study. The projection data are simulated in a XRM system with a source-to-isocenter distance 10 mm and a source-to-detector distance 25 mm. The detector has 2000×2000 pixels with a pixel size of $2.0\,\mu$m. Poisson noise is simulated considering an initial exposure of 5×10^6 photons at each detector pixel without any filters, i.e. $I_0 = 5 \times 10^6$. In this work, only monoenergetic X-rays are considered. The reconstruction volume has a size of $1024 \times 1024 \times 300$ voxels with an isotropic voxel size of $1.34\,\mu$m.

For reconstruction, the parameter e_n is set to 5×10^{-5} for Poisson noise tolerance. The other noise tolerance parameter e_c is set to 5×10^{-5}, 2×10^{-4}, 5×10^{-4}, 10^{-3} and 5×10^{-3} for $\alpha = 1, 25\%, 10\%, 5\%$ and 1%, respectively. For the wTV regularization, 10 iterations of SART + wTV are applied to get the final reconstruction.

3 Results

The reconstruction results of one example slice without any filter or with an opaque filter are displayed in Fig. 3. With the current intensity $I_0 = 5 \times 10^6$, FDK reconstructs the bone very well from non-filtered data. The zoom-in ROI in Fig. 2(b) illustrates that although the image suffers from noise, the major lacunae can still be recognized. For wTV and PWLS, they can reconstruct the bone better with a higher SSIM value of 0.996 and 0.961 respectively, since both of them can suppress Poisson noise. The lacunae in the wTV and PWLS ROIs are also recognized better than those in FDK.

Due to the missing data when using the opaque filter, streak artifacts occur in the cortical bone tissue in Figs. 2(e)-(g). In addition, some regions have apparent wrong intensity values, appearing over bright or dark. No matter which algorithm is used, the majority of lacunae are not reconstructed.

The reconstruction results of the example slice with filters of different transmission rates are displayed in Fig. 3. When the transmission rate $\alpha = 0.25\%$, Poisson noise is observed in reconstruction in Fig. 3(a), especially at the bone marrow area. Consequently, only the locations and sizes of large lacunae can be determined. For $\alpha \leq 10\%$, the lacunae in the zoom-in ROIs are hardly visible in Figs. 3(b)-(d).

For wTV, in Figs. 3(e)-(h) where α varies from 25% to 1%, Poisson noise pattern is not observed in any of the images. Moreover, the lacunae can still be distinguished even though α is as low as 5%. When $\alpha = 1\%$, the lacunae in the ROI lack contrast, although they can be seen to some degree.

PWLS reduces Poisson noise in measured projections. Therefore, in the reconstructed images for α between 25% and 5%, lacunae are observed well. However, for $\alpha = 1\%$, the lacunae in the ROI are only partially visible (Fig. 3(l)).

4 Discussion

With an opaque filter, independently from the reconstruction algorithm, most lacunae are not reconstructed. Using FDK with a transmission rate α smaller than 25%, most lacunae are obscured by Poisson noise. PWLS and wTV are both able to reconstruct lacunae well even when α is as small as 5%. However, PWLS is more efficient than wTV. Therefore, using PWLS with a 5% filter is an optimal option in terms of computation efficiency and image quality.

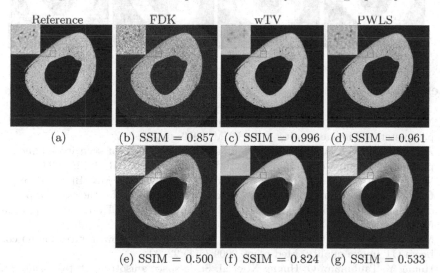

Fig. 2. Reconstruction results of one example slice without any filter (top row) and with an opaque filter (bottom row) using different reconstruction algorithms, window: $[0, 6.25 \times 10^{-5}]/\mu m$. A square ROI containing 6 lacunae is zoomed in.

Fig. 3. Reconstruction results of the example slice with filters of different transmission rates, window: $[0, 6.25 \times 10^{-5}]/\mu m$. The top, middle and bottom rows are for FDK, wTV and PWLS, respectively.

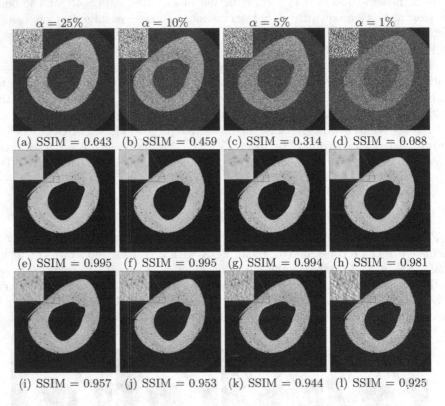

$\alpha = 25\%$ $\alpha = 10\%$ $\alpha = 5\%$ $\alpha = 1\%$

(a) SSIM = 0.643 (b) SSIM = 0.459 (c) SSIM = 0.314 (d) SSIM = 0.088

(e) SSIM = 0.995 (f) SSIM = 0.995 (g) SSIM = 0.994 (h) SSIM = 0.981

(i) SSIM = 0.957 (j) SSIM = 0.953 (k) SSIM = 0.944 (l) SSIM = 0.925

References

1. Mill L, Kling L, Grüneboom A, et al. Towards in-vivo x-ray nanoscopy: Acquisition parameters vs. image quality. Proc BVM. 2019; p. 251–256.
2. Auvinen A, Bridges J, Dawson K, et al. Health effects of security scanners for passenger screening (based on X-ray technology). SCENIHR. 2012; p. 24.
3. Wang G, Yu H. The meaning of interior tomography. Phys Med Bio. 2013;58(16).
4. Guo Y, Zeng L, Wang C, et al. Image reconstruction model for the exterior problem of computed tomography based on weighted directional total variation. Appl Math Model. 2017;52:358–377.
5. Mail N, Moseley D, Siewerdsen J, et al. The influence of bowtie filtration on cone-beam CT image quality. Med phys. 2009;36(1):22–32.
6. Huang Y, Taubmann O, Huang X, et al. Scale-space anisotropic total variation for limited angle tomography. IEEE Trans Radiat Plasma Med Sci. 2018;2(4):307–314.
7. Wang J, Li T, Lu H, et al. Penalized weighted least-squares approach to sinogram noise reduction and image reconstruction for low-dose X-ray computed tomography. IEEE Trans Med Imaging. 2006;25(10):1272–1283.

An Optical Colon Contour Tracking System for Robot-aided Colonoscopy

Localization of a Balloon in an Image using the Hough-transform

Giuliano Giacoppo[1], Anna Tzellou[1], Joonhwan Kim[2], Hansoul Kim[2],
Dong-Soo Kwon[2,3], Kent W. Stewart[1], Peter P. Pott[1]

[1]Institute of Medical Device Technology, University Stuttgart, Germany
[2]Department of Mechanical Engineering, Korea Advanced Institute of Science and
Technology, Daejeon, Republic of Korea
[3]EasyEndo Surgical Inc., Daejeon, Republic of Korea
giuliano.giacoppo@imt.uni-stuttgart.de

Abstract. During colonoscopy there is a risk that the intestinal wall may
be injured or may pain occur by the insertion of an endoscope. Surgery
through endoscopes must be learned by physicians through extensive
training. To simplify the insertion of endoscopes, research is being carried
out on robotic-aided systems. Here, a sensor is needed to detect the
contour of the intestine in order to enable an injury-free and painless
insertion of the endoscope. In this paper a tube-balloon is designed
for a gentle contour tracking of the intestinal anatomy. This is inserted
through the working channel of the endoscope and placed in the intestinal
lumen in front of the endoscope's head in the field of view of the camera.
A Matlab-algorithm is used to detect the balloon in each image. The
balloon appears as a two-dimensional circle, which can be detected using
a Hough-Transformation. The displacement of balloon after touching
the intestine wall is calculated as a vector between the circle's center
and the image center. This ensures that the robot-aided endoscope can
follow the intestinal contour.

1 Introduction

Colonoscopy is used to detect colorectal cancer at an early stage in the average-
risk population [1, 2]. The conventional method is established on a large scale
in everyday clinical practice. In Germany, 58.5 % of women and men over the
age of 55 have had such an examination carried out within the last 10 years
[3]. However, pain or even injuries at the intestinal wall can occur [4]. In
order to compensate for these disadvantages, innovative approaches are under
development to improve the requirements in terms of clinical applicability, user-
friendliness, and functionality of the instruments. A trend towards robot-aided
flexible endoscopes with multiple working channels, called overtubes, is emerging
[5, 6, 7, 8, 9]. Nevertheless, the insertion of such endoscopes into the body can

be difficult and time consuming. Thus, an integration of a precise, automated insertion instrument as a sensor or reference point to determine the individual anatomy should facilitate a simplified insertion. This should increase usability and user-friendliness of such a device and reduce the operating time. In this paper an optical colon contour tracking system for robot-aided colonoscopy is presented. To achieve this a balloon as a sensor for determining the contour and thus the curved pathway of the intestine with real-time image analysis is investigated. It is examined how long the image evaluation takes with regard to the calculation time and whether the balloon as sensing element is detected reliably.

2   Material and methods

To capture the information of the curved pathway of the intraluminal individual anatomy of the intestine, a balloon is placed in front of the overtube in the camera's field of view via the working channel of the overtube (Fig. 1). This balloon is flexibly attached on a tube, which is bent away by the intestinal wall. Using image processing, the balloon can be detected and its position relative to the overtube can be determined. If the balloon is moved away by the intestinal wall, the position relative to the overtube also changes. Since the image center is known and the robot-aided overtube is bendable in $x-$ and $y-$directions, it is able to follow the balloon. Thereby, the overtube follows the individual anatomy of an intestine.

2.1   Mechanical setup

The complete system consists of a balloon prototype, a camera module, a single-board computer for image acquisition, and a PC for image analysis (Fig. 1). In the prototype the balloon is made of natural rubber. It is fixed to a polyurethane tube $\emptyset_{Out} = 2\,mm$, series PUN-H (Festo SE & Co. KG, Germany) using heat-shrinkable tubing. Radial holes allow air to enter and inflate the spherical balloon. The balloon is filled with 10 to 20 ml ambient air and reaches a diameter

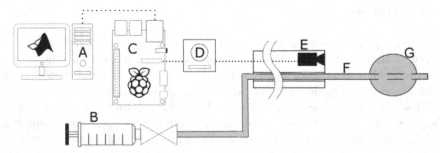

Fig. 1. Schematic of the test bench (A: PC running Matlab, B: syringe and valve, C: Raspberry Pi 3 model B, D: camera module, E: overtube with camera, F: tube, G: Balloon).

of about 27 mm. Air is supplied via a Omnifix® Solo disposable syringe 30 ml (B. Braun AG, Melsungen, Germany) and a Luer Luck valve (three-way valve from Teqler, NetMed S.à.r.l., Wecker, Luxembourg).

For image recording a Raspberry Pi 3 model B with a camera module RASP CAM 2 (Raspberry Pi Foundation, UK) is used, on which a mini camera RPI V22 with 8 MP, 77,6 ° (Denash, Chengdu, China) is connected. This camera is placed at the head of the overtube (Fig. 1 – E). The Raspberry Pi is connected via Ethernet to a PC (ASUS UX310U, Intel® Core™ i7-6500U CPU @ 2.50 GHz, 16 GB RAM), on which image processing is performed by MATLAB® R2019a (The MathWorks, Inc.).

2.2 Algorithm

The aim of the algorithm is to identify the inflated balloon as a circle and its center in an image. For this purpose, the camera takes images, which are loaded as PNG files into the Matlab workspace. Subsequently, each image is pre-processed to finally identify a circle. The first steps are to convert the original image into a grayscale image and increase the contrast as well as to limit the image size to 640x480 pixels to create an defined starting position (Fig. 2). The coordinate origin is located in the upper left corner. Afterwards, the Hough-Transformation (HT) [10, 11] is used to detect the balloon as circle in an image.

The HT is a standard procedure for the detection of parameterized curves and very robust but also very complex to calculate [12]. Even if the circle is covered, e.g. supply tube for the balloon, the HT can be successful. It is assumed that only the balloon with a specific radius range is detected as a circle with the correct settings, since other circular patterns such as circular cross-sections in the intestine or shadows lie outside the radius of the searched circle.

A circle is described as a function of $r^2 = (x_i - a)^2 + (y_i - b)^2$ in a two-dimensional space. Where r is the radius, a and b are the center of the circle. From the input image (Fig. 2c, increased contrast) an edge image is generated (Fig. 3a) via a binary image depending on the threshold. In the image, edges are represented as black pixels and the remaining pixels are shown white. The HT has to recognize which edges form a circle. For this purpose, a circle with the predefined radius r is drawn at each edge point and its circle points are temporarily stored in an accumulator field (Fig. 3b). Since in an accumulator

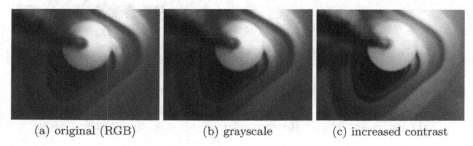

(a) original (RGB)   (b) grayscale   (c) increased contrast

Fig. 2. Pre-processing of images in steps (a),(b),(c).

field several circle points can be found at the same place, this place is counted up, similar to a voting. Once all edge points in the algorithm have passed through, the accumulator field is evaluated. The point that has the highest value (most votes) or exceeds a certain threshold is the center of the identified circle (Fig. 3c). If the radius r of the circle to be searched is not known, the radius can be variable within a certain range and runs through the algorithm several times with the different radii.

Once the center of the circle has been determined, a vector can be calculated to the image center. The image center represents the point where the overtube will move by a straight movement. The vector indicates where the camera or overtube should move to.

2.3   Experimental setup

To validate the algorithm, 400 images were acquired in a colon model (M40 Colonoscope Training Model, Kyoto Kagaku Co., LTD, Japan). The settings in the algorithm, in which range the searched radius lies, was for a minimum radius of 100 px and maximal radius of 110 px.

Calculation time is of interest and has been investigated offline. The function stopwatch (tic toc) was used in Matlab. It was examined how long it takes to find one circle, as well as the cases when no or several circles are found.

3   Results

The construction allows a flexible placing of the balloon in front of the camera. The balloon is pushed away from the intestinal wall and consequently changes its position relative to the overtube. Using the system of a camera, Raspberry Pi, and Matlab, 5 images per second could be processed. The visualization of the image with the determined circle and values are shown on a monitor. Fig. 4 shows a sample image as it appears on the PC screen, with the identified circle, its coordinates and vector v for the direction of movement.

A total of 400 images were evaluated to determine the balloon as expected as a circle. In 353 images (88 %) only the balloon was detected. In the remaining images 38 times (10 %) no circle was identified and 9 times (2 %) more than

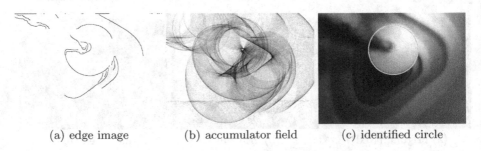

(a) edge image   (b) accumulator field   (c) identified circle

Fig. 3. Working principle Hough-transform (HT).

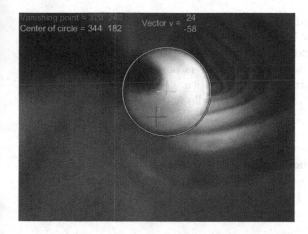
Vanishing point = 320 240
Center of circle = 344 182
Vector v = 24 / -58

Fig. 4. Visualization of identified circle and calculated vector.

one circle was identified. The analysis of the calculation time of the Hough-Transformation was 125 ms (standard deviation (SD) = 17 ms). The calculation time was an average of 122 ms (SD = 14 ms) if one circle was detected, an average of 130 ms (SD = 20 ms) if no circle was detected and an average of 119 ms (SD = 16 ms) if more than one circle was detected.

4   Discussion

With this setup, it is possible to obtain information on the curved pathway of the intestine. The use of a balloon as a sensor or reference point is possible. It can be easily integrated in robot-aided overtubes. With the Hough-Transformation the balloon can be recognized as a circle in an image. Thereby, the balloon is localized in an image and thus also in the intestine and a robot-aided contour tracking can be realized. To generate a higher probability of success, several approaches were investigated. It turned out that the edge of the balloon is often only partially recognized. In order to clearly discriminate the balloon from the rest of the image and thus enable sufficient edge detection, it should be well illuminated. For this reason the balloon should be clearly distinguished in the image and no shadows should appear which are falsely detected as circles.

It should also be mentioned that the images were taken on a phantom. In reality, soiling is to be expected, which can have a negative effect on the detection.

To ensure that it can be used in the medical field in the future, the process time should be reduced. Currently, the calculation time of the Hough-Transformation is at 125 ms (SD = 17 ms). It is clear that the high computational effort of the Hough-Transformation is accompanied by a loss of speed.

Looking closer at the images it becomes apparent that the balloon occludes a considerable part of the image. Since this visual impairment can lead to a lack of acceptance by some of the personnel, a solution should be sought that limits the visual impairment to a minimum.

The balloon can be removed through the working channel after reaching the desired sites. The field of view is therefore not restricted during actual surgery. Furthermore, through the working channel other instruments can be applied.

To conclude, a proof of concept is shown. It is possible to use a balloon to sense the contour of the intestinal wall and capture it in images. This allows a localization of the overtube relative to the balloon and thus to the intestinal wall.

Acknowledgement. This work was supported by Federal Ministry of Education and Research of Germany (Grant #: 01DR19002A) and by International Joint Technology Development Project funded by the Korean Ministry of Trade, Industry and Energy (Grant #: P0006718).

References

1. Quintero E, Castells A, Bujanda L, et al. Colonoscopy versus fecal immunochemical testing in colorectal-cancer screening. N Engl J Med. 2012;366(8):697–706.
2. Levin B, Lieberman DA, McFarland B, et al. Screening and surveillance for the early detection of colorectal cancer and adenomatous polyps, 2008: a joint guideline from the american cancer society, the US multi-society task force on colorectal cancer, and the american college of radiology. Gastroenterology. 2008;134(5):1570–1595.
3. Robert Koch-Institut. Inanspruchnahme der Darmspiegelung in Deutschland. RKI-Bib1 (Robert Koch-Institut);. Available from: https://www.rki.de/DE.
4. Reckter B. VDI nachrichten, editor. Robotergestützte magnetische Endoskopie. Online; 2020. Available from: https://www.vdi-nachrichten.com/technik/robotergestuetzte-magnetische-endoskopie/.
5. Burgner-Kahrs J, Rucker DC, Choset H. Continuum robots for medical applications: a survey. IEEE Trans Robot. 2015;31(6):1261–1280.
6. Patel N, Seneci C, Yang GZ, et al. Flexible platforms for natural orifice transluminal and endoluminal surgery. Endoscopy international open. 2014;2(2):E117–23.
7. Kume K. Flexible robotic endoscopy: current and original devices. Computer assisted surgery (Abingdon, England). 2016;21(1):150–159.
8. Abbott DJ, Becke C, Rothstein RI, et al. Design of an endoluminal NOTES robotic system. In: IEEE/RSJ International Conference on Intelligent Robots and Systems, 2007. Piscataway, NJ: IEEE Service Center; 2007. p. 410–416.
9. Hwang M, Kwon DS. K-FLEX: a flexible robotic platform for scar-free endoscopic surgery. Int J Med Robot. 2020;16(2):e2078.
10. Yuen HK, Princen J, Dlingworth J, et al. A comparative study of hough transform methods for circle finding. In: Baker KD, editor. Procedings of the Alvey Vision Conference 1989. Alvey Vision Club; 1989. p. 29.1–29.6.
11. Pedersen SJK. Circular hough transform. In: Encyclopedia of Biometrics; 2009. .
12. Nischwitz A, Fischer M, Haberäcker P. Bildverarbeitung: Band II des Standardwerks Computergrafik und Bildverarbeitung. 4th ed. Springer Vieweg; 2020.

Externe Ventrikeldrainage mittels Augmented Reality und Peer-to-Peer-Navigation

Simon Strzeletz[1], José Moctezuma[2], Mukesch Shah[3], Ulrich Hubbe[3], Harald Hoppe[1]

[1]Hochschule Offenburg, Labor für Computerassistierte Medizin
[2]Stryker Leibinger GmbH & Co. KG, Freiburg
[3]Universitätsklinikum Freiburg, Klinik für Neurochirurgie
simon.strzeletz@hs-offenburg.de

Zusammenfassung. Das hier vorgestellte System verbindet das neue Konzept der Peer-to-Peer-Navigation mit dem Einsatz von Augmented Reality zur Unterstützung von bettseitig durchgeführten externen Ventrikeldrainagen. Das sehr kompakte und genaue Gesamtsystem beinhaltet einen Patiententracker mit integrierter Kamera, eine Augmented-Reality-Brille mit Kamera und eine Punktionsnadel bzw. einen Pointer mit zwei Trackern, mit dessen Hilfe die Anatomie des Patienten aufgenommen wird. Die exakte Position und Richtung der Punktionsnadel wird unter Zuhilfenahme der aufgenommenen Landmarken berechnet und über die Augmented-Reality-Brille für den Chirurgen sichtbar auf dem Patienten dargestellt. Die Methode zur Kalibrierung der statischen Transformationen zwischen Patiententracker und daran befestigter Kamera beziehungsweise zwischen den Trackern der Punktionsnadel sind für die Genauigkeit sehr wichtig und werden hier vorgestellt. Das Gesamtsystem konnte in vitro erfolgreich getestet werden und bestätigt den Nutzen eines Peer-to-Peer-Navigationssystems.

1 Einleitung

Der Einsatz herkömmlicher Navigationssysteme für externe Ventrikeldrainagen (EVD) ist in dringlichen Situationen zu aufwendig, wenngleich dies aus Gründen der Genauigkeit, insbesondere für Ungeübte, wünschenswert wäre. AlAzri et al. haben in [1] gezeigt, dass externe Ventrikeldrainagen, die ohne Navigationsunterstützung durchgeführt werden, sehr ungenau sind. Zwar ist die Sterblichkeitsrate gering, doch mit jeder weiteren fehlgeschlagenen Platzierung steigt das Risiko einer Verletzung des Gewebes. Ferner sind Augmented-Reality-Brillen (AR-Brillen) zur Einblendung von Einstichpunkt und -richtung noch nicht in der klinischen Routine angekommen. Beide Aspekte werden in dem hier vorgestellten Konzept kostengünstig adressiert. Bisherige Konzepte dieser Art benötigen bildgebende Verfahren und sind bzgl. ihrer Genauigkeit nicht validiert [2].

Herkömmliche Navigationssysteme weisen eine eindeutige Trennung zwischen nachverfolgender Kamera und nachverfolgtem Tracker auf. Das Konzept der

Springer Fachmedien Wiesbaden GmbH, ein Teil von Springer Nature 2021
C. Palm et al. (Hrsg.), *Bildverarbeitung für die Medizin 2021*,
Informatik aktuell, https://doi.org/10.1007/978-3-658-33198-6_18

Peer-to-Peer-Navigation (P2P) hebt diese Trennung auf [3]: Präzise kalibrierte Kameras befinden sich unmittelbar im Operationssitus – insbesondere integriert in Trackern, die ihrerseits andere Tracker nachverfolgen. Die Anordnung der Tracker-LEDs ist so gewählt, dass eine monokulare Kamera ausreicht, um Transformationen schnell und präzise mittels Point-to-Line-Matching berechnen zu können. Neben weiteren Details wurde in [4] gezeigt, dass die dabei erzielte Genauigkeit den Anforderungen im chirurgischen Bereich genügt.

2 Material und Methoden

Im hier vorliegenden Anwendungsbeispiel der EVD trägt der Operateur eine AR-Brille mit integrierter Kamera W, die sowohl den Patiententracker T als auch den auf der Punktionsnadel bzw. dem Pointer S befestigten Tracker A nachverfolgt (Abb. 1). Die in T integrierte Kamera K verfolgt einen zweiten an S angebrachten Tracker B. Dieser Punktions-Tracker kann von K und W beidseitig nachverfolgt werden. Präkalibriert sind die rigiden Transformationen T ↔ K, S ↔ A sowie S ↔ B. Die entscheidende Transformation S → W entsteht wahlweise über die Kette S → A → W oder S → B → K → T → W. Die Punktionsnadel bzw. der Pointer bleiben auch dann sichtbar, wenn einer dieser Pfade unterbrochen ist. Punktionsnadel, Pointer sowie Patiententracker sind als sterile Einwegartikel konzipiert.

Abb. 1. Das Gesamtsystem besteht aus AR-Brille, Peer-to-Peer Patiententracker und Punktionsnadel bzw. Pointer.

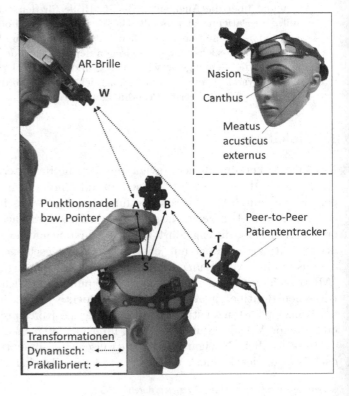

2.1 Algorithmus

Nach Befestigen des Patiententrackers und Aufsetzen der AR-Brille führen folgende Schritte zum Kocher-Punkt c und der Punktionsrichtung d (nach Seeger [5]):

1. Digitalisierung von ipsilateralem m_I und kontralateralem m_K Meatus acusticus externus.
2. Digitalisierung von Nasion n und ipsilateralem Epicanthus e_I. Die sagittale Mittelebene M verläuft durch n und steht senkrecht auf $m_I - m_K$.
3. Vom Nasion ausgehend: Digitalisierung von Punkten q_i entlang der Sagittalebene in Richtung Bregma. Durch Projektion der q_i auf M ergeben sich die projizierten Punkte p_i, entlang derer der Punkt p_M bestimmt wird, der sich 120 mm vom Nasion entfernt befindet.
4. Digitalisierung von Punkten r_j des ipsilateralen Bereichs, der sich circa 25 mm entfernt von p_M und M befindet. Der Punktionspunkt c wird so berechnet, dass sich dieser in der Ebene E befindet, die durch m_I, m_K und p_M verläuft und 25 mm (gemessen entlang der gekrümmten Oberfläche r_j) von p_M entfernt ist.
5. Bestimmung des Lotfußpunktes e_L des ipsilateralen Epicanthus e_I auf der Ebene E. Die Punktionsrichtung ist $d = e_L - c$.

Sowohl die digitalisierten Punkte als auch die aus diesen Punkten berechnete Punktionsstelle und Punktionsrichtung werden ortsgenau als Überlagerung in der AR-Brille dargestellt. Die Digitalisierung selbst erfolgt mittels Fußpedal.

2.2 Kalibrierung der statischen Transformationen

Die Genauigkeit des Gesamtsystems hängt entscheidend davon ab, dass die statischen Transformationen zwischen Kamera K und Tracker T sowie zwischen den beiden Trackern A und B der Punktionsnadel bzw. des Pointers exakt kalibriert sind.

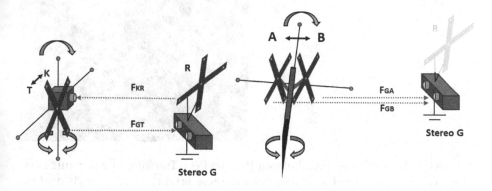

Abb. 2. Schematische Darstellung des Aufbaus zur Bestimmung der Transformation F_{KT} bzw. F_{AB}.

Zur Kalibrierung der Transformation F_{KT} wird der Verbund aus Kamera K und Tracker T auf einem Kalibrierkreuz befestigt, an dessen Enden sich jeweils eine Kugel befindet (Abb. 2 links). Nun werden die Mittelpunkte dieser vier Kugeln im Koordinatensystem T bestimmt, indem diese in einer Mulde pivotiert und dabei von einem Stereokamerasystem G beobachtet werden. Nach jeweils 1000 aufgenommenen Transformationen F_{GT_i} aus möglichst vielen Blickwinkeln werden die Kugelmittelpunkte m_{T_j} mit $1 \leq j \leq 4$ optimiert. In gleicher Weise werden die Mittelpunkte der Kugeln auch im Koordinatensystem K der Kamera bestimmt, wobei nun ein fester Tracker R als Referenz dient. Wiederum durch Pivotieren und Aufnahme von jeweils 1000 Transformationen F_{KR_i} können die Mittelpunkte m_{K_j} optimiert werden. F_{KT} ergibt sich nun mittels Least-Square-Fit der Punkte m_{T_j} auf die Punkte m_{K_j} (Point-to-Point-Matching).

Vollkommen analog wird auch der Verbund aus den Trackern A und B auf einem Kalibrierkreuz befestigt und zunächst Tracker A, dann Tracker B um jede der vier Kugeln pivotiert und dabei vom Stereokamerasystem G beobachtet (Abb. 2 rechts). Aus den jeweils 1000 Transformationen F_{GA_i} bzw. F_{GB_i} werden wiederum die Mittelpunkte der Kugeln m_{A_j} bzw. m_{B_j} optimiert, und die Transformation F_{AB} ergibt sich nun mittels Least-Square-Fit der Punkte m_{B_j} auf die Punkte m_{A_j}.

3   Ergebnisse

Das Gesamtsystem konnte inzwischen erfolgreich in vitro (Abb. 1) getestet werden. Dabei wurde, wie in Kapitel 2 beschrieben, vorgegangen, um die Anatomie des Patienten aufzunehmen. Einstichstelle und Punktionsrichtung konnten problemlos in der AR-Brille auf dem Patienten überlagert dargestellt werden (Abb. 3).

Abb. 3. Blick durch ein Display der AR-Brille auf den Patienten.

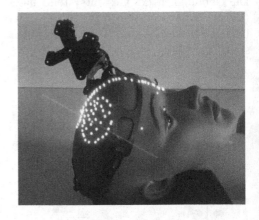

Dass das Konzept des monokularen Peer-to-Peer-Trackings die Genauigkeits-anforderungen chirurgischer Navigationssysteme erfüllt, konnte in [3] nachgewiesen werden. Für die Kalibrierung der statischen Transformationen wurde gezielt eine Stereo-Kamera eingesetzt, um eine noch höhere Genauigkeit zu erzielen. Das Tracking mit einer Stereo-Kamera ist im Vergleich zu monokularem Pose-Estimation im Schnitt um den Faktor 2,5 genauer. In Abbildung 4 (links) sind die Abweichungen der mit Stereo- und Monokular-Tracking pivotierten Punkte mit je 1000 Transformationen für eine Kalibrierung des Peer-to-Peer-Patiententrackers aufgelistet. Abbildung 4 (rechts) zeigt die statistische Verteilung der Abweichungen in mm für jeden pivotierten Punkt.

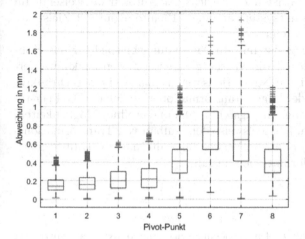

Abb. 4. Vergleich der Berechnung von jeweils vier pivotierten Punkten mittels Stereo- und Monokular-Tracking bei der P2P-Tracker-Kalibrierung. Die Daten zu diesem Boxplot sind in Tabelle 1 zusammengefasst.

| Tracking | Abweichung in mm | |
	Median	Maximum
Stereo 1	0,14	0,45
Stereo 2	0,15	0,51
Stereo 3	0,20	0,61
Stereo 4	0,21	0,71
Monokular 5	0,41	1,22
Monokular 6	0,73	1,91
Monokular 7	0,64	1,93
Monokular 8	0,39	1,20

Tabelle 1. Ergebnisse von jeweils vier pivoten Punkten.

4   Diskussion

Vergleichbare Systeme für navigierte Eingriffe sind meist mit hohen Kosten verbunden. Das hier vorgestellte System ist sehr kostengünstig und ermöglicht dennoch das genaue Auffinden und präzise Einblenden der Anatomie auf dem Patienten. So kann ein Eingriff ohne lange Wartezeiten bettseitig auch von nicht erfahrenen Chirurgen durchgeführt werden. Anatomische Strukturen aus bildgebenden Verfahren können, sofern diese bezüglich des Patiententrackers registriert wurden, direkt in der AR-Brille eingeblendet werden. Das Gesamtsystem wird an einem Laptop betrieben und kostet lediglich circa 1350 Euro (600 Euro für die AR-Brille, 600 Euro für die Kameras, circa 150 Euro für die übrigen Komponenten), wobei der batteriebetriebene Pointer- bzw. Punktionsnadel-Tracker und der Patienten-Tracker T als Einwegartikel konzipiert sind. Die hier vorgestellte Möglichkeit, kostengünstig, schnell und genau eine navigierte externe Ventrikeldrainage durchzuführen ist nach Ansicht der Autoren wegweisend. Im nächsten Schritt wird das Gesamtsystem an einem Phantomkopf mit Zielstrukturen durch Neurochirurgen evaluiert.

Die externe Ventrikeldrainage ist nur ein Anwendungsbeispiel für das Konzept der Peer-to-Peer-Navigation, die vielseitig eingesetzt werden kann. Herkömmliche, platzintensive optische Navigationssysteme sind bei eingeschränkter Sicht auf ihre Tracker nicht in der Lage, Transformationen zu liefern. Die Peer-to-Peer-Navigation erlaubt Tracking auf engstem Raum und eröffnet Möglichkeiten, die bisher nicht möglich waren, beispielsweise den Aufbau von Transformationsketten (Tracken um die Ecke) oder die Verwendung alternativer Transformationspfade, falls einzelne Transformationen ausfallen.

Literatur

1. AlAzri A, Mok K, Chankowsky J, et al. Placement accuracy of external ventricular drain when comparing freehand insertion to neuronavigation guidance in severe traumatic brain injury. Acta Neurochir. 2017; p. 0942–0940.
2. Kunz C, Hlavac M, Schneider M, et al. A system for augmented reality guided ventricular puncture using a holoLens: design implementation and initial evaluation. In: T Neumuth et al (eds) CURAC 2018. 2018; p. 132–137.
3. Strzeletz S, Hazubski S, Moctezuma JL, et al. Peer-to-peer-navigation in der computerassistierten Chirurgie. T Neumuth et al (eds) CURAC 2018. 2018; p. 119–124.
4. Strzeletz S, Hazubski S, Moctezuma JL, et al. Fast, robust, and accurate monocular peer-to-peer tracking for surgical navigation. Int J Comput Assist Radiol Surg. 2020; p. 479–489.
5. Seeger W. Atlas of topographical anatomy of the brain and surrounding structures for neurosurgeons, neuroradiologists, and neuropathologists. 1978; p. 420–323.

Abstract: Contour-based Bone Axis Detection for X-ray-guided Surgery on the Knee

Florian Kordon[1,2,3], Andreas Maier[1,3,4], Benedict Swartman[5],
Maxim Privalov[5], Jan Siad El Barbari[5], Holger Kunze[2,1]

[1]Pattern Recognition Lab, Universität Erlangen-Nürnberg (FAU), Erlangen
[2]Siemens Healthcare GmbH, Forchheim
[3]Erlangen Graduate School in Advanced Optical Technologies (SAOT), Universität
Erlangen-Nürnberg (FAU), Erlangen
[4]Machine Intelligence, Universität Erlangen-Nürnberg (FAU), Erlangen
[5]Department for Trauma and Orthopaedic Surgery, BG Trauma Center
Ludwigshafen, Ludwigshafen
florian.kordon@fau.de

The anatomical axis of long bones is an important reference line for guiding fracture reduction and assisting in the correct placement of guide pins, screws, and implants in orthopedics and trauma surgery. While planning such axes can be easily done on pre-operative static data, doing so consistently on live images during surgery is inherently more complex due to motion and a limited field of view. In addition, non-sterile interaction with a planning software is unwanted. To circumvent these limitations, we propose a simple and clinically motivated image-guided approach for detection of the anatomical axis of long bones on 2D X-ray images. We translate the established two-line/two-circle manual method to a learning based extraction of anatomical features and subsequent geometric construction. A multi-task neural network first predicts a bone segmentation mask as well as region of interest (ROI) encodings of the relevant shaft sections of the bone. A segmentation contour is then computed using a logical XOR operation with a morphologically eroded version of the segmentation mask. Lastly, the relevant sections of this contour are extracted by evaluating the predicted ROIs and are subsequently used as auxiliary lines to derive the anatomical axis with the 2-line/2-circle method. The approach is evaluated for the femur and tibia in the knee joint and achieves a median angulation error of 0.19° and 0.33° respectively. An inter-rater study with three trauma surgery experts confirms reliability of the method and recommends further clinical application [1].

References

1. Kordon F, Maier A, Swartman B, et al. Contour-based bone axis detection for X-ray guided surgery on the knee. Proc MICCAI. 2020; p. 671–680.

Springer Fachmedien Wiesbaden GmbH, ein Teil von Springer Nature 2021
C. Palm et al. (Hrsg.), *Bildverarbeitung für die Medizin 2021*,
Informatik aktuell, https://doi.org/10.1007/978-3-658-33198-6_19

Novel Evaluation Metrics for Vascular Structure Segmentation

Marcel Reimann, Weilin Fu, Andreas Maier

Pattern Recognition Lab, FAU Erlangen-Nürnberg
`marcel.reimann@fau.de`

Abstract. For the diagnosis of eye-related diseases segmentation of the retinal vessels and the analysis of the tortuousness, completeness, and thickness of these vessels are the fundamental steps. The assessment of the quality of the retinal vessel segmentation, therefore, plays a crucial role. Conventionally, different evaluation metrics for retinal vessel segmentation have been proposed. Most of them are based on pixel matching. Recently, a novel non-global measure has been introduced. It focuses on the skeletal similarity between vessel segments rather than the pixel-wise overlay and redefines the terms of the confusion matrix. In our work, we re-implement this evaluation algorithm and discover the design flaws in the algorithm. Therefore, we propose modifications to the metric. The basic structure of the algorithm, which combines the thickness and curve similarity is preserved. Meanwhile, the calculation of the curve similarity is modified and extended. Furthermore, our modifications enable us to apply the evaluation metric to three-dimensional data. We show that compared to the conventional pixel matching-based metrics our proposed metric is more representative for cases where vessels are missing, disoriented, or inconsistent in their thickness.

1 Introduction

The analysis of fundus images plays an important role in the diagnosis of many eye-related diseases, such as Diabetic Retinopathy (DR), Glaucoma and age-related macular degeneration, which are the leading causes of vision loss according to [1]. Segmentation of the retinal vessels is the fundamental step for fundus image analysis, and provides the physician with information on the thickness, tortuousness, and completeness of the retinal vessels [2]. During the past decades, many algorithms have been developed to generate accurate, fast, and robust retinal vessel segmentation. However, the evaluation metrics to assess the quality of these segmentation results are mainly based on pixel-wise overlapping and fail to capture the vascular structures of the vessels [2].

Recently, a new metric which utilizes the skeletal similarities between vessel segments to redefine each term in the confusion matrix has been proposed by Yan et al. [3]. The metric is a weighted combination of the thickness and curve similarity between the vessel segments of the ground truth and the test segmentation. Their metric overcomes the inter-observer problems of ground truths in evaluation data sets and ensures the completeness of the vessel tree in the test segmentation. These are significant improvements compared to traditional metrics. However, when re-implementing their algorithm, several design flaws are observed. In this work, we closely examine the algorithm by Yan *et al.*, point out their mathematical shortcomings, and propose solutions to the discovered problems. In this way, we can obtain a correct 2-D skeletal similarity-based evaluation metric and potentially lift the algorithm into 3-D. This enables the usage for more applications, such as the evaluation of airway segmentation.

2   Materials and methods

2.1   Existing algorithm

In the algorithm by Yan *et al.* the test and reference segmentations are skeletonized and the thickness of the vessel at each point of the skeleton is computed. Afterwards, the skeleton of the reference is cut into smaller components with a length in the range of $[4, 15]$ pixels. In the next step, each of the components gets assigned a searching range of $[1, 2]$ pixels and the average vessel thickness of the component is computed. Afterwards, a third order polynomial is fitted to the points of the reference skeleton and the points of the test skeleton within the searching range. Next, the first three coefficients of the cubic functions are compared using the cosine similarity which results in the curve similarity of that component. The thickness similarity can be evaluated by comparing the average thickness of the vessels in that part of the segmentation. The curve and thickness similarity are then balanced by the parameter $\alpha \in [0, 1]$ resulting in the skeletal similarity of the components mentioned above. The overall score is computed by summing up the individual scores weighed by the length of the corresponding reference component. Eventually, the values for true positives, false negatives, false positives, and true negatives are redefined using the searching range and the computed skeletal similarity.

While reviewing their algorithm, we discovered the computation of the curve similarity to be inaccurate. The coefficients of cubic functions may describe the curvature globally. However, looking at small intervals of the function, the coefficients alone cannot be used to calculate the curve similarity. As an example, we demonstrate the obvious similarity in curvature of $f(x) = x^3 + x^2 + \sqrt{2}x$ and $g(x) = x^3 + x^2 - \sqrt{2}x$ on the interval $[34, 48]$ compared to the dissimilarity for values close to the origin (Fig. 1).

However, if we compute the cosine similarity of the coefficients, the similarity results to 0.0. In conclusion, even though the algorithm by Yan *et al.* seems to provide accurate results, the metric is mathematically inaccurate.

2.2   Modification of the algorithm

Even though there is an error in the algorithm, we follow the idea behind it and try to modify the computation to yield correct and reasonable results.

2.2.1 Piece-wise curvature of retinal vessel trees. Firstly, we had a look at the curvature of all components of the skeleton, to check whether a third order polynomial as an approximation is necessary. We tried cubic, quadratic, and linear approximations to the components and evaluated the Mean Squared Error (MSE). As expected, the MSE decreased by an increasing order of the polynomial. However, a linear approximation yields a MSE of 3.389 pixels on average. We consider this a negligible error, which is underlined by Heneghan *et al.* [4], stating that retinal vessel trees are piece-wise linear. Therefore, we are able to proceed with linear instead of cubic approximations.

2.2.2 Modifications based on singular value decomposition. To make our metric expandable to three-dimensional data, we choose to perform a singular value decomposition on the mean subtracted data and select the first eigenvector as the orientation vector of the linear approximation. The curve similarity is then calculated using the cosine similarity of the two corresponding orientation vectors.

2.2.3 Modifications based on directed Hausdorff distance. Another option to replace the curve similarity cs is a point-wise comparison of the components A of the reference and B of the test segmentation. The maximum distance $\check{H}(A,B)$ is then weighed by the length l_{ref} of the reference component and subtracted from 1 in order to receive similarity scores in the interval $[0,1]$

$$cs = 1 - \frac{\check{H}(A,B)}{l_{ref}} \tag{1}$$

As comparison metric we choose the directed Hausdorff distance, because it is commonly known, and used for the evaluation of image segmentation, even for three-dimensional data [5].

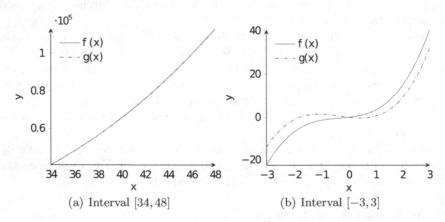

(a) Interval $[34, 48]$ (b) Interval $[-3, 3]$

Fig. 1. Curvature of the functions $f(x)$ and $g(x)$ on different intervals.

2.3 Database

In this work, the STARE database [6] is utilized to evaluate the proposed metric. The STARE database contains 20 fundus images of shape 605 × 704 pixels. Each image is provided with two manually annotated label maps. The manual annotations from the first expert is utilized as the ground truth. Different modifications, such as morphological operations and small vessel removal are applied on the ground truth to generate test images. In this work we show exemplary results for erosion, erosion plus skeleton and deletions as shown in Figure 2.

3 Results

In the evaluation process we compare the scores of specificity, sensitivity, and accuracy of the traditional computation, the algorithm by Yan *et al.* and the two proposed modifications. To assess the performance of the curve and the thickness similarity, we set the parameter α to 0 and 1, respectively. In addition to the results (Tab. 1, 2, 3), we first verify the metric by comparing the ground truth image with itself, receiving higher scores than the existing algorithm. For Hausdorff we receive an average sensitivity of 99.98%, for SVD 99.99% and for Yan's algorithm 97.66% with α set to 0. When α is set to 1 the score of the modifications with 99.739% is almost indiscernible higher than of Yan's metric with an average sensitivity of 99.738%. The difference is caused by the restriction in Yan's metric that the test component of the skeleton must be at least 0.6 times the size of the reference, otherwise the similarity score is directly set to 0. In our metric we do not impose this restriction leading to higher scores and a better comparison of all the pixels in the segmentation.

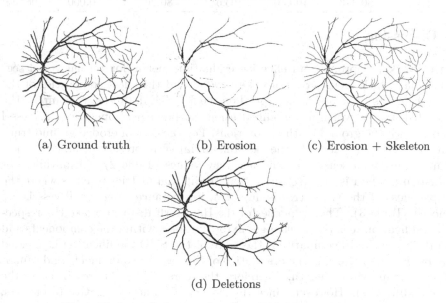

(a) Ground truth   (b) Erosion   (c) Erosion + Skeleton

(d) Deletions

Fig. 2. Evaluation data set based on STARE image no. 162.

Table 1. Erosion evaluation of STARE image No. 162.

	alpha = 0.0			alpha = 1.0		
	Se	Sp	Acc	Se	Sp	Acc
Traditional	29.529	100.000	94.979	29.529	100.000	94.979
Yan *et al.*	31.828	100.000	84.759	14.640	100.000	80.917
Hausdorff	35.393	100.000	85.556	26.934	100.000	83.665
SVD	43.851	100.000	87.447	26.934	100.000	83.665

Table 2. Erosion + Skeleton evaluation of STARE image No. 162.

	alpha = 0.0			alpha = 1.0		
	Se	Sp	Acc	Se	Sp	Acc
Traditional	52.706	100.000	96.630	52.706	100.000	96.630
Yan *et al.*	97.597	100.000	99.463	78.263	100.000	95.140
Hausdorff	99.617	100.000	99.914	78.263	100.000	95.140
SVD	99.945	100.000	99.988	78.263	100.000	95.140

Table 3. Deletion evaluation of STARE image No. 162.

	alpha = 0.0			alpha = 1.0		
	Se	Sp	Acc	Se	Sp	Acc
Traditional	88.746	100.000	99.198	88.746	100.000	99.198
Yan *et al.*	74.303	100.000	94.255	75.885	100.000	94.609
Hausdorff	76.716	100.000	94.794	80.266	100.000	95.588
SVD	80.473	100.000	95.634	80.266	100.000	95.588

4 Discussion

In this work, we propose an effective evaluation metric for retinal vessel segmentation, which focuses on both the skeletal and thickness similarities of the
vessel segments. The metric is applied on the STARE database, to compare the
annotated images which are modified using morphological operations or vessel
removal with the ground truth annotations. For the case of eroded ground truth
combined with the skeleton, the skeletal similarity is preserved, and our metric maintains high sensitivity and accuracy values (Table 2). Meanwhile, our
evaluation method is more sensitive than traditional metrics to cases where the
completeness of the vessel tree is impaired, for instance when small vessels are
removed (Table 3). The properties of the Hausdorff distance make the respective modification sensitive to changes in tortuousness within the components and
also their length. In comparison, the score of the SVD modification is affected
only by changes regarding the orientation of the vessels' components and cannot
reflect their individual length. Therefore, the scores (Table 1) are higher for the
SVD modification. However, since the Hausdorff value is sensitive to outliers,
it is observed that additive noise greatly affects the Hausdorff metric (Table 4).

Table 4. Noise evaluation of STARE image no. 162.

	alpha = 0.0			alpha = 1.0		
	Se	Sp	Acc	Se	Sp	Acc
Traditional	97.660	100.000	99.833	97.660	100.000	99.833
Yan *et al.*	98.026	100.000	99.559	89.875	100.000	97.736
Hausdorff	96.383	100.000	99.191	89.875	100.000	97.736
SVD	99.859	100.000	99.969	89.875	100.000	97.736

This is a disadvantage of that modification. In Table 1 we give an example for a combination of thickness and skeleton variation. In general, we recommend looking at different values for α, as low values introduce the curve similarity and high values the thickness similarity into the overall scores.

For future work, a user study could be carried out to confirm the effectiveness and superiority of the proposed metrics in a clinical environment. The proposed evaluation metrics could be directly applied on assessing the quality of the segmentation of other 2D vascular structures. More experiments could be conducted to extend our method into 3D and apply it on assessing the quality of more complicated tasks, such as airway segmentation.

References

1. Cheloni R, Gandolfi SA, Signorelli C, et al.   Global prevalence of diabetic retinopathy: protocol for a systematic review and meta-analysis.   BMJ Open. 2019;9(3):e022188.
2. Chetan L Srinidhi, P Aparna, Jeny Rajan. Recent advancements in retinal vessel segmentation. J Med Syst. 2017;41(4):1–22.
3. Yan Z, Yang X, Cheng KT. A skeletal similarity metric for quality evaluation of retinal vessel segmentation. IEEE Trans Med Imaging. 2018;37(4):1045–1057.
4. Heneghan C, Flynn J, O'Keefe M, et al. Characterization of changes in blood vessel width and tortuosity in retinopathy of prematurity using image analysis. Med Image Anal. 2002;6(4):407–429.
5. Taha AA, Hanbury A. Metrics for evaluating 3D medical image segmentation: analysis, selection, and tool. BMC Med Imaging. 2015;15.
6. Hoover AD, Kouznetsova V, Goldbaum M. Locating blood vessels in retinal images by piecewise threshold probing of a matched filter response. IEEE Trans Med Imaging. 2000;19(3):203–210.

A Machine Learning Approach Towards Fatty Liver Disease Detection in Liver Ultrasound Images

Adarsh Kuzhipathalil[1], Anto Thomas[1], Keerthana Chand[1],
Elmer Jeto Gomes Ataide[2], Alexander Link[4], Annika Niemann[3,5],
Sylvia Saalfeld[3,5], Michael Friebe[2], Jens Ziegle[2]

[1]Faculty of Computer Science, University of Magdeburg, Germany
[2]INKA-Application Driven Research, University of Magdeburg, Germany
[3]Department of Simulation and Graphics, University of Magdeburg, Germany
[4]Department of Gastroenterology, Hepatology and Infectious Diseases, University of Magdeburg
[5]STIMULATE Research Campus, University of Magdeburg
adarsh.kuzhipathalil@st.ovgu.de

Abstract. Fatty liver disease (FLD) is one of the prominent diseases which affects the normal functionality of the liver by building vacuoles of fat in the liver cells. FLD is an indicator of imbalance in the metabolic system and could cause cardiovascular diseases, liver inflammation, cirrhosis and furthermore neoplasm. Detection and specification of a FLD are beneficial to arrange an early and best adapted treatment. We present a computer aided diagnostic (CAD) tool for FLD detection using ultrasound images. The developed pipeline consists of separate segmentation and classification modules. During the development phase these modules were trained on 6 patient cases and validated with 2. The whole model was evaluated on a totally different set of data with 5 patient cases and performed with an overall classification accuracy of 0.84. The model showed impressive performance considering the size of training data. Also the multi-module architecture enables the predictions from the model to be better explainable.

1 Introduction

The liver has a significant role in detoxification protein synthesis and production of chemicals that helps in proper digestion. There are few diseases which affects its notmal functionality. Examples of liver disease include: Fatty liver disease (FLD), cirrhosis and cancer. Our study mainly concentrates on FLD. Blood tests, liver ultrasound (US) imaging, computed tomography and liver biopsy can be employed to detect and diagnose FLD [1].

US imaging is more common due to its lower cost and its non-invasive nature. FLD diagnosis often depends of the subjective judgement of the physicans due to differences in US equipment, poor image quality and the physical differences of patients. As physicians depend on different aspects of the US image for diagnosis, there are high variations in diagnosis which often depends on the experience of the physicians. Incorrect diagnosis could lead to wrong and contra-productive treatment, e.g. wrong concentration of medication may harm the patient. Previously published works on FLD [2] and diffused liver disease [3] detection in US images was successful in developing computer aided diagnostic (CAD) tools which aided the physicians in the diagnosis. Both of these works gives out one single prediction for the whole US image. We developed the tool which help in detecting fatty tissue in the US image and generate the prediction in such a way that it is better explainable for physicians with different levels of experience.

2   Material and methods

The major distinguishing character is the difference in texture patterns between fatty and non-fatty liver observed from US images. The FLD detection problem can essentially be modelled as a pattern recognition problem by extracting the texture features from respective classes and further building the classifier. There are previous efforts in developing similar pipelines for liver US images. Fractal Dimension Texture Analysis (FDTA), the Spatial Gray Level Dependence Matri-ces (SGLDM), the Gray Level Difference Statistics (GLDS), the Gray Level Run Length Statistics (RUNL), First Order Gray Level Parameters (FOP), Gray level Co-occurrence matrix (GLCM) and Wavelet Transforms (WT) are some commonly used texture feature extraction techniques [3, 4].

For developing the FLD detection pipeline, we have generated a dataset consisting of 13 patient cases in total. In the course of development 8 out of 13 were used and the remaining 5 were used to test the system at the fully developed stage. The study was performed according to the "World Medical Association Declaration of Helsinki - Ethical Principles for Medical Research Involving Human Subjects." All subjects included in the study provided written informed consent and the study protocol was approved by the local Institutional Review Board of Otto von Guericke University, Magdeburg. All images were anonymized prior to analysis.

The dataset was generated by two US systems (Philips iU22 and GE LOGIQ E10) consisting 964 images in total in fatty class and 1060 images in non-fatty class. The images were stored in JPEG format. The datasets were labelled according to the clinical diagnostic outcome. Segmentation ground truths were generated with the help of an experienced hepatologist. These were chosen in such a way that these contained only the characteristic liver texture excluding vessels and border tissues. This means that the segmentation masks did not necessarily contain the whole liver parts in the US image. Also the non fatty regions inside the fatty liver samples were not considered differently while gen-erating the segmentation masks. This was done to enable a pipeline to classify similar regions without explicitly training on such regions. Furthermore, this dataset was used in the machine learning (ML) pipeline for feature extraction and classification.

2.1   Training and output pipelines

The training phase of the pipeline is split in two different branches (Fig 1). The input dataset consists of fatty and non-fatty liver US images and the corresponding segmentation masks. The first branch takes the data and converts it to liver and background classes. The liver and background classes along with the labels makes up the training data for the first module. One the other branch, just the region of interest is extracted using the segmentation masks. Which means only the liver portion of the US image is selected and grouped as fatty and non-fatty class. These two classes along with the corresponding labels are used as the training data for the second module.

Before the feature extraction was performed on the US images, the images were converted into patches. The texture features were extracted from these generated patches since a global feature vector from the whole image is inefficient in case of US image texture, as the texture has large variations throughout the image. Overlapping patches were used in this case. This helped in better usage of the available data. The optimal patch size was found out to be 30×30 pixels. This was evaluated by experimenting with multiple patch sizes ranging from 10×10 till 50×50 pixels. Smaller patches failed to extract the texture characteristics and on the other hand larger patches resulted in extracting features from a mix of different textures.

For the prediction and visualization (Fig. 2), the input image is first given to the segmentation module and then to classification module to produce the final prediction results. For both the pipelines, feature importance studies and feature reduction methods using Principal Component Analysis (PCA) were performed. For the segmentation and classification modules random forest classifier was trained with the corresponding set of reduced features.

2.2   Texture feature extraction

Feature extraction step in the pattern recognition problem is the crucial and most influential step of the whole pipeline as it encodes the input image. The encoded features were used in the further decision process. The choice of features directly impacts the accuracy and the generalization of the classes of interest, in this problem the non-fatty and fatty liver tissues. In our approach we used 90 features in total. The majority of features (84) were extracted from Discrete Wavelet Transform (DWT) methods and 6 features from the GLCM.

The discrete wavelet transform (DWT) is performed using a set of 7 discrete wavelets namely Daubechies, Haar, Biorthogonal, Reversebiorthogonal, Symlets, Coiflets, and Mayer wavelets. These wavelets have different scales and translations. DWT decomposes the signal into mutually orthogonal sets of wavelets. The mean, variance and entropy were calculated for each patch decomposed using the seven wavelets, which makes up 84 features of feature vector. The contrast, dissimilarity, homogeneity, Angular Second Moment, energy, and correlation features (6 features in total) were extracted from the GLCM.

Fig. 1. Training pipeline.

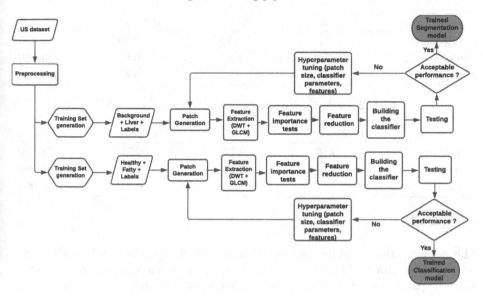

2.3   Model evaluation

Two out of eight patient cases were chosen as validation dataset to evaluate the performance of the model. The modules were evaluated separately using this data. Finally, to check the qualitative performance of the model pipeline and the combined performance of individual modules, 5 patient test cases were given to the pipeline and evaluated. This was done as those 5 cases contained a mix of different FLD stages. The qualitative visual inspection of the predictions mainly concentrated on the accuracy and completeness of segmentation, segmentation performance around the vessels and the classification performance. To evaluate the whole model on the binary classification problem (fatty or non-fatty), a prediction ratio (PR) was generated. PR is the ratio of patches which were classified as fatty to the ones which were classified as non-fatty. This was used as a quantitative measure to test the performance of the whole system.

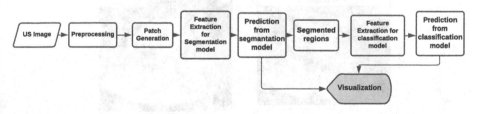

Fig. 2. Prediction pipeline.

Table 1. Performance matrix of the segmentation model.

	Precision	Recall	f1 Score	Support
Background	0.81	0.78	0.80	81,200
Liver	0.79	0.82	0.80	81,200
Accuracy			0.81	162,400

Table 2. Performance matrix of the classification model.

	Precision	Recall	f1 Score	Support
Non-Fatty	0.70	0.72	0.71	36,000
Fatty	0.74	0.74	0.70	45,200
Accuracy			0.71	81,200

3   Results

The segmentation module was tested with 162,400 patches and was able to achieve an accuracy of 0.81 (Table 1). Then the classification module was tested with the patches extracted from the liver sections. The module was tested with 81,200 patches and was able to achieve an average accuracy of 0.71 (Table 2). Equal number of patches were sampled from each of the classes while training and testing. This was necessary since the background is greater in size when compared to the liver sections.

The model was tested with a set of unseen samples for evaluating the qualitative performances. Fig 4 shows the predictions of a fatty sample when tested on the pipeline. The model was able to produce well generalized and accurate results. As seen in the figure, the ground truth contains only a portion of the liver in the US image, but the model was able to segment and classify most of the portions of the liver beyond the ground truth. Similar behavior is shown by the model on all of the testing images. The model performances with different thresholds for PR were evaluated. The model's binary classification accuracy was 0.84 with a PR of 0.60. The model predictions are helpful in locating the fatty regions for further diagnosis.

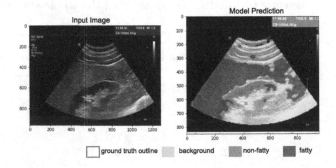

Fig. 3. Model prediction for an input image with a fatty sample.

Fig. 4. Segmentation around the vessels.

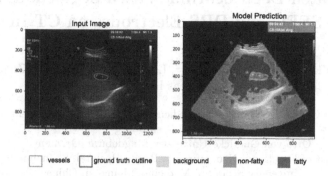

4 Discussions

The fatty tissue classification worked well using a pipeline consisting of segmentation and classification modules. Our proposed multi stage classification solution with the patch based approach was successful in the tissue texture recognition for our datasets. As depicted in Figure 4, the model was capable of successfully processing images that include vessels and learned to segment liver texture around vessels. Due to the adopted strategy in selection of ground truth, the quantitative model evaluation doesn't consider the regions which were predicted outside the ground truth. To evaluating model performance on these regions, a different set of ground truth with the segmentation masks covering the whole liver portion has to be generated. Due to the adopted strategy in generating the segmentation masks, model is not explicitly trained on minor variations in the texture. Hence the chances of overfitting is minimized.

There are few drawbacks for the developed model. Both the segmentation and classification modules were sensitive to the image scale. The used dataset was a mix of different scaled images. But rescaling the images to a single size resulted in loosing the details as our datasets were in JPEG format. Using DICOM or TIFF files would give better results.

References

1. Langer SG, Carter SJ, Haynor DR, et al. Image acquisition: ultrasound, computed tomography, and magnetic resonance imaging. World J Surg. 2001;25:1428–1437.
2. Fu M, D S, Hussain. Automated classification of liver disorders using ultrasound images. J Med Syst. 2012;36(5):3163–3172.
3. Kyriacou E, Pavlopoulos S, et al. Computer assisted characterization of diffused liver disease using image texture analysis techniques on B-scan images. IEEE Nucl Sci Symp Conf Rec (1997). 1997;2:1479–1483.
4. Kyriacou E, Pavlopoulos S, et al. Fuzzy neural network-based texture analysis of ultrasonic images. IEEE Eng Med Biol Mag. 2000;19:39–47.

Automated Deep Learning-based Segmentation of Brain, SEEG and DBS Electrodes on CT Images

Vanja Vlasov[1], Marie Bofferding[2], Loïc Marx[1], Chencheng Zhang[3], Jorge Goncalves[1], Andreas Husch[1], Frank Hertel[1,4]

[1]Luxembourg Centre for Systems Biomedicine (LCSB), University of Luxembourg, Belvaux, Luxembourg
[2]Otto von Guericke University Magdeburg, Germany
[3]Department of Functional Neurosurgery, Ruijin Hospital, Shanghai Jiao Tong University School of Medicine, Shanghai, China
[4]National department of Neurosurgery, Hospital Centre of Luxembourg (CHL), Luxembourg
vanja.vlasov@uni.lu

Abstract. Stereoelectroencephalography (sEEG) and deep brain stimulation (DBS) are effective surgical diagnostic and therapeutic procedures of the depth electrodes implantation in the brain. The benefit and outcome of these procedures directly depend on the electrode placement. Our goal was to accurately segment and visualize electrode position after the sEEG and DBS procedures. We trained a deep learning network to automatically segment electrodes trajectories and brain tissue from postsurgical CT images. We used 90 head CT scans that include intracerebral electrodes and their corresponding segmentation masks to train, validate and test the model. Mean accuracy and dice score in 5-fold cross-validation for the 3D-cascade U-Net model were 0.99 and 0.92, respectively. When the network was tested on an unseen test set, the dice overlap with the manual segmentations was 0.89. In this paper, we present a deep-learning approach for automatic patient-specific delineation of the brain, the sEEG and DBS electrodes from different varying quality of CT images. This robust method may inform on the postsurgical electrode positions fast and accurately. Moreover, it is useful as an input for neurosurgical and neuroscientific toolboxes and frameworks.

1 Introduction

With advances in stereotactic techniques, robotics and neuroimaging, there has been a worldwide increase in the use of stereoelectroencephalography (sEEG) [1]. SEEG is a surgical diagnostic procedure that helps to find brain areas responsible for the epileptogenic activity in the complex cases of epilepsy. During the sEEG surgery, 4 to 18 depth electrodes are implanted in the patient's brain to record local field potentials from several brain structures. Depth electrode recordings are sampled from the electrode entry site along the trajectory to the final target

Springer Fachmedien Wiesbaden GmbH, ein Teil von Springer Nature 2021
C. Palm et al. (Hrsg.), *Bildverarbeitung für die Medizin 2021*,
Informatik aktuell, https://doi.org/10.1007/978-3-658-33198-6_22

point. Therefore, fast and accurate 3D visualization of the implanted electrodes is crucial for the outcome of the procedure and the following therapeutic decision.

Automated, accurate deep brain stimulation (DBS) electrode delineations toolboxes have been used in neurosurgical and scientific practice [2, 3]. However, there is a lack of available, successful tools for sEEG electrode segmentation and state-of-the-art in postsurgical electrode evaluation is still done visually by clinicians. This approach is based on the co-registration of patient image modalities, it is prone to errors and time-consuming. Due to extensive metal artefacts, electrodes thin nature, banding and overlapping, the simple thresholding of appropriate Hounsfield units is not satisfactory to segment implanted electrodes from a CT volume. Recently published semi-automated toolboxes for sEEG segmentation are an improvement of the state-of-the-art, but not validated on a larger heterogeneous data-sets [4, 5, 6, 7]. Arnulfo et al. segment sEEG contacts from a thresholded cone-beam homogeneous voxel space CT images based on presurgical planned trajectories [4]. However, the error might arise with this approach since sEEG electrodes are bending and overlapping and their postoperative trajectories are not as planned before the surgery. Novel methods are also mostly based on patient MRI and CT co-registration and not on deep learning [5, 6]. These methods require manual corrections and annotations when patients unilateral or bilateral electrodes are overlapping.

Novel advances in deep learning provided frameworks for training a convolutional neural network (CNN) specialized for medical imaging [8]. We trained such a network in order to develop a robust, automated and a fast electrode and brain segmentation tool for CT imaging. Our solution is not requiring any additional imaging modality and preprocessing. By including post-operative DBS imaging, we increase a dataset and ensure to learn a solution that is robust towards all kinds of depth electrodes.

2   Materials and methods

2.1   Dataset description

A total of 90 anonymised head CT image data set from patients that underwent routine clinical planning of stereotactic surgery procedures was available for this study. The data set contained post-operative CT imaging with one or more electrodes implanted in the brain as part of a DBS or SEEG procedure and additional pre-operative T1- weighted MRIs. Post-DBS scans were acquired at the Centre Hospitalier de Luxembourg (40 images, 81 DBS electrodes) and post-sEEG scans at the Shanghai Rujin Hospital (50 images, 334 sEEG electrodes). Among the data-set were CT images obtained in different centres using three CT scanner vendors, images of different quality and reconstructed with other than soft-tissue filters, for example, bone-filter CT scans. Images with implant- and patient-based artifacts, such as beam hardening and metal or motion artifacts, were included in the study. For training the network, 35 post DBS and 45 post sEEG CT volumes were randomly selected. The remaining 10 CT images were used as a network performance test set. To generate CT image labels for training, firstly, the brain was extracted and DBS electrodes were segmented with a previously published pipeline [2]. Secondly, across the post sEEG CT scans the fitting high Hounsfield Unit (HU) intensity threshold was used to extract all the electrodes and wires. Finally, all electrodes and brain labels in CT space were manually corrected and unnecessary wires and bone structures were removed using ITK-SNAP.

The training data was split into five random cross-validation sets. Training CT images and corresponding labels were resampled to the median voxel dimension of the image volumes, $0.48 \times 0.48 \times 0.66$ mm.

2.2   Network architecture

As CT volumes are impractical and memory expensive to train the full 3D resolution, with the input size of $512 \times 512 \times X$, the 3D-cascade U-net model enables the network to accumulate contextual and spatial information. The 3D cascade U-net model architecture, used in this work for segmentation, has been designed from the nnU-Net framework [8]. The architecture of the network is shown in Fig. 1., where first a 3D-low-resolution U-net is employed followed by a

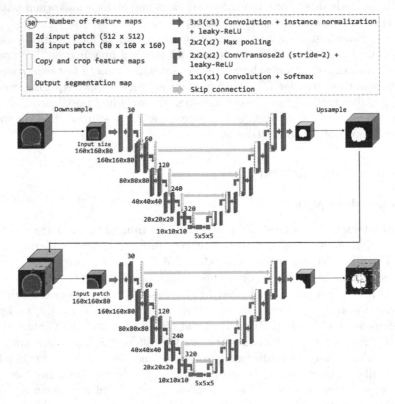

Fig. 1. Two parts of the 3D Cascade U-Net model network architecture: low resolution 3D U-Net following with patch based 3D U-Net.

full high-resolution 3D U-net on smaller image patches. Random rotations and translations were used to augment the training data.

The framework utilizes a loss-function combining dice-loss and cross-entropy loss to mitigate class imbalance problems. The initial learning rate of the stochastic gradient descent was 10^{-2} with a decay of 3×10^{-5}. Learning was terminated due to no further improvement of the validation loss.

Data processing was carried out on the High-Performance-Computing (HPC) cluster of the University of Luxembourg, utilizing four Tesla V100 GPU with 16GB GPU Memory.

2.3 Performance assessment

In addition to the cross-validation, we evaluated the trained network on the independent test set. Within the test set, there was a CT scan with a bone reconstruction kernel instead of the typical soft tissue filter allowing insights on performance on different CT reconstruction noise. The segmentation performance was assessed using the Sørensen-Dice similarity coefficient.

3   Results

The mean accuracy for the model in the cross-validation was > 0.99 and mean Dice Coefficient was 0.921. In the analysis on the independent test set, comparing network segmentation of both brain and electrodes label with manual segmentation, the mean dice score with standard deviation was 0.897 ± 0.043 and average computation time of 230.2 ± 65.4 seconds.

Figure 2 illustrates the qualitative visualisation of the method segmentations. Segmentation's are shown for post-operative CT scans with implanted DBS and SEEG electrodes. Figure 3 shows an example of the network performance for CT image with bone reconstruction filter. Our U-Net achieved plausible segmentations in postsurgical images for both procedures. The nnU-net-based 3D Cascade model showed convincing performance. Furthermore, our method correctly labelled brain shift observed in frontal areas as background class.

4   Discussion

This paper introduced a nnU-net-based approach for depth electrode and brain segmentation from CT head scans.

One of the main concerns regarding using deep learning is a lack of generalisation: a network losing the ability to yield satisfactory results on input data with different properties than the training data. By including training data from two centres, different image quality and reconstruction filters, as well as the brain with SEEG and DBS electrode implants our network was able to learn to appropriately segment electrodes trajectories within and outside the brain parenchyma. Moreover, our network delineated the sEEG electrodes and brain in very bad soft tissue contrast example in CT scan reconstructed with the bone kernel.

To our knowledge, this is the first deep-learning automated network that can robustly segment patient-specific depth electrodes after sEEG and DBS proce-

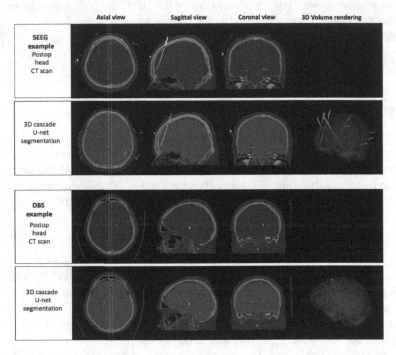

Fig. 2. Electrode and brain segmentation results of CT postsurgical imaging visualized in synchronized axial, sagittal, coronal planes and 3D patient specific surface rendered partly transparent volume. The extracted brain mask is presented in red and segmented electrodes in green.

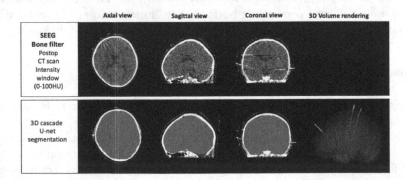

Fig. 3. Visual representation of the post-op head CT scan reconstructed using bone filter and electrode and brain segmentations obtained our network. The extracted brain mask is presented in red and segmented electrodes in green.

dures and brain from CT scans. Our approach may inform on the postsurgical electrode contacts positions fast and accurate and be an input for neurosurgical and neuroscientific toolboxes and frameworks.

5   Acknowledgement

The experiments presented in this paper were carried out using the HPC facilities of the University of Luxembourg (Varrette, Bouvry, Cartiaux, & Georgatos, 2014) – see https://hpc.uni.lu.

We thank Dr. Krasimir Minkin and the Department of Neurosurgery, University Hospital "Saint Ivan Rilski", Sofia, Bulgaria, for providing single anonymised postsurgical sEEG CT volume for testing here presented models.

References

1. Katz JS, Abel TJ. Stereoelectroencephalography Versus Subdural Electrodes for Localization of the Epileptogenic Zone: What Is the Evidence? Neurotherapeutics. 2019;16(1):59–66.
2. Husch A, Petersen MV, Gemmar P, et al. Post-operative deep brain stimulation assessment: Automatic data integration and report generation. Brain Stimul. 2018;11(4):863–866. Available from: https://doi.org/10.1016/j.brs.2018.01.031.
3. Horn A, Li N, Dembek TA, et al. Lead-DBS v2: Towards a comprehensive pipeline for deep brain stimulation imaging. NeuroImage. 2019 jan;184:293–316.
4. Arnulfo G, Narizzano M, Cardinale F, et al. Automatic segmentation of deep intracerebral electrodes in computed tomography scans. BMC Bioinformatics. 2015;16(1):1–12.
5. Blenkmann AO, Phillips HN, Princich JP, et al. Ielectrodes: A comprehensive open-source toolbox for depth and subdural grid electrode localization. Front Neuroinform. 2017;11(March):1–16.
6. Granados A, Vakharia V, Rodionov R, et al. Automatic segmentation of stereoelectroencephalography (SEEG) electrodes post-implantation considering bending. Int J Comput Assist Radiol Surg. 2018;13(6):935–946. Available from: https://doi.org/10.1007/s11548-018-1740-8.
7. Narizzano M, Arnulfo G, Ricci S, et al. SEEG assistant: A 3DSlicer extension to support epilepsy surgery. BMC Bioinformatics. 2017;18(1):1–13.
8. Isensee F, Petersen J, Klein A, et al. nnU-Net: Self-adapting Framework for U-Net-Based Medical Image Segmentation. Informatik aktuell. 2019; p. 22.

Segmentation of the Fascia Lata in Magnetic Resonance Images of the Thigh

Comparison of an Unsupervised Technique with a U-Net in 2D and Patch-wise 3D

Lis J. Louise P[1], Klaus Engelke[1,2], Oliver Chaudry[1,2]

[1]Institute of Medical Physics, Friedrich-Alexander-Universität Erlangen-Nürnberg
[2]Department of Medicine 3, Friedrich-Alexander-Universität Erlangen-Nürnberg and University Hospital Erlangen
oliver.chaudry@imp.uni-erlangen.de

Abstract. To quantify muscle properties in the thigh, the segmentation of the fascia lata is crucial. For this purpose, the U-Net architecture was implemented and compared for 2D images and patched 3D image stacks in magnetic resonance images (MRI). The training data consisted of T_1 MRI data sets from elderly men. To test the performance of the models, they were applied on other data sets of different age groups and gender. The U-Net approaches were superior to an unsupervised semiautomatic method and reduced post-processing time.

1 Introduction

Quantification of adipose tissue (AT) in skeletal muscle is of growing interest to understand mechanisms of muscle weakness during ageing and in diseases such as sarcopenia and cachexia. The mid-thigh is the preferred anatomical location for such measurements. It was recently shown that intermuscular adipose tissue (IMAT), the combination of AT among muscles and the agglomeration of larger adipocytes within muscles is a very sensitive parameter to monitor exercise effects, the most widely used intervention to prevent muscle weakness with increasing age [1]. The assessment of IMAT requires an accurate segmentation of the fascia lata (FL), an envelope of fibrous tissue separating subcutaneous adipose tissue from muscles and IMAT (Fig. 1). Several unsupervised semiautomatic algorithms for FL segmentation of MRI images of the thigh have been developed, however, due to poor contrast of the FL in MRI images, corrective operator interactions are frequently required [2]. Segmentation of 3D MRI data sets of the thigh consisting of 20 to 30 slices requires a large effort as studies in the field typically consist of hundreds of patient visits. Therefore, the aim of this study was to use a convolutional neural network to reduce the overall segmentation and analysis time. The network should be applicable to populations of men and women of different ages. It was not the aim to fully automate

C. Palm et al. (Hrsg.), *Bildverarbeitung für die Medizin 2021*,
Informatik aktuell, https://doi.org/10.1007/978-3-658-33198-6_23

the process, but to achieve a segmentation accuracy comparable to our current gold standard [2], which includes a supervision of the semiautomatic process and necessary manual corrections by a medical expert.

2   Methods

We used four different MRI datasets (D1-D4) from three different longitudinal exercise intervention trials in subjects with and without sarcopenia. D1 was taken from the FROST study [3] consisting of 43 elderly men (age $\geq$ 72 years, BMI 24.5±1.9 kg/m^2), including two visits and 70 scans in total. From the FRANSO study [4], 17 young men (age $\geq$ 25 years, BMI 23.4±1.9 kg/m^2) were taken to form D2 and 17 elderly men (age $\geq$ 72 years, BMI 27.3±2.2 kg/m^2) to form D3. D4 consisted of 16 elderly women (age $\geq$ 71 years, BMI 24.9±1.4 kg/m^2), from the FORMOSA study [5]. All datasets comprised a wide range of muscle fat content.

2.1   Data acqusition

Whole MR image acquisition was performed using a 3T scanner (MAGNETOM Skyra^{fit}, Siemens Healthineers AG, Erlangen, Germany) and an 18-channel body receive array coil (Fig. 1). The images were aquired by a T_1 weighted Turbo Spin Echo sequence: TR: 844 ms, TE: 14 ms, voxel size: 0.5×0.5×3.0 mm^3 (no slice gap), matrix size: 512×512 in 28 slices, bias field was corrected by the N4ITK algorithm [6].

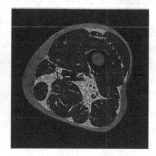

Fig. 1. Typical T_1 MR image of the thigh, 3D segmented fascia lata visible as thin line of fibrous tissue around the muscles (magenta), segmented IMAT within the fascia (yellow).

2.2   Deep learning architecture and training

The FL segmentation was performed by the U-Net deep neural network. The implementation followed the original publication [7], except for the padding per convolution, which did not change the input dimensions. To overcome the class imbalance between the thin FL contour around the muscles and the background, the region bordered by the FL volume was segmented instead of the contour. In order to analyze performance, we compared an implementation in 2D with a patched 3D U-Net. The 2D model received the full image resolution while for the 3D approach the images were downsampled to 256×256 pixels, without downsampling in through plane direction. The input consisted of patches of 4 slices each, both approaches were trained only on D1. Dropout regularization was applied at the end of every convolutional block. The training also included data augmentation, adding random spatial transformations (like shear, rotation, shifts and flips) to data samples. Subsequently, the model was tested on D2, D3 and D4.

The networks were trained to optimize a loss function defined as a linear combination of the dice loss (DL) and the weighted cross entropy (WCE)

$$\text{Loss}(y, p) = \alpha WCE + (1 - \alpha)DL \tag{1}$$

With DL defined as $1 - DSC$ and DSC being the dice similarity coefficient

$$DSC(y, p) = \frac{2\sum_i y_i p_i + s}{\sum_i y_i + \sum_i p_i + s} \tag{2}$$

With y being the true image and p the predicted segmentation map. The term s denotes a smoothing factor which was set to 0.0001. Analogously, WCE is defined as

$$WCE(y, p) = -(\beta \cdot y log(p) + (1 - y) log(1 - p)) \tag{3}$$

with β empirically determined to be 0.4 in order to penalize false positive predictions. The total number of 2D samples was 1960 individual slices (28 slices per 3D volume), which were shuffled, normalized and split into training (70 %), validation (15 %) and test (15 %) sets. The models were implemented using tensorflow and trained on a Nvidia Geforce GTX 1060 6GB GPU, using the Adam optimizer. Due to GPU memory limitations, the batch size for the 2D model was restricted to 2. For the 3D model, the data set was split at patient level into 57 for training, 7 for validation and 6 patients for testing. For the 3D model the patch size was restricted to 4 slices with a batchsize of 1. The optimum values for α=0.2 and the learning rate of 2e-4 were found by a grid search in combination with a ten-fold cross validation. Training the 2D model took 2 hours for 12 epochs. The last 6 epochs were trained at a learning rate of 2e-5 to refine the results, initial weights came from pretraining the model on the segmentation of the cross sectional thigh area. Additional parameters were: dropout rate 0.5, augmentation: horizontal flip and nearest neighbor interpolation, with rotation range 20, width shift range 0.2 and height shift range 0.2.

2.3   Evaluation of the results

For the comparison of the segmentation results between the U-Net and the gold standard, the DSC and the Hausdorff distance (HD) of images were used. HD computes the maximum distance between the sets of non-zero pixels A and B

$$HD(A, B) = \max(h(A, B), h(B, A)) \tag{4}$$

Table 1. Accuracy of the 2D U-Net and unsupervised method against gold standard.

Group	D1	D2	D3	D4
DSC unsup.	0.975±0.075	0.984±0.024	0.993±0.002	0.971±0.018
DSC U-Net 2D	0.996±0.002	0.991±0.008	0.995±0.002	0.985±0.008
HD [pixel] unsup.	15.02±16.76	14.18±14.38	7.344±4.557	23.49±14.83
HD [pixel] U-Net 2D	3.417±1.564	8.575±7.092	5.289±2.418	11.67±5.707
Number of samples	196	442	442	416

Table 2. Accuracy of the 3D U-Net against gold standard.

Group	D1	D2	D3	D4
DSC (upsampled)	0.994±0.002	0.992±0.002	0.994±0.004	0.982±0.001
HD [pixel] (upsampled)	4.224±1.719	6.459±3.813	5.179±3.514	21.698±48.458
Number of patients	7	17	17	16

with h being the directed distance

$$h(A, B) = \max_{a \in A} \min_{b \in B} \|a - b\| \tag{5}$$

DSC was used in order to leave out the background, as this takes up approximately 80 % of the image. Additionally the HD was computed to quantify the offset between the boundaries of the prediction and the gold standard mask, because DSC is not sensitive enough against small differences at the borders of the masks. Before calculating the test accuracies, the prediction was thresholded, counting every pixel <0.1 as background.

3   Results

3.1   2D U-Net model

Final training accuracy for DSC was 0.9950, with a validation accuracy of 0.9955 (before thresholding). Tab. 1 shows the results of the 2D U-Net and the results of the unsupervised segmentation technique before the manual correction process. Fig. 2 shows the 2D U-Net results (after thresholding) and difference images in relation to the gold standard.

As expected, DSC of the 2D U-Net was highest in D1, the dataset used for training. In comparison to D1, DSC was similar for D2 and D3, with D3 being higher than D2. Lowest DSC was found for D4, the cohort of elderly women, which compared to D1 and D2 show a larger amount of IMAT and subcutaneous adipose tissue (SAT). Images of D4 also show more connective tissue, visible in the SAT. The young men of D3 with the least amount of AT, showed the best results. A similar trend was observed for the unsupervised segmentation technique. Numerically, the 2D U-Net results for DSC and HD were always superior.

Fig. 2. Top row: MR image with overlay of the prediction mask (magenta). Bottom row: gold standard mask (red), prediction mask (cyan) and intersection of both masks (gray).

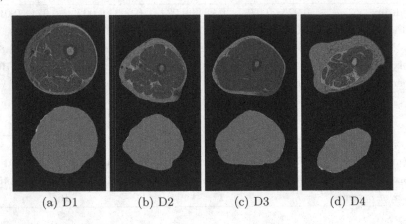

(a) D1   (b) D2   (c) D3   (d) D4

3.2   3D U-Net model

3D U-Net results are shown in Tab. 2. Accuracy is measured in the upsampled prediction masks, after applying a median filter to smoothen the edges.

Results for the 3D model were similar to 2D results, but details around the fascia contour were less accurate in 3D, which can be seen in the HD values. In rare cases, in particular for very high levels of fat infiltration, the 2D U-Net model performed poorly and created holes or segmented too much of the SAT (Fig. 3 bottom row, left and right).

3.3   Post-processing time

Compared to the unsupervised segmentation, manual post-processing times were significantly reduced by the 2D U-Net model (Tab. 3.)

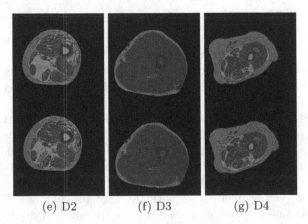

(e) D2   (f) D3   (g) D4

Fig. 3. Comparison of the 3D segmentation (upper row) with the 2D segmentation (bottom row) for the same patients in D2, D3 and D4.

Table 3. Manual post-processing time.

Group	D2	D3	D4
Unsupervised [min]	4.3±1.7	2.4±1.1	6.8±2.9
2D U-Net [min]	1.8±0.9	1.0±0.4	4.6±2.5

4 Discussion and conclusion

Two different U-Net models for the segmentation of the FL were implemented. Although the models were only trained on images of elderly men, both approaches also delivered excellent results for young men. The models were able to predict the FL segmentation with higher accuracy than the unsupervised method, which halved the time for final manual corrections. The patched 3D approach overall showed sligthly lower accuracy in the test datasets but produced smoother, less convex segmentations. Results for D4 indicated that higher subcutaneous and intramuscular AT content caused poorer segmentation. Data from both genders and 3D information should be included in the training data to gain best results.

References

1. Grimm A, Nickel MD, Chaudry O, et al. Feasibility of dixon magnetic resonance imaging to quantify effects of physical training on muscle composition—a pilot study in young and healthy men. Eur J Radiol. 2019;114:160–166.
2. Chaudry O, Friedberger A, Grimm A, et al. Segmentation of the fascia lata and reproducible quantification of intermuscular adipose tissue (IMAT) of the thigh. Magn Reson Mater Phy. 2020;.
3. Kemmler W, Kohl M, Jakob F, et al. Effects of high intensity dynamic resistance exercise and whey protein supplements on osteosarcopenia in older men with low bone and muscle mass. Final results of the randomized controlled FrOST study. Nutrients. 2020;12(8):2341.
4. Kemmler W, Grimm A, Bebeneck M, et al. Effects of combined whole-body electromyostimulation and protein supplementation on local and overall muscle/fat distribution in older men with sarcopenic obesity: the randomized controlled franconia sarcopenic obesity (FranSO). Calcif Tissue Int. 2018;103:266–277.
5. Kemmler W, Teschler M, Goisser S, et al. Prevalence of sarcopenia in Germany and the corresponding effect of osteoarthritis in females 70 years and older living in the community: results of the FORMoSA study. Clin Interv Aging. 2015;10:1565–1573.
6. Tustison NJ, Avants BB, Cook PA, et al. N4ITK: improved N3 bias correction. IEEE Trans Med Imaging. 2010;29:1310–1320.
7. Ronneberger O, Fischer P, Brox T. U-Net: convolutional networks for biomedical image segmentation. Proc MICCAI. 2015;9351:234–241.

Abstract: Automatic CAD-RADS Scoring using Deep Learning

Felix Denzinger[1,2], Michael Wels[2], Katharina Breininger[1], Mehmet A. Gülsün[2], Max Schöbinger[2], Florian André[3], Sebastian Buß[3], Johannes Görich[3], Michael Sühling[2], Andreas Maier[1]

[1] Pattern Recognition Lab, Universität Erlangen-Nürnberg, Erlangen, Germany
[2] Siemens Healthcare GmbH, Computed Tomography, Forchheim, Germany
[3] Das Radiologische Zentrum - Radiology Center, Sinsheim-Eberbach-Erbach-Walldorf-Heidelberg, Germany
felix.denzinger@fau.de

Coronary CT angiography (CCTA) has established its role as a non-invasive modality for the diagnosis of coronary artery disease (CAD). The CAD-Reporting and Data System (CAD-RADS) has been developed to standardize communication and aid in decision making based on CCTA findings. The CAD-RADS score is determined by manual assessment of all coronary vessels and the grading of lesions within the coronary artery tree. We propose a bottom-up approach for fully-automated prediction of this score using deep-learning operating on a segment-wise representation of the coronary arteries. The method relies solely on a prior fully-automated centerline extraction and segment labeling and predicts the segment-wise stenosis degree and the overall calcification grade as auxiliary tasks in a multi-task learning setup. We evaluate our approach on a data collection consisting of 2,867 patients. On the task of identifying patients with a CAD-RADS score indicating the need for further invasive investigation our approach reaches an area under curve (AUC) of 0.923 and an AUC of 0.914 for determining whether the patient suffers from CAD. This level of performance enables our approach to be used in a fully-automated screening setup or to assist diagnostic CCTA reading, especially due to its neural architecture design–which allows comprehensive predictions [1].

References

1. Denzinger F, Wels M, Breininger K, et al. Automatic CAD-RADS scoring using deep learning. Proc MICCAI. 2020; p. 45–54.

© Der/die Autor(en), exklusiv lizenziert durch
Springer Fachmedien Wiesbaden GmbH, ein Teil von Springer Nature 2021
C. Palm et al. (Hrsg.), *Bildverarbeitung für die Medizin 2021*,
Informatik aktuell, https://doi.org/10.1007/978-3-658-33198-6_24

Towards Deep Learning-based Wall Shear Stress Prediction for Intracranial Aneurysms

Annika Niemann[1,2], Lisa Schneider[1], Bernhard Preim[1], Samuel Voß[2,3], Philipp Berg[2,3], Sylvia Saalfeld[1,2]

[1]Department of Simulation and Graphics, Otto-von-Guericke University of Magdeburg
[2]Forschungscampus STIMULATE, Otto-von-Guericke University of Magdeburg
[3]Department of Fluid Dynamics and Technical Flows, University of Magdeburg
annika.niemann@ovgu.de

Abstract. This work aims at a deep learning-based prediction of wall shear stresses (WSS) for intracranial aneurysms. Based on real patient cases, we created artificial surface models of bifurcation aneurysms. After simulation and WSS extraction, these models were used for training a deep neural network. The trained neural network for 3D mesh segmentation was able to predict areas of high wall shear stress.

1 Introduction

Intracranial aneurysm growth and rupture is strongly associated with the blood flow inside the aneurysm and its parent vessel. Assessment of individual rupture risk can be supported by hemodynamic simulations [1]. These are time-consuming and need expert knowledge. For the integration of wall shear stress (WSS) information into clinical routine a deep learning method might be used. In this work we explore how areas of high wall shear stress can be predicted using deep learning on surface meshes.

Recently, Gharleghi et al. [2] presented deep learning WSS prediction for the left main coronary artery bifurcation. They splitted the bifurcation into separate vessels. For each part, a 2D representation with several geometrical parameters was generated. Then, deep learning was applied to the 2D representation. Their results had an average mean absolute error of 0.0407 Pa.

Based on 4000 artificially created abdominal aortic aneurysms, Jordanski et al. [3] compared several machine learning approaches to model the relationship between geometric parameters and WSS distribution. The best results were achieved by Gaussian conditional random fields. In this study we generated artificial intracranial aneurysms and performed deep learning mesh segmentation to predict areas of high WSS.

C. Palm et al. (Hrsg.), *Bildverarbeitung für die Medizin 2021*,
Informatik aktuell, https://doi.org/10.1007/978-3-658-33198-6_25

Table 1. Parameters of real world aneurysms that were characterised by a roundly shaped saccular aneurysm at vessel bifurcation. Provided are min, max and average values (in degree respectively mm) for the parameters described in Fig. 1.

	r_i	r_1	r_2	r_a	d	α	β
average	2.53	1.87	1.75	2.09	3.67	97.31	93.77
min	1.81	0.96	1.04	1.11	1.65	64.00	60.00
max	3.38	2.48	2.58	3.44	6.15	157.00	120.00

2   Materials and methods

For this study we chose a simplified configuration consisting of a bifurcation aneurysm with one inlet and two outlets of the parent artery. Based on the results of hemodynamic simulations, regions of high WSS were segmented and serve as ground truth.

2.1   Artificial aneurysm configuration

The simplified, artificial bifurcation aneurysms were created with CAD software. Each geometry consists of three cylinders, representing one inlet vessel and two outlets and a sphere for the saccular bifurcation aneurysm. The aneurysm creation has seven adjustable parameters (Fig. 1): the radius of the inlet (r_i), the radius of the first outlet (r_1), the radius of the second outlet (r_2), the radius of the aneurysm (r_a), the distance between aneurysm center and bifurcation (d), the angle between the first outlet and the inlet (α), and the angle between the second outlet and the inlet (β). In order to extract realistic default values for these parameters, we analyzed 200 patient-specific 3D aneurysm models from our previous work. We then selected cases which have a high agreement w.r.t.

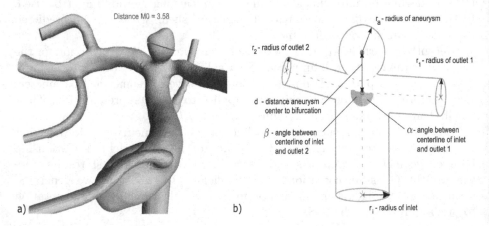

Fig. 1. Overview of parameters for artificial aneurysm creation; a) example of reference aneurysm with measure of aneurysm diameter; b) concept of artificial aneurysm creation with seven parameters.

our artificial configuration (i.e. spherical, saccular bifurcation aneurysm) yielding 13 reference cases. Their average, minimum and maximum values are shown
in Table 1. The artificial aneurysms were created with randomly generated parameters in the same range of the values of the reference aneurysms.

2.2 Hemodynamic simulations

Hemodynamic simulations were performed in order to assess the WSS of the
artificial aneurysm geometries. These simulations are based on computational
fluid dynamics, which is a numerical approach to solve fluid flow problems using
Navier-Stokes equations. For this purpose, each flow domain, containing vessels
and aneurysm, was spatially discretized into volumetric cells (1.2 to 2.4 million
cells for each configuration depending on the domain size). Blood was modeled
as incompressible and laminar fluid with a density of $1055\,\mathrm{kg/m^3}$ and dynamic
viscosity of $0.004\,\mathrm{Pa\,s}$. Boundary conditions of the domain were modeled as follows: Constant velocity of $0.3\,\mathrm{m/s}$ as inflow into the parent artery, rigid vessel
walls with no-slip condition, and zero-pressure assumption at the outlets. The
total simulation time was $5\,\mathrm{s}$ (quasi-steady, time step of $0.01\,\mathrm{s}$) while only the
time range of $[3\text{-}5]\,\mathrm{s}$ was used for temporal averaging the WSS field. In total, 145 artificial aneurysms were simulated with STAR-CCM+ 13.06 (Siemens
PLM Software Inc., Plano, TX, USA). Finally, aneurysm surface and temporal
averaged WSS magnitude values were exported for further analysis.

2.3 Deep learning segmentation

The aneurysm surfaces are remeshed using the ACVD algorithm [4] to obtain
a similar number of edges. The deep learning approach requires label per edge
while the WSS magnitude values from the flow simulation were obtained at
vertices. Thus, we calculate the edge labels as average WSS of the associated
vertices. Areas of high WSS are defined based on a reference value.This reference
value is obtained by listing the maximum WSS of each aneurysm and calculating
the median of it. Areas, where the WSS is larger than 0.4 times the reference
value, are defined as areas of high WSS. An example is shown in Figure 2.

We trained a deep learning mesh segmentation using the *medMeshCNN* architecture [5]. For the first experiment, we used a small dataset consisting of 24
training meshes and 3 test meshes. The second experiment included 123 training
and 10 test meshes. Due to problems in feature calculation, the last experiment
comprised 118 training and 9 test meshes.

Instead of transforming the mesh information to 2D, we directly work with 3D
surface meshes. Deep learning segmentation is used to predict areas of high WSS.
Further experiments included variation of the edge features used.*medMeshCNN*
calculates angles and ratio between edges of adjacent faces. In experiments 3,4
and 5 we added curvature [6] and in experiment 5 mesh thickness [7] (defined as
diameter of the maximum inscribed sphere) to the feature calculation. Both features were first calculated for each vertex and than mapped to the corresponding

Table 2. Parameters of the experiments, where # denotes the experiment number, GC the Gaussian curvature and MC the mean Gaussian curvature.

#	training	test	additional features	pooling resolution						batch size	weighted loss	
1	15	3	-	2500	2000	1500	1000	750		10	0.2	0.8
2	123	10	-	2500	2000	1500	1000	750		10	0.2	0.8
3	123	10	GC	2500	2000	1500	1000	750		10	0.2	0.8
4	123	10	GC & MC	2500	2000	1500	1000	750	500	5	0.01	0.99
5	118	9	GC & thickness	2500	2000	1500	1000	750	500	5	0.01	0.99

edges. In the following, selected experiments are presented. The parameters of each experiment are summarised in Table 2.

3   Results

The training accuracy of the first experiment was constantly increasing and approaching 100 %. This proved that the *medMeshCNN* architecture is able to learn the presented mesh attributes. However, the test accuracy was far worse (between 61 and 68 %) and decreasing after 50 epochs.

Increasing the number of training meshes did improve the test accuracy, as shown by the second experiment (Fig. 3). Again, overfitting occurred and the test accuracy decreased after epoch 40. In Figure 4, the result for one of the test meshes is shown. The corresponding simulation result and ground truth are shown in Figure 2. While an accuracy over 85 % is reached, the visual inspection shows some differences. Only a small part of the large WSS area is predicted by the net. But additional spots on the wall are falsely predicted.

For the third experiment the Gaussian curvature was included in the feature list. As visible in Figure 3, this leads to a test accuracy of over 91 %. Unfortunately, this accuracy was reached by labelling most edges as normal WSS, omitting the high WSS class.

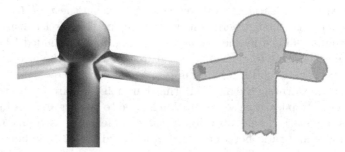

Fig. 2. Depiction of the resulting WSS (left) and a corresponding ground truth segmentation for training (right).

To overcome the problem of the vanishing high WSS class, the weights of the loss function were adjusted. Experiment 4 additionally included the mean Gaussian curvature as a feature. Thus, an accuracy of 85% was reached (Fig. 3). Figure 4 shows the prediction of the net. Compared to experiment 2, there are less but larger predicted high WSS areas. The net from experiment 4 predicts a larger area as high WSS than the ground truth segmentation for the deep learning shows. Compared with the original simulation result, both areas of high WSS are segmented by the net. The high WSS in the lager vessel is not completely segmented.

In experiment 5, additional to the curvature features, the mesh thickness was included. This did not improve the results. The test accuracy stayed below 80% and WSS areas were scattered over the whole mesh (Fig. 4).

Prediction of high WSS areas with the trained net needed 43 seconds on average per mesh.

4   Discussion

Areas of high WSS can be predicted by deep learning mesh segmentation methods. In all presented experiments, the training accuracy converged to 100%.

While high training accuracy was reached, the test accuracy showed limitations. A major limitation is the used dataset. As seen in the first two experiments, increasing the number of training examples does improve the test accuracy. We used artificially created intracranial aneurysms. These shared the same basic geometry, a bifurcation aneurysm with proximal parent and two distal outflow vessels. *medMeshCNN* is able to learn the geometry based on meshes and mesh features. While the geometries of the meshes are similar, the variance

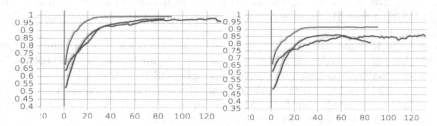

Fig. 3. Training (left) and test (right) accuracy per epoch of experiment 2 (without additional features; red), experiment 3 (GC; green), experiment 4 (GC&MC; blue).

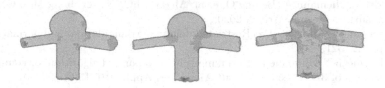

Fig. 4. Result of experiment 2 (left), 4 (middle) and 5 (right).

in the segmentation is higher. This might hinder the training and complicate generalization. Including the curvature and adjusting the weights of the loss function does improve the results.

Another factor which needs further research is the choice of suitable thresholds for generation of the segmentation ground truth data. In experiment 4, a larger high WSS area around the junction was predicted than shown in the ground truth. A modified threshold value (lower reference value) might result in a better agreement between ground truth segmentation, deep learning high WSS prediction and simulation results.

In the presented work, only two WSS classes were segmented. Further research should include several classes to produce more detailed WSS predictions. Increasing the number of classes also requires careful adjustment of the training parameters, especially the weights for the loss function.

While finding suitable parameters for the net is a challenging and time-consuming task, the prediction of WSS with deep learning is considerably faster than traditional hemodynamic simulation and does not require expert knowledge.

In conclusion, we analyzed the potential of deep learning mesh segmentation for the fast prediction of WSS in intracranial bifurcation aneurysms. This approach provides fast results, which could be included into clinical routine. The quality of the results depends on several parameters. A weighted loss function with focus on the high WSS areas and the inclusion of the mesh curvature improved the prediction results.

References

1. Berg P, Voß S, Janiga G, et al. Multiple aneurysms anatomy challenge 2018 (MATCH) phase II: rupture risk assessment. Int J Comput Assist Radiol Surg. 2019 05;14.
2. Gharleghi R, Samarasinghe G, Sowmya A, et al. Deep learning for time averaged wall shear stress prediction in left main coronary bifurcations. In: 2020 IEEE 17th International Symposium on Biomedical Imaging (ISBI); 2020. p. 1–4.
3. Jordanski M, Radovic M, Milosevic Z, et al. Machine learning approach for predicting wall shear distribution for abdominal aortic aneurysm and carotid bifurcation models. IEEE J Biomed and Health Inform. 2016 12;PP:1–1.
4. Valette S, Chassery JM, Prost R. Generic remeshing of 3D triangular meshes with metric-dependent discrete voronoi diagrams. IEEE Trans Vis Comput Graph. 2008 03;14:369–381.
5. Schneider L, Niemann A, Beuing O, et al. MedMeshCNN – enabling MeshCNN for medical surface models. ArXiv. 2020;.
6. Cohen-Steiner D, Morvan JM. Restricted delaunay triangulations and normal cycle; 2003. p. 312–321.
7. Inui M, Umezu N, Shimane R. Shrinking sphere: a parallel algorithm for computing the thickness of 3D objects. Comput Aided Des Appl. 2016;13(2):199–207.

Evaluating Design Choices for Deep Learning Registration Networks
Architecture Matters

Hanna Siebert[1,2], Lasse Hansen[1], Mattias P. Heinrich[1]

[1]Institute of Medical Informatics, University of Lübeck
[2]Graduate School for Computing in Medicine and Life Sciences, University of Lübeck
siebert@imi.uni-luebeck.de

Abstract. The variety of recently proposed deep learning models for deformable pairwise image registration leads to the question how beneficial certain architectural design considerations are for the registration performance. This paper aims to take a closer look at the impact of some basic network design choices, i.e. the number of feature channels, the number of convolutions per resolution level and the differences between partially independent processing streams for fixed and moving images and direct concatenation of input scans. Starting from a simple single-stream U-Net architecture, we investigate extensions and modifications and propose a model for 3D abdominal CT registration evaluated on data from the Learn2Reg challenge that outperforms the baseline network VoxelMorph used for comparison.

1 Introduction

Deformable image registration aims to align pairs of images or image volumes by predicting non-linear transformations that optimises an appearance or shape-based metric. Registration of medical images helps to analyse large image datasets for research purposes and plays an important role in clinical practice, including diagnostic tasks, image-guided interventions, and motion tracking [1]. Recent deep learning-based image registration methods [2, 3, 4, 5, 6] show the potential to outperform conventional methods in terms of improved registration speed and accuracy. However, the estimation of large deformations is still considered challenging. Meanwhile there is a large variety of publications presenting different deep learning networks for image registration offering multiple suggestions for the design of architectures consisting of different architectural modules.

We take up the idea of several registration networks which include an U-Net architecture to learn deformations [2, 4]. The idea of not directly concatenating fixed and moving image before feature extraction is examined as well and has been used in [7] where fixed and moving images are analyzed in separate pipelines for affine registration or in the dual-stream registration network proposed in [8].

This paper aims to take a closer look at the impact of different architectural design ideas on the registration performance in order to finally propose an architecture for abdominal CT registration that combines the most convincing of the considerations examined. We compare our results to the simple baseline network for unsupervised pairwise image registration VoxelMorph [2].

2 Materials and methods

We examine four different architectural designs for pairwise image registration, starting from a simple single-stream U-Net architecture, which is then extended and further modified. All considered architectures are visualised in Fig. 1.

Our investigations start with a registration model that is from its basic structure similar to VoxelMorph [2], but with one difference that it contains fewer skip connections. The model concatenates fixed and moving images at the beginning and uses sequences of convolution followed by instance normalisation and leaky ReLU. The resolution of the spatial dimensions is first successively decreased by strided convolutions to $\frac{1}{24}$ of the input image dimensions and then

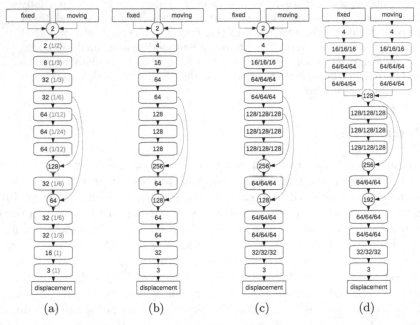

(a)   (b)   (c)   (d)

Fig. 1. Overview of the different considered architectures with given number of feature channels being output from the convolutions (rounded rectangles) and concatenations (circles). The initial architecture (a) is modified so that first the number of feature channels (b) and then the number of convolutions (c) is increased. The last modification (d) results in a two-stream architecture that starts with separate encoder blocks for fixed and moving image. Modifications to the previous architecture are marked in red respectively. The corresponding output resolutions are indicated in blue within the visualisation of model (a) and apply to all of the models.

increased again by upconvolutions. The central part of the architecture consists of an U-Net like part using two skip connections [9]. Conversely to the reduction in resolution, the number of feature channels from the convolution layers is firstly increased up to 64 and then decreased (Fig. 1 (a)) until the output yields 3 feature channels that correspond to the 3 displacement dimensions. As the displacements are considered to be within the the range of $[-1, 1]$, the last convolution layer is followed by a *tanh* activation function and the obtained output is used for warping with the moving input image.

The first modification we make to this initial architecture is to double the number of feature channels (quadrupling the parameters) of all convolution layers of the network (Fig. 1 (b)). We then extend the number of Convolution-InstanceNorm-ReLU sequences per resolution level to three (Fig. 1 (c)). Finally, we propose a two-stream architecture with separate encoder blocks for fixed and moving image and their concatenated output as input for the U-Net part of the architecture (Fig. 1 (d)). Different from [8], which introduces a continuous dual-stream architecture, we concatenate the two streams within the encoder part of the network at a spatial resolution of $\frac{1}{6}$ of the input dimensions. As we use monomodal data for our experiments, the weights are shared between the two encoders of this two-stream architecture. In Fig. 2, our final image registration approach is illustrated.

We train our models using a loss function which ensures similarity of fixed and warped moving image and smooth deformation fields. Modality independent neighbourhood descriptors (MIND) with self-similar context (SSC) [10] are extracted from fixed and warped moving image and the mean squared error between them is calculated. Additionally, we apply diffusion regularisation to

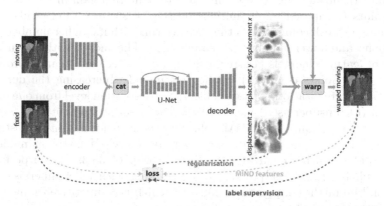

Fig. 2. Our model for pairwise image registration with label supervision: Fixed and moving images are given into separate encoder blocks for the extraction of features that are then concatenated and passed to an U-Net and following decoder block for the estimation of displacements. The obtained displacement fields are used to warp the moving image. The loss function is designed so that the warped moving image and labels resemble the fixed image and labels (similarity of MIND features and label supervision) and furthermore the deformation fields are smooth (diffusion regularisation).

achieve smooth and plausible deformation fields. For our proposed two-stream architecture, we furthermore investigate the benefits of label supervision by further extending the loss function by computing the mean squared error between fixed an warped moving one-hot encoded label maps (background excluded) weighted inversely proportional to the square root of the class frequency.

For our experiments we use the Learn2Reg challenge [11] dataset containing 30 abdominal CT scans with thirteen manually labeled abdominal organs, including spleen ■, right kidney ■, left kidney ■, gall bladder ■, esophagus ■, liver ■, stomach ■, aorta ■, inferior vena cava ■, portal and splenic vein ■, pancreas ■, left adrenal gland ■, and right adrenal gland ■ [12]. The data has been linearly pre-registered and we re-sample the data to dimensions of $144 \times 112 \times 192$ to reduce computational complexity. The dataset is split into 20 training cases and 10 test cases. For evaluation we consider all possible pairwise combinations of the test cases (leading to 45 unique pairs). We train our networks using Adam and a learning rate of 0.001 (0.0001 for the baseline network of VoxelMorph) for 50,000 iterations. Diffusion regularisation is weighted in such a way that the standard deviation of the Jacobian determinant stays below 1.0 on the training set and for label supervision we chose a weighting of $\lambda_{ls} = 2$.

3   Results

In Tab. 1, we report the average Dice overlap and properties of the Jacobian determinant as well as the inference time on GPU and the number of trainable parameters. Comparing the registration performance, the first model examined (1-stream (a), unsupervised) was only able to achieve a gain in Dice overlap of 2.5 % points (compared to the initially overlap of 25.15 %) and yields a worse performing network compared to the VoxelMorph with its higher number of skip connections and lower number of parameters. The model with an increased number of feature channels (1-stream (b), unsupervised) led to an improvement of about 2 % points compared to the first model. Increasing the number of convolution-normalisation-activation blocks per resolution level from one to three (1-stream (c), unsupervised) increased the Dice overlap by another 2 % points leading to a score similar to VoxelMorph, whereas the deformation field estimated by VoxelMorph is less smooth. With our unsupervised 2-stream model (d), we were able to achieve an average Dice overlap of 35.39 %, outperforming VoxelMorph by nearly 4% points. When training with label supervision, this score could be further improved to 43.85 %, which is competitive to many other approaches (cf. learn2reg.grand-challenge.org).

Tab. 2 shows Dice scores for the different considered label classes pointing out that the registration methods showed the best improvement of Dice overlap for comparably large and medium-sized organs. For these organs, also label supervision during training showed the highest improvement of registration performance compared to unsupervised training. These findings are also exemplary visually confirmed by Fig. 3.

Table 1. Evaluation results using Dice scores and Jacobian determinant, average inference time on GPU (Quadro P6000), and number of parameters. Dice scores are averaged over all thirteen label classes (background excluded). Initial refers to average values before registration. The quality of the deformation field is evaluated through the Jacobian determinant. Small standard deviations indicate smooth deformation fields and values below 0 indicate singularities, i.e. foldings.

	avg Dice [%]	std $det(J)$	$det(J) < 0$ [%]	inf. time/ pair [ms]	param. count
initial	25.14 ± 12.85	-	-	-	-
VoxelMorph unsuperv.	31.70 ± 13.75	0.5853	3.61	117.58	396451
1-stream (a), unsuperv.	27.85 ± 12.56	0.4096	0.89	44.09	746467
1-stream (b), unsuperv.	29.78 ± 12.60	0.4600	1.10	50.17	2985251
1-stream (c), unsuperv.	31.72 ± 13.01	0.4184	0.96	75.09	6814499
2-stream (d), unsuperv.	$\mathbf{35.39 \pm 14.05}$	0.4681	1.38	102.32	7449123
2-stream (d), superv.	$\mathbf{43.85 \pm 11.33}$	0.5012	1.37	102.32	7449123

Table 2. Dice overlap in % for the 13 different label classes (see text for colour coding).

	■	■	■	■	■	■	■	■	■	■	■	■	■
initial	42	34	35	2	23	62	24	33	36	5	15	8	9
VM unsuperv.	53	45	45	3	28	72	29	47	44	7	17	12	10
1-stream (c), unsuperv.	54	41	44	4	29	73	31	44	45	8	16	13	10
2-stream (d), unsuperv.	60	49	50	4	28	78	35	50	46	11	19	17	12
2-stream (d), superv.	73	69	71	7	37	83	47	59	52	12	26	20	15

fixed   moving   warped VM   warped (c)   warped (d)u.   warped (d)s.

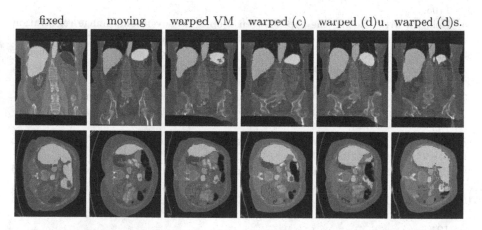

Fig. 3. Result visualization (coronal/axial) of different architectures (VoxelMorph (VM), 1-stream (c), unsupervised 2-stream (d)u., supervised 2-stream (d)s.) for one test pair: fixed and moving image and warped moving images output from the different models.

4 Discussion

We investigated several architectures for deep-learning based deformable image registration. Besides the expected observations that increased numbers of feature channels and convolution-normalisation-activation sequences led to improved registration results, we found out that concatenating the features extracted by separate encoder blocks for moving and fixed image achieved better results than directly concatenating the input images. With this two-stream architecture, we were able to outperform the simple baseline network for unsupervised pairwise image registration VoxelMorph. Due to the fact that we performed our experiments on a labeled dataset, we could further show that - starting from the initial untrained case - including label supervision when training our model led to a further substantial increase of Dice overlap of 8 % points compared to unsupervised training.

References

1. Hill DL, Batchelor PG, Holden M, et al. Medical image registration. Physics in medicine & biology. 2001;46(3):R1.
2. Balakrishnan G, Zhao A, Sabuncu MR, et al. Voxelmorph: a learning framework for deformable medical image registration. IEEE Trans Med Imag. 2019;38(8):1788–1800.
3. Mok TC, Chung AC. Large deformation diffeomorphic image registration with laplacian pyramid networks. Proc MICCAI. 2020; p. 211–221.
4. Eppenhof KAJ, Pluim JPW. Pulmonary CT registration through supervised learning with convolutional neural networks. IEEE Trans Med Imag. 2019;38(5):1097–1105.
5. Heinrich MP. Closing the gap between deep and conventional image registration using probabilistic dense displacement networks. Proc MICCAI. 2019; p. 50–58.
6. Eppenhof KAJ, Lafarge MW, Veta M, et al. Progressively trained convolutional neural networks for deformable image registration. IEEE Trans Med Imag. 2020;39(5):1594–1604.
7. de Vos BD, Berendsen FF, Viergever MA, et al. A deep learning framework for unsupervised affine and deformable image registration. Med Image Anal. 2019;52:128–143.
8. Hu X, Kang M, Huang W, et al. Dual-stream pyramid registration network. Proc MICCAI. 2019; p. 382–390.
9. Ronneberger O, Fischer P, Brox T. U-net: convolutional networks for biomedical image segmentation. Proc MICCAI. 2015; p. 234–241.
10. Heinrich MP, Jenkinson M, Papiez BW, et al. Towards realtime multimodal fusion for image-guided interventions using self-similarities. Proc MICCAI. 2013; p. 187–194.
11. Hansen L, Hering A, Heinrich MP, et al.. Learn2Reg: 2020 MICCAI registration challenge; 2020. https://learn2reg.grand-challenge.org.
12. Xu Z, Lee CP, Heinrich MP, et al. Evaluation of six registration methods for the human abdomen on clinically acquired CT. IEEE Trans Biomed Eng. 2016;63(8):1563–1572.

Learning the Update Operator for 2D/3D Image Registration

Srikrishna Jaganathan[1,2], Jian Wang[2], Anja Borsdorf[2], Andreas Maier[1]

[1]Pattern Recognition Lab, FAU Erlangen-Nürmberg, Erlangen, Germany.
[2]Siemens Healthineers AG, Forchheim, Germany.
srikrishna.jaganathan@fau.de

Abstract. Image guidance in minimally invasive interventions is usually provided using live 2D X-ray imaging. To enhance the information available during the intervention, the preoperative volume can be overlaid over the 2D images using 2D/3D image registration. Recently, deep learning-based 2D/3D registration methods have shown promising results by improving computational efficiency and robustness. However, there is still a gap in terms of registration accuracy compared to traditional optimization-based methods. We aim to address this gap by incorporating traditional methods in deep neural networks using known operator learning. As an initial step in this direction, we propose to learn the update step of an iterative 2D/3D registration framework based on the Point-to-Plane Correspondence model. We embed the Point-to-Plane Correspondence model as a known operator in our deep neural network and learn the update step for the iterative registration. We show an improvement of 1.8 times in terms of registration accuracy for the update step prediction compared to learning without the known operator.

1 Introduction

In minimally invasive interventions, live 2D X-ray imaging is prominent for providing image guidance. The information available from 2D imaging alone is limited and can be augmented by overlaying the preoperative 3D volume over the 2D images. To obtain this overlay, the 3D volume needs to be accurately positioned such that, the corresponding structures are aligned between the 2D image and 3D volume. The optimal positioning of the 3D volume is accomplished using 2D/3D registration. A 2D/3D registration aims to find an optimal 3D transformation such that the misalignment between the 2D image and the 3D volume is minimized. Traditionally, to find this optimal transformation, the 2D/3D registration problem is formulated as an optimization problem. Depending on the application, 2D/3D registration can be classified into different sub-classes like modality of the images, the number of 2D views available, and constraints on the estimated transformation. A complete overview of the different traditional 2D/3D registration techniques and its different sub-class are

Springer Fachmedien Wiesbaden GmbH, ein Teil von Springer Nature 2021
C. Palm et al. (Hrsg.), *Bildverarbeitung für die Medizin 2021*,
Informatik aktuell, https://doi.org/10.1007/978-3-658-33198-6_27

summarized in [1]. Recently, end-to-end Deep Learning (DL)-based solutions have also been proposed for both single-view [2, 3] and multi-view 2D/3D registration [4] which shows significant improvement in terms of robustness and computational efficiency but often suffer in terms of registration accuracy.

In this work, we address single-view rigid 2D/3D registration between pre-operative CT volume $\mathbf{V}$ and live fluoroscopic X-ray images I_{Flr}. Generally, in single-view 2D/3D registration, the 3D CT volume is rendered using Digitally Reconstructed Radiograph (DRR) to obtain a simulated X-ray image I_{DRR}. A similarity measure is defined to find the correspondences between the I_{DRR} and I_{Flr}. Using this similarity measure, classical techniques model the 2D/3D registration as an optimization problem to find the optimal transformation such that the registration error is minimized. However, in single-view 2D/3D registration, due to the aperture problem, the 2D misalignment between the structures (obtained by finding 2D correspondences) gives only the observable 2D motion error. To find the 3D misalignment (thus the optimal 3D transformation), the unobservable motions in 2D should also be accounted for. This can be effectively constrained using the Point-to-Plane Correspondence (PPC) model [5]. With the PPC model, a dynamic 2D/3D registration framework was proposed in [5], which performs iterative 2D/3D registration by solving the PPC model at each iteration. It achieves state-of-the-art performance in terms of both registration accuracy and robustness. However, the framework relies on having accurate 2D correspondences between I_{Flr} and I_{DRR}, which makes it sensitive to outliers in the estimated 2D correspondences. To make the framework robust against outliers, a DL-based attention model was proposed [6].

In this work, we extend the PPC-based registration framework to use a learned update operator. The update operator consists of 2D matching, weighing of the matches, and estimating the 3D rigid transformation such that it satisfies the PPC constraint. Since the PPC model is differentiable, it can be directly used as a known operator [7] and can be embedded as a layer in Deep Neural Network (DNN). Learning with the PPC model as a known operator has shown promising results when it was applied to learn correspondence weights for the 2D matches [6]. We propose to learn all the three steps of the PPC update operator fused into a single DNN, contrary to the previous attempts which only learned parts of the update operator [6, 8].

2   Methods

2.1   PPC-based 2D/3D registration framework

The PPC-based registration framework proposed in [5] is an iterative registration scheme and depends on the PPC constraint to estimate the optimal transformation at each iteration. Registration is performed between 3D CT volume $\mathbf{V}$ and 2D X-ray image I_{Flr} which are provided as inputs to the framework. Along with it, an initial transformation $\mathbf{T}_{\mathrm{init}}$ is required which provides a rough initial alignment.

The framework consists of an initialization step where the surface points along with their gradients are extracted from $\mathbf{V}$ using a 3D Canny edge detector, and the gradient of X-ray image (∇I_{Flr}) is computed from I_{Flr}. The initialization step is performed only once, and the values are cached. After the initialization step, the update operation is performed iteratively until convergence. The update operation consists of the following steps. Based on the current transformation estimate, the gradient image of DRR (∇I_{DRR}) is rendered. Surface points with gradients perpendicular to the current viewing direction are selected as contour points $\mathbf{w}_i$ where $i \in 1, \ldots, N$ with N contour points. The contour points $\mathbf{w}_i$ are projected into ∇I_{DRR} to get the projected contour points $\mathbf{p}_i$. Now, 2D matching is performed to find the corresponding projected contour points $\mathbf{p}'_i$ in ∇I_{Flr}. The correspondence set $(\mathbf{p}_i, \mathbf{p}'_i)$ along with contour points $\mathbf{w}_i$, and its gradients $\mathbf{g}_i$ are used to compute the 3D motion update based on the PPC model. If the 2D matches are noisy, a weighted version of the PPC model is used to reduce the effect of the noisy matches. The weighted PPC model gives a linear constraint $\mathbf{WAdv} = diag(\mathbf{W})\mathbf{b}$, where $\mathbf{A}$ and $\mathbf{b}$ are the data terms which are computed based on the estimated 2D correspondences. $\mathbf{W}$ is a diagonal matrix which consists of weights for each correspondences. Each correspondence contributes one row of $\mathbf{A}, \mathbf{b}$ and $\mathbf{W}$. Closed form solution $\mathbf{dv} = (\mathbf{WA}^+)(diag(\mathbf{W})\mathbf{b})$ using the pseudo inverse of $\mathbf{A}$ is used for computing the 3D motion. The rigid 3D transformation matrix $\mathbf{T}_{\text{est}}$ is computed from the 3D motion vector $\mathbf{dv}$, which serves as an input for the next update step.

2.2   Learnable update operator for PPC-based 2D/3D registration framework

The update operator in PPC-based registration framework finds $\mathbf{T}_{\text{est}}$ given a set of inputs $(\nabla I_{\text{Flr}}, \nabla I_{\text{DRR}}, \mathbf{w}_i, \mathbf{g}_i, \mathbf{p}_i)$. Fig. 1 shows the network architecture used for training the update operator. The FlowNet C architecture [9] is used for estimating 2D matches between ∇I_{Flr} and ∇I_{DRR} by predicting optical flow

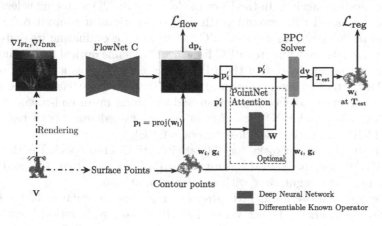

Fig. 1. Schematic of the proposed update operator for PPC based iterative registration framework.

$\mathbf{dp}_i$ at projected contour points $\mathbf{p}_i$ similar to [8]. Using $\mathbf{p}'_i = \mathbf{p}_i + \mathbf{dp}_i$ and the 3D information $(\mathbf{w}_i, \mathbf{g}_i)$, correspondence weighting matrix $\mathbf{W}$ is predicted using PointNet Attention model similar to [6]. This step is optional and we define two architectures PPC Flow and PPC Flow Attention, where we use the PointNet Attention only for the later. The 3D motion $\mathbf{dv}$ is computed using the PPC Solver which gives us the current estimated 3D transformation $\mathbf{T}_{\mathrm{est}}$. Applying $\mathbf{T}_{\mathrm{est}}$, the contour points $\mathbf{w}_i$ are updated. We use the mean Target Registration Error (mTRE) as registration loss $\mathcal{L}_{\mathrm{reg}}$. It is computed using $\frac{1}{N}\sum_i^N \|\mathbf{T}_{\mathrm{est}}(\mathbf{w}_i) - \mathbf{T}_{\mathrm{gt}}(\mathbf{w}_i)\|$ for a set of N contour points and ground truth transformation $\mathbf{T}_{\mathrm{gt}}$. Additionally, we also use optical flow loss $\mathcal{L}_{\mathrm{flow}}$ by computing average End Point Error (EPE) at projected contour points $\mathbf{p}_i$ as proposed in [8], to make the network training more stable.

2.3 Experimental setup

The data set used for training and evaluation is from reconstruction data of Cone Beam CT (CBCT) for the vertebra region [6]. The data set consists of 56 acquisitions from 55 patients. The data is split into 38 patients for training, 5 patients for validation, and 12 patient for testing. The training samples are created using random initial transformation from the ground truth registration using different viewing directions from the volume similar to [8]. We generate random initial transformations with an initial mTRE in the range of $[0, 45]$ mm. Each sample consists of $(\nabla I_{\mathrm{Flr}}, \nabla I_{\mathrm{DRR}}, \mathbf{w}_i, \mathbf{g}_i, \mathbf{p}_i)$ along with $\mathbf{T}_{gt}$. There are about 18,000 such samples for training and validation, and 8,000 samples for testing.

The update operator of the PPC-based registration framework performs one registration iteration. We train and evaluate the performance of the update operator using three different models namely Flow, PPC Flow, and PPC Flow Attention. The Flow and PPC Flow models are used to compare the effects of known operator learning. In the Flow model, only the 2D matching is learned by training the model with ground truth flow annotations at contour points $\mathbf{p}_i$ as proposed in [8]. Here, we use the PPC solver only for evaluating its registration performance after one update. PPC Flow uses the same optical flow architecture as the Flow model along with the PPC model embedded as a known operator. PPC Flow Attention integrates the PPC Flow with the attention model [6] to learn both correspondence estimation and weighing in an end-to-end manner. Both PPC Flow and PPC Flow Attention are trained using both registration loss (mTRE) and optical flow loss (average EPE).

We train all the networks for 200,000 iterations (100 epochs) with a batch size of 16. We use the ADAM optimizer with a learning rate of 1e-4 and weight decay is used as a regularizer with a decay rate of 1e-6.

For evaluation, we use mTRE after one registration update which measures the registration error. Lower values indicate better registration accuracy. In addition, we also use reduction factor which is computed for samples whose $\mathrm{mTRE}_{i+1} < \mathrm{mTRE}_i$ as $(1 - \frac{\mathrm{mTRE}_{i+1}}{\mathrm{mTRE}_i})$ where mTRE_i is the error before update step and mTRE_{i+1} is the error after the application of the update step. It is

Table 1. Registration error measured using mTRE in [mm] of different networks after one update operation, evaluated on test data set. The initial mTRE indicates the initial registration error. The $50^{th}, 75^{th}, 95^{th}$ percentile errors are provided to indicate percentage of samples having an error $\leq$ the indicated value. The mTRE ($\mu \pm \sigma$) and the reduction factor ($\mu \pm \sigma$) summarizes the model performance over all the samples.

| | Percentile mTRE [mm] | | | mTRE [mm] | Reduction Factor |
	50th	75th	95th	$\mu \pm \sigma$	$\mu \pm \sigma$
Initial	20.18	30.09	39.75	20.59 ± 11.76	
Flow	7.45	15.20	34.59	11.27 ± 11.66	0.47 ± 0.38
PPC Flow	5.03	8.80	15.41	6.21 ± 4.70	0.68 ± 0.17
PPC Flow Attention	**4.70**	**8.31**	**14.68**	$\mathbf{5.88 \pm 4.50}$	$\mathbf{0.69 \pm 0.17}$

set to 0.0 for samples whose error increases after the update. It takes a value between 0.0 to 1.0 where higher values are better. The reduction factor indicates how much of the error can be reduced with one update step.

3 Results

The performance of the different models evaluated on the test data set is summarized in Table 1. The Flow, PPC Flow, and PPC Flow Attention models achieve a mTRE ($\mu \pm \sigma$ computed over all samples) of 11.27 ± 11.66 mm, 6.21 ± 4.70 mm and 5.88 ± 4.50 mm respectively. The reduction factor for Flow, PPC Flow, and PPC Flow Attention is ($\mu \pm \sigma$ computed over all samples) 0.47 ± 0.38, 0.68 ± 0.17, 0.69 ± 0.17 respectively. Fig. 2 compares the change in registration error after one update for all the models used.

4 Discussion and conclusion

We proposed a DL-based extension to learn the update operation of the PPC-based iterative 2D/3D registration framework. PPC Flow learns the 2D match-

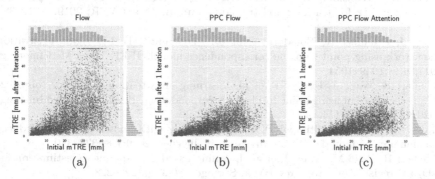

Fig. 2. Error distribution for the test data set, showing registration errors before and after one update operation for (a) Flow, (b) PPC Flow, and (c) PPC Flow Attention. For better visualization, the values of mTRE after 1 iteration are clipped at 50mm.

ing operation with PPC model as a known operator. It improves the performance of the update operation by a factor of 1.8 compared to Flow model in terms of mean reduction in registration error as shown in Table 1. Our intuition is that, the PPC model enforces constraints to learn correspondences that are relevant for the registration thus improving the performance. PPC Flow Attention learns 2D matching and weighting together in an end-to-end manner. This improves the performance over the PPC Flow model as it can effectively discard the outliers that might still be present in the correspondences predicted using PPC Flow.

The proposed update operator serves as an initial step in extending the PPC-based registration framework to a DL-based module which retains the strength of classical 2D/3D registration techniques while also providing all the benefits of DL-based methods. However, there are still some areas that need to be addressed for achieving this goal. Especially, in cases where we start with small registration errors, the learned update operator has minimal influence. We plan to address this issue in our future work either by unrolling the iterative registration or with multiple learned update operators. Additionally, one can explore how to make the update operator tailor-made for specific clinical applications.

Disclaimer. The concepts and information presented in this paper are based on research and are not commercially available.

References

1. Markelj P, Tomaževič D, Likar B, et al. A review of 3D/2D registration methods for image-guided interventions. Med Image Anal. 2012;16(3):642–661.
2. Miao S, Wang ZJ, Zheng Y, et al. Real-time 2D/3D registration via CNN regression. In: Proc ISBI; 2016. p. 1430–1434.
3. Miao S, Piat S, Fischer P, et al. Dilated FCN for multi-agent 2D/3D medical image registration. In: Proc AAAI; 2018. p. 4694–4701.
4. Liao H, Lin WA, Zhang J, et al. Multiview 2D/3D rigid registration via a point-of-interest network for tracking and triangulation. In: Proc CVPR; 2019. p. 12638–12647.
5. Wang J, Schaffert R, Borsdorf A, et al. Dynamic 2-D/3-D rigid registration framework using point-to-plane correspondence model. IEEE Trans Med Imaging. 2017;36(9):1939–1954.
6. Schaffert R, Wang J, Fischer P, et al. Learning an attention model for robust 2-D/3-D registration using point-to-plane correspondences. IEEE Trans Med Imaging. 2020;39(10):3159–3174.
7. Maier AK, Syben C, Stimpel B, et al. Learning with known operators reduces maximum error bounds. Nature machine intelligence. 2019;1(8):373–380.
8. Schaffert R, Weiß M, Wang J, et al. Learning-based correspondence estimation for 2-D/3-D registration. In: Proc BVM. Springer; 2020. p. 222–228.
9. Dosovitskiy A, Fischer P, Ilg E, et al. FlowNet: learning optical flow with convolutional networks. In: Proc ICCV; 2015. p. 2758–2766.

Abstract: Generation of Annotated Brain Tumor MRIs with Tumor-induced Tissue Deformations for Training and Assessment of Neural Networks

Hristina Uzunova[1], Jan Ehrhardt[1], Heinz Handels[1]

[1]Institute of Medical Informatics, University of Lübeck
uzunova@imi.uni-luebeck.de

Machine learning methods, especially neural networks, have proven to excel at many image processing and analysis methods in the medical image domain. Yet, their success strongly relies on the availability of large training data sets with high quality ground truth annotations, e.g. expert segmentation of anatomical/pathological structures. Therefore, generating realistic synthetic data with ground truth labels has become crucial to boost the performance of neural networks. Most of the large publicly available datasets containing some type of pathologies are commonly designed for the segmentation (detection/ localization) of the particular pathological structure and thus only contain expert segmentations of the latter. On the other hand, datasets containing ground truth annotations of normal anatomy are usually generated from healthy populations. This leads to a lack of ground truth annotation to evaluate the accuracy of standard algorithms on pathological data, and a lack of data to train algorithms that target anatomical structures in pathological data. In this work, we propose a method for the generation of realistic pathological data with ground truth labels of both anatomical and pathological structures [1]. This is achieved by a GAN-based domain translation approach, that retains the topology of a healthy source domain, whereas the appearance of a target pathological domain is recreated. This way, the anatomic annotations of the source domain, can be directly applied to the generated images. Our method also includes an explicit pathology injection with available ground truth segmentations. Furthermore, we propose a novel inverse probabilistic approach to simulate tumor-induced deformations of the surrounding tissue. For our experiment brain tumor MRIs are generated and used for training and evaluation of segmentation and registration neural networks, proving the feasibility of our approach.

References

1. Uzunova H, Ehrhardt J, Handels H. Generation of annotated brain tumor MRIs with tumor-induced tissue deformations for training and assessment of neural networks. Proc MICCAI. 2020; p. 501–511.

© Der/die Autor(en), exklusiv lizenziert durch
Springer Fachmedien Wiesbaden GmbH, ein Teil von Springer Nature 2021
C. Palm et al. (Hrsg.), *Bildverarbeitung für die Medizin 2021*,
Informatik aktuell, https://doi.org/10.1007/978-3-658-33198-6_28

Abstract: Multi-camera, Multi-person, and Real-time Fall Detection using Long Short Term Memory

Christian Heinrich[1], Samad Koita[2], Mohammad Taufeeque[2], Nicolai Spicher[1], Thomas M. Deserno[1]

[1]Peter L. Reichertz Institute for Medical Informatics of TU Braunschweig and Hannover Medical School, Germany
[2]Indian Institute of Technology Bombay, India
christian.heinrich@plri.de

Falls occurring at home are a high risk for elderly living alone. Several sensor-based methods for detecting falls exist and – in majority – use wearables or ambient sensors. Video-based fall detection is emerging. However, the restricted view of a single camera, distinguishing and tracking of persons, as well as high false-positive rates pose limitations. We have proposed the following [1]: We augment the human pose estimation algorithm openpifpaf for fall detection by adding multi-camera and multi-person tracking support. For each person, five temporal and spatial features are extracted and processed by a long short-term memory (LSTM) network, classifying each frame as a fall or no fall event. We use the UP-fall detection dataset for evaluation and achieve a F1-score of 92.5%. Still, we observe a trend of false-positives, which might result from the imbalance in the data (36% videos showing falls) with respect to their rare occurrences in real life. For improvement, we will acquire a multi-camera dataset in our smart home environment that represents falls and everyday activities.

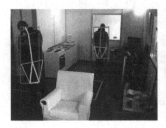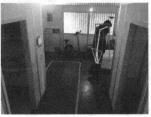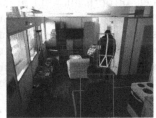

Fig. 1. Initial results acquired in the smart home lab from three cameras capturing two persons. Each person is surrounded by a red bounding box and pose key points are visualized by colored lines. Right panel: The view is restricted which underlines the need for multi-camera support. Faces are masked due to the COVID-19 pandemic.

References

1. Taufeeque M, Koita S, Spicher N, et al. Multi-camera, multi-person, and real-time fall detection using long short term memory. Proc SPIE. 2021;Accepted.

Abstract: Probabilistic Dense Displacement Networks for Medical Image Registration

Contributions to the Learn2Reg Challenge

Lasse Hansen, Mattias P. Heinrich

Institut für Medizinische Informatik, Universität zu Lübeck
hansen@imi.uni-luebeck.de

Medical image registration plays a vital role in various clinical workflows, diagnosis, research studies and computer-assisted interventions. Currently, deep learning based registration methods are starting to show promising improvements that could advance the accuracy, robustness and computation speed of conventional algorithms. However, until recently there was no commonly used benchmark dataset available to compare learning approaches with each other and their conventional (not trained) counterparts. To overcome this shortcoming the 2020 MICCAI registration challenge, Learn2Reg (L2R), was initiated [1]. L2R comprises four complementary registration sub-tasks (brain MRI/US, inhale/exhale lung CT, abdominal CT, hippocampus MRI), that tackle the imminent challenges of medical image registration: learning from small datasets, estimating large deformations, dealing with multi-modal scans and learning from weak labels. At the same time L2R lowers the entry barrier for new groups in this emerging field with a simplified challenge design by providing pre-processed data (resampled, cropped, pre-aligned) and expects only voxel displacement fields. Our methodical contribution to the L2R challenge is the adaptation of the probabilistic dense displacement (pdd) network to all tasks [2, 3]. Features (handcrafted MIND-SSC or learned Obelisk) are extracted from the fixed and moving image. Next, a feature correlation layer evaluates a dense displacement space for each grid point. A final displacement field is obtained by encouraging smoothness with alternating filters that act on spatial (mean-field inference) and displacement dimensions (approx. min-convolutions) using unsupervised learning with a nonlocal metric loss. With our challenge entry we were able to rank first in two sub-tasks (brain MRI/US and respiratory lung CT), and second in the overall challenge and thus, could establish the (probabilistic dense displacement) network as a fast and accurate general purpose registration framework for medical 3D scans.

References

1. Hansen L, Hering A, Heinrich M, et al.. Learn2Reg: 2020 MICCAI registration challenge; 2020. https://learn2reg.grand-challenge.org.
2. Heinrich MP. Closing the gap between deep and conventional image registration using probabilistic dense displacement networks. Proc MICCAI. 2019; p. 50–58.

3. Heinrich MP, Hansen L.   Highly accurate and memory efficient unsupervised
   learning-based discrete CT registration using 2.5 D displacement search. Proc MIC-
   CAI. 2020; p. 190–200. github.com/multimodallearning/pdd2.5.

Abstract: Joint Imaging Platform for Federated Clinical Data Analytics

Jonas Scherer[1,3,6], Marco Nolden[1,4,6], Jens Kleesiek[2,5,6], Jasmin Metzger[1,6],
Klaus Kades[1,3,6], Verena Schneider[2,6], Hanno Gao[1,6], Peter Neher[1,6],
Ralf Floca[1,4,6], Heinz-Peter Schlemmer[2,3,6], Klaus Maier-Hein[1,3,4,6],
and the DKTK JIP Consortium[6]

[1]Division of Medical Image Computing, German Cancer Research Center (DKFZ)
[2]Division of Radiology, German Cancer Research Center (DKFZ)
[3]Medical Faculty Heidelberg, University of Heidelberg
[4]Pattern Analysis and Learning Group, Heidelberg University Hospital
[5]Institute for Artificial Intelligence in Medicine (IKIM), University Hospital Essen
[6]German Cancer Consortium (DKTK)
k.maier-hein@dkfz-heidelberg.de

Image analysis is one of the most promising applications of artificial intelligence (AI) in healthcare, potentially improving prediction, diagnosis and treatment of diseases. While scientific advances in this area critically depend on the accessibility of large-volume and high-quality data, sharing data between institutions faces various ethical and legal constraints as well as organizational and technical obstacles. The Joint Imaging Platform (JIP) of the German Cancer Consortium (DKTK) addresses these issues by providing federated data analysis technology in a secure and compliant way [1]. Using the JIP, medical image data remains in the originator institutions, but analysis and AI algorithms are shared and jointly used. Common standards and interfaces to local systems ensure permanent data sovereignty of participating institutions. The JIP is established in the radiology and nuclear medicine departments of 10 university hospitals in Germany (DKTK partner sites). In multiple complementary use cases we show that the platform fulfills all relevant requirements to serve as a foundation for multicenter medical imaging trials and research on large cohorts: the harmonization and integration of data, interactive analysis, automatic analysis, federated machine learning as well as extensibility and maintenance processes, which are elementary for the sustainability of such a platform. The results demonstrate the feasibility of employing the JIP as a federated data analytics platform in heterogeneous clinical IT and software landscapes, solving an important bottleneck for the application of AI to large-scale clinical imaging data.

References

1. Scherer J, Nolden M, Kleesiek J, et al. Joint imaging platform for federated clinical data analytics. JCO Clinical Cancer Informatics. 2020;(4):1027–1038.

Towards Mouse Bone X-ray Microscopy Scan Simulation

Weilin Fu[1,2], Leonid Mill[1], Stephan Seitz[1,2], Tobias Geimer[1], Lasse Kling[4], Dennis Possart[4], Silke Christiansen[4], Andreas Maier[1,3]

[1]Pattern Recognition Lab, Friedrich-Alexander Universtiy
[2]International Max Planck Research School for Physics of Light (IMPRS-PL)
[3]Erlangen Graduate School in Advanced Optical Technologies (SAOT)
[4]Fraunhofer-Institut für Keramische Technologien und Systeme (IKTS)
weilin.fu@fau.de

Abstract. Osteoporosis occurs when the body loses too much bone mass, and the bones become brittle and fragile. In the aging society of Europe, the number of people with osteoporosis is continuously growing. The disease not only severely impairs the life quality of the patients, but also causes a great burden to the healthcare system. To investigate on the disease mechanism and metabolism of the bones, X-ray microscopy scans of the mouse tibia are taken. As a fundamental step, the micro-structures, such as the lacunae and vessels of the bones, need to be segmented and analyzed. With the recent advances in the deep learning technologies, segmentation networks with good performance have been proposed. However, these supervised deep nets are not directly applicable for the segmentation of these micro-structures, since manual annotations are not feasible due to the enormous data size. In this work, we propose a pipeline to model the mouse bone micro-structures. Our workflow integrates conventional algorithms with 3D modeling using Blender, and focuses on the anatomical micro-structures rather than the intensity distributions of the mouse bone scans. It provides the basis towards generating simulated mouse bone X-ray microscopy images, which could be used as the ground truth for training segmentation neural networks.

1 Introduction

Osteoporosis means "porous bone", and is a systemic skeletal disorder. Under a microscope, a bone looks like a honeycomb, where healthy bones have small holes, and osteoporotic bones have large ones. The loss of bone mass weakens the bones and makes bones prone to breaking. Osteoporosis is the most common reason for bone fractures among the elderly [1]. From the macroscopic aspects, osteoporosis can be caused by hormone change, various diseases or medication treatments [2]. From the microscopic aspects, all osteoporosis cases are caused by an imbalanced bone resorption and formation process. Two types of cells are involved in this procedure: when the speed of bone matrix degeneration by

Springer Fachmedien Wiesbaden GmbH, ein Teil von Springer Nature 2021
C. Palm et al. (Hrsg.), *Bildverarbeitung für die Medizin 2021*,
Informatik aktuell, https://doi.org/10.1007/978-3-658-33198-6_32

osteoclasts is faster than the regeneration by osteoblasts, bone mass loss and osteoporosis occurs. In the aging European society, osteoporosis is causing both pain to the patients and financial burden to the health care system [1].

To investigate on the metabolism and disease mechanism of bones, the mouse tibia which resemble human bones are utilized as the experimental targets. In one experiment protocol, the sample mouse bones are processed and scanned with the X-ray Microscope (XRM) [3] to achieve huge data volumes with the resolution up to $0.7 \times 0.7 \times 0.7 \mu m^3$. Inside the bone mass, the lacunae where the osteoclasts and the osteoblasts dwell, and vessels which provide for the cells, are of our interest. Segmentation and further statistical analysis of the lacunae and vessels from the bones in the XRM data are crucial steps towards understanding the micro-structures and metabolism of the bones. With the recent advances of the deep learning technology, various successful segmentation networks have been proposed. However, supervised nets require labeled training data, which is unfeasible to obtain via manually annotation for our task.

In this work, we propose a pipeline to generate binary models of the mouse bone XRM data with the help of Blender [4]. Blender is an open-source computer graphics software which can be used for 3-D modeling. Twelve mouse bone XRM datasets are provided to support the simulation procedure. Our pipeline consists of four main steps. Firstly, the shape of the bone is simulated using a combination of classical algorithms. Secondly, irregularly shaped bone cracks created using Blender are indented onto the outer surface of the bone mass. Thirdly, the lacunae inside the bone mass are simulated by seeding several manually created primitives in random locations. Fourthly, the vessels inside the bone mass are simulated by placing manually modeled vessel primitives using a set of rules. The proposed pipeline is straight-forward and can grasp the characteristics of the bone micro-structures. The generated bone models make the fundamental step to simulate training data for supervised deep learning-based methods.

2   Materials and methods

2.1   Database

A database composed of 12 X-ray Microscopy (XRM) scans of the mouse tibia is provided. These scans are acquired on a Xradia Versa 520 XRM system. Among them, 6 bone segments are from healthy mice, and the other 6 are from osteoporosis mice. Each mouse tibia has the length of around 2 cm in real, while the XRM volume has the shape of $1980 \times 2024 \times 1999$ pixels with the isotropic resolution of $1.34 \mu m^3$. The raw data is stored in 16 bit unsigned format, and each volume has the size of around 2 GB.

The XRM scans are used as the modeling targets for the simulation process. In this work we focus on the shape simulation of the mouse bone, thus the high resolution and intensity ranges of the scans are not demanded. To save memory and computation cost, a preprocessing pipeline is applied. Firstly, a volume of interest (VOI) from each scan is extracted by a medical scientist to remove both ends of the tibia which are not of interest and are often corrupted due to the cone beam artefacts. Secondly, the VOI is binarized using the Otsu's [5] threshold. Thirdly, the binarized VOI is automatically cropped into stacks of shape $1000 \times 1000 \times 200$ pixels. Note that the center of each stack is the weighing center of each bone segment, and we assume that the centerline of the bone segment is parallel to the z-axis within the 200 slices.

2.2   Simulation for data augmentation

In this work, we aim to generate bone shape models with the size of $1000 \times 1000 \times 200$ pixels. The simulation of the bone model is composed of four steps, namely bone shape modeling, bone crack indentation, lacunae simulation and vessel simulation. A combination of classical algorithms are used for bone mass simulation, while the Blender [4] is utilized for the bone crack, lacunae and vessel simulation process.

2.2.1   Bone shape simulation.

To obtain binary masks of the bone shape, the Gradient Vector Flow (GVF) [6] method is applied to obtain an anisotropically diffused gradient vector field such that the gradient vectors of the edge map can reach into non-informative homogeneous regions. Then the active contour model [6], which is also regarded as the Snakes algorithm, is employed to extract the inner and the outer bone shape descriptors. Finally the Statistical Shape Model (SSM) [7] is trained to generate diversed new shapes.

The GVF method aims for an anisotropically diffused gradient vector field $\mathbf{v} = [u(x,y), v(x,y)]$ of the edge map ∇f by minimizing the energy function

$$E = \iint \mu(u_x^2 + u_y^2 + v_x^2 + v_y^2) + |\nabla f|^2 |\mathbf{v} - \nabla f|^2 \mathrm{d}x\mathrm{d}y \qquad (1)$$

Minimization of $(u_x^2 + u_y^2 + v_x^2 + v_y^2)$, requires the vector $\mathbf{v}$ to vary slowly; while minimization of $|\nabla f|^2 |\mathbf{v} - \nabla f|$ enforces the resulting field to resemble the gradient of the edge field, especially in regions with high edge responses.

The Snakes algorithm is employed to locate the points on the inner and outer contours of each 2-D slice of the mouse bone. A snake is a flexible 2-D discrete line c, and evolves towards the contours along the gradient directions in the GVF field by minimizing the following energy function

$$E(c) = E_{\text{internal}}(c) + E_{\text{external}}(c) \qquad (2)$$

$$E_{\text{internal}}(c) = \sum \alpha \left\| c' \right\|^2 + \beta \left\| c'' \right\|^2 \qquad (3)$$

$$E_{\text{external}}(c) = \sum - \left\| \mathbf{v}(c) \right\|^2 \qquad (4)$$

The internal energy term E_{internal} is the weighted summation of the magnitudes of the first and second derivatives of the snake curve c, where α, β are the weighing factors. It controls the length and the curvature of the curve c. The external energy term E_{external} is the negative summation of the GVF field gradient magnitudes at the snake points. Minimization of E_{internal} constrains that the snake curve is short and smooth; minimization of E_{external} pushes the snake points towards the contours where the GVF field has the maximum values.

The Snakes algorithm keeps the order and the number of the initialized snake points, thus generates ideal inputs to train the SSM. On each 2-D x-y slice, 1 332 and 400 snake points are utilized to characterize the outer and inner contours respectively. In other words, each bone segment shape is represented as a $(1\,332 + 400) \times 200 \times 3 = 1\,039\,200$ dimensional shape descriptor x_i. The mean vector $\bar{x}$ of these descriptors is computed and the shape matrix D is constructed

$$\bar{x} = \frac{1}{N} \sum_{i=1}^{N} x_i \tag{5}$$

$$D = (x_1 - \bar{x}, ..., x_N - \bar{x}) \tag{6}$$

Singular Value Decomposition (SVD) is then applied on the matrix D to obtain the eigenvectors ϕ and eigenvalues λ, which are then utilized to create models with new shapes

$$x = \bar{x} + b \cdot \phi \tag{7}$$

where b is the multiplicative factor with each element ranging from $-2\sqrt{\lambda_i}$ to $2\sqrt{\lambda_i}$.

2.2.2 Bone crack simulation. Due to the preparing procedure of the tibia sample, the outer surface of the mouse bones often has cracks (Fig. 1). Here we create indentations onto the outer surface of the bone mass with the help of Blender. Firstly, primitives for the cracks are created manually in Blender (Fig. 2). The primitive templates are designed to be irregular and asymmetric such that the indented cracks are as diversed as possible. Secondly, 20 seeding points on the outer contour of the bone mass are randomly selected. Thirdly, for each position, a random primitive is chosen, rescaled and rotated within a certain range. Then augmented primitive is used as a structuring element to erode the bone mass.

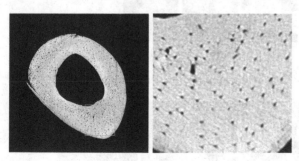

Fig. 1. 2-D x-y slice from a healthy mouse XRM scan in (left), enlarged ROI in (right).

2.2.3 Lacunae simulation. In bone XRM scans, lacunae are represented as dark cavities that can be approximated using balls, ellipses, or combinations of them. Four particle primitives are designed in Blender (Fig. 3). In each generated bone mass segment, around $150\,k$ center point positions are selected according to prior anatomical knowledge. For each centering point, a lacuna primitive is chosen and augmented with random rotation and scaling.

2.2.4 Blood vessel simulation. The blood vessels in the XRM stacks are modeled as tree branches with the Sapling Tree Gen plugin of Blender. In a 200-slice stack, the vessels have at most one bifurcation. Thus the sapling primitives are designed to have simple structures (Fig. 4). We also contrain that two vessels are at least (100, 100, 20) pixels apart from each other, and should be roughly aligned, deviating i.e. maximum ±30° from the direction of the bone axial. In a healthy bone segment sample, the number of unconnected vessels ranges from three to eight.

3   Results

The inner and outer contour surfaces of the bone shapes simulated with different settings of the multiplicative factor **b** in Eq. 7 are rendered in Paraview [8] (Fig. 5(a)). The eigen contour surfaces when **b = 0** are highlighted in red color. A patch from a 2-D slice of the simulation result is presented in Fig. 5(b), and the 3-D render of the color-coded lacunae and vessels is shown in Fig. 5(c).

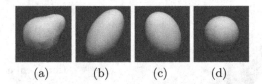

(a)   (b)   (c)   (d)   (e)

Fig. 2. Bone crack simulation. Crack templates rendered in Paraview [8].

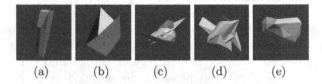

(a)   (b)   (c)   (d)

Fig. 3. Lacunae simulation. Lacunae templates rendered in Paraview [8].

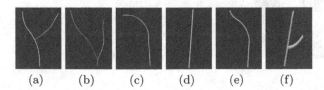

(a)   (b)   (c)   (d)   (e)   (f)

Fig. 4. Blood vessel simulation. Vessel templated rendered in Paraview.

Fig. 5. Simulated bone contours in (a), an example patch from a 2-D slice of a simulation result in (b), red lacunae and green vessels in (c). (a) rendered in Paraview [8].

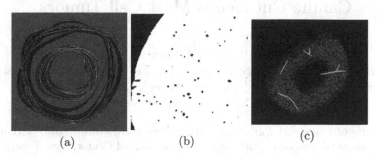

(a)   (b)   (c)

4 Discussion

In this work, we propose a pipeline to model the mouse tibia segments and the micro-structures inside. We use the statistical shape model to generate bones of different shapes, and employ Blender to simulate the bone cracks, the lacunae and the vessels. Comparing the 2-D x-y slice of the simulation result in Fig. 5(b) and that of the the real XRM data in Fig. 1, a close similarity is observed. The proposed pipeline provides an approach to generate unlimited amount of binarized bone XRM masks, which make the fundamental step towards training data simulation for segmentation networks. In the future, domain adaptation approaches could be applied to train network models with the simulated data; more complicated primitives could be designed to model osteoporosis bones.

References

1. Borgström F, Karlsson L, Ortsäter G, et al. Fragility fractures in Europe: burden, management and opportunities. Arch Osteoporos. 2020;15:1–21.
2. Svedbom A, Hernlund E, Ivergård M, et al. Osteoporosis in the European Union: a compendium of country-specific reports. Arch Osteoporos. 2013;8(1):1–218.
3. Mill L, Bier B, Syben C, et al. Towards in-vivo X-ray nanoscopy. In: Bildverarbeitung für die Medizin 2018. Springer; 2018. p. 115–120.
4. Community BO. Blender - a 3D modelling and rendering package. Stichting Blender Foundation, Amsterdam; 2018. Available from: http://www.blender.org.
5. Otsu N. A threshold selection method from gray-level histograms. IEEE transactions on systems, man, and cybernetics. 1979;9(1):62–66.
6. Xu C, Prince JL. Snakes, shapes, and gradient vector flow. IEEE Trans Image Process. 1998;7(3):359–369.
7. Dryden IL, Mardia KV. Statistical shape analysis: Wiley series in probability and statistics. New York, NY: John Wiley & Sons, Ltd; 1998.
8. Ahrens J, Geveci B, Law C. Paraview: An end-user tool for large data visualization. The visualization handbook. 2005;717.

Dataset on Bi- and Multi-nucleated Tumor Cells in Canine Cutaneous Mast Cell Tumors

Christof A. Bertram[1], Taryn A. Donovan[2], Marco Tecilla[3],
Florian Bartenschlager[1], Marco Fragoso[1], Frauke Wilm[4], Christian Marzahl[4],
Katharina Breininger[4], Andreas Maier[4], Robert Klopfleisch[1],
Marc Aubreville[5,4]

[1]Institute of Veterinary Pathology, Freie Universität Berlin, Berlin, Germany
[2]Department of Anatomic Pathology, Animal Medical Center, New York, USA
[3]Roche Pharma Research and Early Development (pRED), Pharmaceutical Sciences,
BIOmics and Pathology - Roche Innovation Center Basel, Switzerland
[4]Pattern Recognition Lab, Computer Sciences, Friedrich-Alexander-Universität
Erlangen-Nürnberg, Erlangen, Germany
[5]Technische Hochschule Ingolstadt, Ingolstadt, Germany
christof.bertram@fu-berlin.de

Abstract. Tumor cells with two nuclei (binucleated cells, BiNC) or more nuclei (multinucleated cells, MuNC) indicate an increased amount of cellular genetic material which is thought to facilitate oncogenesis, tumor progression and treatment resistance. In canine cutaneous mast cell tumors (ccMCT), binucleation and multinucleation are parameters used in cytologic and histologic grading schemes (respectively) which correlate with poor patient outcome. For this study, we created the first open source data-set with 19,983 annotations of BiNC and 1,416 annotations of MuNC in 32 histological whole slide images of ccMCT. Labels were created by a pathologist and an algorithmic-aided labeling approach with expert review of each generated candidate. A state-of-the-art deep learning-based model yielded an F_1 score of 0.675 for BiNC and 0.623 for MuNC on 11 test whole slide images. In regions of interest ($2.37mm^2$) extracted from these test images, 6 pathologists had an object detection performance between 0.270 - 0.526 for BiNC and 0.316 - 0.622 for MuNC, while our model archived an F_1 score of 0.667 for BiNC and 0.685 for MuNC. This open dataset can facilitate development of automated image analysis for this task and may thereby help to promote standardization of this facet of histologic tumor prognostication.

1 Introduction

Microscopic evaluation of tumor biopsies can yield important information pertaining to the biological behaviour of a tumor obtained from a patient. Depending upon the tumor type, different microscopic characteristics are combined to grading schemes, which are useful estimators of patient outcome. For canine cutaneous mast cell tumors (ccMCT), a frequent skin tumor of dogs, the current grading system encompasses counting the number of mitosis (cells undergoing division), number of multinucleated cells (MuNC) and cells with aberrant nuclear size and shape in an tumor area of $2.37mm^2$ [1]. As opposed to a single nucleus in most mast cells, MuNC contain three or more nuclei. Tumor cells with two nuclei (binucleated cells, BiNC) have not been evaluated as an prognostic parameter in histologic sections in previous studies, however, studies on cytologic specimens of ccMCT revealed a negative correlation to patient outcome [2].

Formation of BiNC and MuNC results in increased numbers of chromosomes (genetic material) per cell (polyploidy). This augments the metabolic capacities of the cell, which is an effective strategy in coping with escalating requirements for tumor growth. Polyploidy is considered to be key actuator of oncogenesis, tumor progression, and chemotherapy resistance [3, 4]. Additional nuclei can be acquired by 1) fusion with other neoplastic or non-neoplastic cells (syncytia) or 2) by an incomplete cell cycle (endoreplication) in the absence of cell division (failure of cytokinesis). During normal mitosis, the chromosomes are duplicated and divided into two nuclei, which are further separated into two daughter cells. If this last step is aborted then both nuclei will remain in the cell of origin.

Deep learning-based algorithms are considered a powerful tool for reproducible automated image analysis (for example for mitotic figures), however, they require large amounts of labeled data for training and testing models [5, 6]. In the present work we present the first open dataset on BiNC and MuNC in ccMCT, establish a baseline performance for deep-learning based pipeline and compare algorithmic performance to six veterinary pathologists.

2   Materials and methods

For this study we developed a novel set of labels for 32 publicly available whole slides images (WSI, resolution of 0.25 microns per pixel) of ccMCT. WSI were initially provided by Bertram et al. [6] for a mitotic figure dataset, which included 44,880 mitotic figure labels, on the same images.

2.1   Labeling of bi- and multi-nucleated tumor cells

One pathologist screened the 32 WSI using the annotation software SlideRunner [7] and labeled BiNC and MuNC as separate label classes. Thereby, 10,381 labels of BiNC and 775 labels of MuNC were obtained. Because omission of target cells during manual screening was considered a major limitation, we decided to additionally use an algorithmic-aided pipeline to identify potential target cells. Each of the candidates was subsequently reviewed by a pathologist. Using the labeling protocol described in Bertram et al. [6], we split the manual database into three folds and used each fold to train a deep learning-based network (Sec. 2.2) in order to detect overlooked candidates. A high sensitivity of finding additional BiNC and MuNC candidates was reached by using a low detection cutoff, which intentionally resulted in in many false positive detections in order to reduce a confirmation bias of the reviewing pathologist. A total of 66,585 potential BiNC and 6,958 MuNC candidates with model scores between 0.3 and 1.0 were retrieved and extracted as 128×128 px images for expert review. Of these, 9,602 (14.4 %) were classified as BiNC and 641 (9.2 %) as MuNC, which increased the label classes by 92.5 % and 82.7 %, respectively, compared to the manual database. Patches that were not assigned to these two classes were useful as hard negatives in training a classification network (Fig. 1). The final algorithmic-augmented datasets includes 19,983 labels of BiNC and 1,416 labels of MuNC. All code and the labels can be accessed on our github project page: https://github.com/DeepPathology/CCMCT_Bi_Multinucleated.

2.2 Dataset validation

In order to establish a baseline for automatic detection, we trained a customized deep learning model. WSI were split into training (N = 21) and test cases (N = 11) according to the original publication of the images [6]. Our model consists of two stages as previously described for automated mitotic figure detection [5]. The primary object detection stage is a customized RetinaNet [8] with a pre-trained ResNet-18 stem [9]. The second stage is a patch classifier, which was also derived from a pre-trained ResNet-18 architecture [9], and was used to differentiate hard negatives with high visual similarity to BiNC and MuNC.

2.2.1 Performance validation on the ground truth dataset. First, our model was validated against the final dataset of the test images. This task evaluated the object detection performance as per the F_1 score on entire histologic sections and can serve as a baseline performance for future research projects.

2.2.2 Performance validation against pathologists. In order to evaluate whether algorithms can approximate the performance of pathologists, we compared object detections from both on smaller tumor areas (region of interest with a size of $2.37mm^2$) from the 11 test WSI. Regions of interest were extracted from the

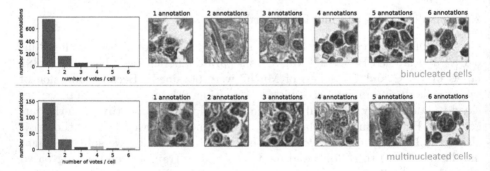

Fig. 1. Number of pathologists agreeing upon an object being a binucleated (upper images) and multinucleated (lower images) tumor cell.

WSI with the following criteria for the tumor region: images containing the most MuNC (as per dataset ground truth), or, if no MuNC were present in the WSI, images containing the most BiNC. For calculation of performance, ground truth (GT) labels comprised of the algorithmically augmented database (dataset ground truth), agreement on labels by 2/6 veterinary pathologists (dual vote ground truth) or agreement by 3/6 veterinary pathologists (three vote ground truth). The F_1 score was used as a metric to compare the algorithmic approaches and six experts to the GT labels. We considered two annotations to be identical if the centers were within a Euclidean distance of 25 px (equivalent to approximately the mean radius of a mast cell).

2.3 Co-localisation of bi-, multi-nucleated and mitotic tumor cells

In order to better understand the pathology task of enumerating BiNC and MuNC, we correlated the density of BiNC and MuNC with mitotic figures (previously published for these WSI [6]). We used a moving window summation with an area of 2.37 mm^2, as described in Auberville et al. [5], to derive the mitotic count (MC), as well as the BiNC count and the MuNC count. To compare those density metrics, we used Pearson's correlation coefficient.

3 Results

Our deep learning-based model yielded an F_1 score of 0.675 for BiNC and 0.623 for MuNC when assessed on the dataset GT of the entire 11 test WSI. Comparing the algorithm to the performance of six veterinary pathologists on regions of interest of the test WSI, the algorithm outperformed all pathologists for detection of BiNC (Tab. 1) and MuNC (Tab. 2) when using the dataset GT definition, but severely deteriorated for multi-expert GT definitions. In our assessment, the expert performance varied significantly (inter-observer variability) regardless of the GT definition, whereas identification of MuNC generally had higher accuracy than identification of BiNC (Fig. 1). This is in contrast to the algorithmic performance which was hampered by lower numbers of labels on MuNC (compared to BiNC) for training the model.

Co-localisation of BiNC cells with MuNC (r = 0.66) had a higher positive correlation than co-localisation of BiNC or MuNC with mitotic density (r = 0.42 and 0.29, respectively).

4 Discussion

With this publication we present a novel open access dataset on BiNC and MuNC in ccMCT. A first deep learning-based model was able to yield an F_1 score of above 0.6 for both label classes and outperformed all pathologists in object detection compared to the dataset GT. The model architecture was based upon previous publications on algorithms for mitotic figure detection [5, 6]. It

Table 1. Performance (F_1 score) of veterinary pathologists (VP 1-6) and our deep learning-based model (DL) for detecting binucleated tumor cells compared to different definitions of ground truth (GT) labels.

	Region of interest test set			WSI test set
	Three-vote GT	Dual-vote GT	Dataset GT	
VP 1	0.513	0.567	0.526	N/A
VP 2	0.524	0.420	0.328	N/A
VP 3	0.392	0.478	0.280	N/A
VP 4	0.424	0.433	0.270	N/A
VP 5	0.261	0.511	0.300	N/A
VP 6	0.470	0.372	0.329	N/A
Median VP 1-6	0.447	0.455	0.314	N/A
DL	0.438	0.424	0.667	0.675

Table 2. Performance (F_1 score) of veterinary pathologists (VP 1-6) and our deep learning-based model (DL) for detecting multinucleated tumor cells compared to different definitions of ground truth (GT) labels.

	Fields of interest test set			WSI test set
	Three vote GT	Dual vote GT	Dataset GT	
VP 1	0.610	0.556	0.622	N/A
VP 2	0.508	0.574	0.513	N/A
VP 3	0.355	0.478	0.361	N/A
VP 4	0.613	0.559	0.545	N/A
VP 5	0.466	0.627	0.441	N/A
VP 6	0.375	0.360	0.316	N/A
Median VP 1-6	0.487	0.558	0.477	N/A
DL	0.481	0.4	0.685	0.628

was beyond the scope of the present study to compare performance of different algorithmic approaches, however, we encourage other research groups to use this publicly available dataset to improve state-of-the-art methods for this task.

Although pathologists are the gold standard for labeling structures in histologic sections, an object detection challenge revealed high inter-rater variability for identifying BiNC and MuNC, which is likely also reflected in label accuracy of the dataset. Obstacles to overcome when classifying BiNC and MuNC include unclear visualization of cell boarders between adjacent cells as well as differentiation from imposters with indented or lobulated nuclear shape. Furthermore, overlooking/omission of objects was a common source of error. Apart from containing additional nuclei, BiNC are often inconspicuous, which makes them difficult to recognize. Enlargement of cell size was more common in MuNC, which could explain somewhat higher sensitivity of identifying these objects. For dataset creation, we therefore decided to use an algorithmic-augmented labeling approach that was able to detect many missed candidates. In order to reduce the bias of this labeling approach we intentionally used a low detection threshold (many false positves) and all labels were reviewed by an expert .

Positive correlation of BiNC and MuNC with mitotic density suggests that endoreplication is a plausible mechanism for their formation in ccMCT. Although the number of MuNC is am important prognostic parameter of ccMCT, the number of BiNC in histologic tumor secions has not been correlated to patient outcome to date (as opposed to cytologic specimens [2]). As the density of BiNC was proportional to that of MuNC and both are evidence of polyploidy, we speculate that histologic assessment of binucleation may have prognostic relevance in ccMCT. Whereas MuNC are very sparse or absent in most ccMCT cases and thus is predictive of poor outcome in only small numbers of cases [1], BiNC are more common in ccMCT and should be considered as a potential prognostic parameter in future studies. Due to the high inter-observer variability observed in this study we highlight that methods of enumeration should be better standardized and we propose that deep learning-based models may be useful to increase reproducibility and possibly accuracy for assessment of this parameter.

Acknowledgement. CAB gratefully acknowledges financial support received from the Dres. Jutta & Georg Bruns-Stiftung für innovative Veterinärmedizin.

References

1. Kiupel M, Webster J, Bailey K, et al. Proposal of a 2-tier histologic grading system for canine cutaneous mast cell tumors to more accurately predict biological behavior. Vet Pathol. 2011;48(1):147–155.
2. Camus M, Priest H, Koehler J, et al. Cytologic criteria for mast cell tumor grading in dogs with evaluation of clinical outcome. Vet Pathol. 2016;53(6):1117–1123.
3. Amend SR, Torga G, Lin KC, et al. Polyploid giant cancer cells: unrecognized actuators of tumorigenesis, metastasis, and resistance. Prostate. 2019;79(13):1489–1497.
4. Chen J, Niu N, Zhang J, et al. Polyploid giant cancer cells (PGCCs): the evil roots of cancer. Curr cancer Drug Targets. 2019;19(5):360–367.
5. Aubreville M, Bertram CA, Marzahl C, et al. Deep learning algorithms out-perform veterinary pathologists in detecting the mitotically most active tumor region. Sci Rep. 2020;10(16447):1–11.
6. Bertram CA, Aubreville M, Marzahl C, et al. A large-scale dataset for mitotic figure assessment on whole slide images of canine cutaneous mast cell tumor. Sci Data. 2019;6(1):1–9.
7. Aubreville M, Bertram C, Klopfleisch R, et al. SlideRunner. In: Bildverarbeitung für die Medizin 2018. Springer; 28. p. 309–314.
8. Lin TY, Goyal P, Girshick R, et al. Focal loss for dense object detection. Proc IEEE ICCV. 2017; p. 2980–2988.
9. He K, Zhang X, Ren S, et al. Deep residual learning for image recognition. Proc IEEE CVPR. 2016; p. 770–778.

Abstract: Data Augmentation for Information Transfer

Why Controlling for Confounding Effects in Radiomic Studies is Important and How to do it

Michael Götz[1], Klaus Maier-Hein[1]

[1]Medical Image Computing Group, Deutsches Krebsforschungszentrum (DKFZ)
m.goetz@dkfz-heidelberg.de

The major goal of radiomics studies is the identification of predictive and reliable markers. It is, therefore, crucial to account for unwanted confounding effects that affect the radiomic features like scanning noise, annotator bias, or the used imaging device and parameter. Usually, these confounding effects are not sufficiently represented in the main cohort of radiomics studies and consequently are investigated in smaller side-studies. Within our study [1], we looked into two questions: a) are those side-studies necessary and b) how to use the information from those studies on the feature stability in the radiomics modelling process. For this, three different methods for incorporating prior knowledge into a radiomics modelling process were compared: the naïve approach (ignoring feature quality), the most common approach consisting of removing unstable features based on correlation ranking, and a novel approach using data augmentation for information transfer (DAFIT). The predictive power and the ability to estimate the predictive power were assessed by looking at the ROC Area under Curve (AUC) and the difference between the AUC from data with and data without confounding effects present. Synthetic and publicly available real lung imaging patient data were used for the experiments. The experiments showed the importance of controlling for confounding effects. Differences between the estimated and true performance of a model of up to 20 and 25 percentage points for real and synthetic data, respectively, showed the possible impact of ignoring confounding effects. Removing unstable features improved the performance estimation, while slightly decreasing the model performance, i.e. decreasing the area under curve achieved with the model. We argue that the reduction of features led to an effective reduction of information that is available to build the model. This point is addressed by the proposed approach, which performed superior both in terms of the estimation of the model performance and the actual model performance.

References

1. Götz M, Maier-Hein KH. Optimal statistical incorporation of independent feature stability information into radiomics studies. Sci Rep. 2020 01;10(737):2045–2322.

© Der/die Autor(en), exklusiv lizenziert durch
Springer Fachmedien Wiesbaden GmbH, ein Teil von Springer Nature 2021
C. Palm et al. (Hrsg.), *Bildverarbeitung für die Medizin 2021*,
Informatik aktuell, https://doi.org/10.1007/978-3-658-33198-6_34

Reduction of Stain Variability in Bone Marrow Microscopy Images

Influence of Augmentation and Normalization Methods on Detection and Classification of Hematopoietic Cells

Philipp Gräbel[1], Martina Crysandt[2], Reinhild Herwartz[2], Melanie Baumann[2], Barbara M. Klinkhammer[3], Peter Boor[3], Tim H. Brümmendorf[2], Dorit Merhof[1]

[1]Institute of Imaging and Computer Vision, RWTH Aachen University, Germany
[2]Department of Hematology, Oncology, Hemostaseology and Stem Cell Transplantation, University Hospital RWTH Aachen University, Germany
[3]Institute of Pathology, University Hospital RWTH Aachen University, Germany
graebel@lfb.rwth-aachen.de

Abstract. The analysis of cells in bone marrow microscopy images is essential for the diagnosis of many hematopoietic diseases such as leukemia. Automating detection, classification and quantification of different types of leukocytes in whole slide images could improve throughput and reliability. However, variations in the staining agent used to highlight cell features can reduce the accuracy of these methods. In histopathology, data augmentation and normalization techniques are used to make neural networks more robust but their application to hematological image data needs to be investigated. In this paper, we compare six promising approaches on three image sets with different staining characteristics in terms of detection and classification.

1 Introduction

Automated analysis of hematological image data is an emerging field in computer vision. Recent technological advances, particularly deep learning, made the classification of hematopoietic cells in bone marrow microscopy images possible. The core steps of an automated system include detection of individual cells, classification of cell type and quantification of entire Whole-Slide Images (WSI). In clinical practice, the analysis of bone marrow samples includes manual screening of selected regions by highly trained medical experts. Deep learning offers, for the first time, the potential to automate this procedure and thereby increase throughput and objectivity.

Bone marrow samples use staining agents to highlight specific properties of the cell. This results in a clearly distinguishable cell nucleus and cytoplasm that is colored according to cell type. While this staining process is standardized and performed following a strictly defined workflow, a certain variability cannot be avoided. In extreme cases, this might lead to slides that are uninterpretable even by human experts, but also slight variations can degrade performance of automated systems.

In the case of histological image analysis, various effects of staining have been extensively researched. In terms of variability of a single stain type, two different kinds of approaches seem prevalent: stain normalization and stain augmentation [1]. The first approach aims at minimizing variance in both training and test images, resulting in simplified network training. Stain augmentation aims at augmenting the training data such that it exhibits a similar distribution (i.e., staining variability) as the test data. Classical approaches for stain normalization are conversion to grayscale, a color-based transform [2] and color deconvolution [3]. Stain augmentation can be performed by altering the different color channels in a transformed image, e.g. using Principal Component Analysis (PCA), the HSV color space or color deconvolution.

Hematology focusses on object (cell) detection and classification. While classification relies on the color of a cell (e.g. basophilic cytoplasm is rather blue while eosinophilic cytoplasm is red) as much as on structure, detection heavily relies on the shape of a cell. This leads to the assumption that classification and detection are affected differently by the aforementioned methods, which can significantly alter the color properties of an image. Consequently, we perform an analysis of several normalization and augmentation techniques on hematological image data with respect to detection and classification separately. To this end, we employ different hematological datasets with varying degrees of staining severity.

2   Materials and methods

2.1   Image data

We use a whole slide microscopy scanner with $63\times$ magnification and automated immersion oiling to obtain high resolution images from bone marrow samples. Each sample is stained in a standardized procedure with Pappenheim staining. Nevertheless, variabilities in the scanned images of stained bone marrow samples occur – both due to effects of the staining but also the subsequent digitalization with automatic focus and illumination setting. We divide the data into three subsets: normal images (NI) in which the staining appears as expected, images that tend towards pink over-staining (OS1) and images that tend towards darker blue over-staining with starker contrast(OS2). Examples are shown in Fig. 1. It needs to be mentioned that not necessarily all extracted patches of a slide with a particular stain exhibit the same stain characteristics as there is also some variation within extracted regions. All three sets have manual annotations from hematological experts.

For the detection task, we divide each set into slightly overlapping patches of size $1600 \times 1600\,\mathrm{px}^2$, resulting in 913 images in NI, 268 images in OS1 and 215 images in OS2. For the classification task, we extract patches of size $244 \times 244\,\mathrm{px}^2$ around individual cells, resulting in 4560 patches in NI, 1385 patches in OS1 and 1075 patches in OS2.

2.2 Normalization methods

The normalization methods are applied to images both in training and in testing and aim at minimizing the variance (caused among others by stain inhomogeneities) that a network is required to learn. Fig. 2 shows some examples for normalization as well as augmentation methods.

2.2.1 Macenko. Based on the color deconvolution method by Macenko et al. [3], two vectors corresponding to the the two different staining components can be extracted. Using these, the image can be decomposed into a stain matrix and a concentration matrix. Images are normalized by replacing the stain matrix of an individual image with a target stain matrix, which can be extracted from a large number of normally stained images.

2.2.2 Grayscale. The image is converted into gray-scale (y) from RGB using the conversion $y = 0.299R + 0.587G + 0.114B$.

2.2.3 LAB. Reinhard et al. [2] proposed a normalization method using image statistics in LAB space. Images in LAB space are adapted so that mean and standard deviation of each of the three channels is the same as in a large number of normally stained images.

2.3 Augmentation methods

Augmentation methods are only applied to images in the training process in order to increase the variance of normally stained images. In this work, we use a parameter x to determine the augmentation strength – higher values for x result in a more perturbed images. Nevertheless, each augmentation has a random element to it, such that the whole spectrum from maximum perturbation to no perturbation is utilized with a given probability. Fig. 2 shows some examples for normalization as well as augmentation methods.

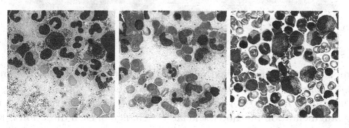

Fig. 1. Three patches from the detection dataset of (from left to right) NI, OS1 and OS2. For classification, patches around each individual cell are extracted.

2.3.1 Macenko. Stain augmentation is performed by perturbing the elements of the concentration matrix extracted based on Macenko et al.'s color deconvolution method. [3]. Preliminary visual analysis showed that a multiplication with a factor from a Gaussian distribution with $\mu = 1$ and $\sigma^2 = \frac{x}{30}$ (with x being the augmentation strength) yields realistic results.

2.3.2 HSV. The augmentation is performed by adding a value drawn from a Gaussian distribution with zero mean and variance x (augmentation strength) to the hue component. The hue component is chosen as most changes in differently stained images show a shift towards pink or blue, which can be represented by a shift in hue.

2.3.3 PCA. Using images from all three datasets, a PCA is performed on the RGB pixel values. Preliminary analysis shows that the first component of PCA corresponds mostly to changes in brightness, while the second component corresponds to the change in color. Consequently, augmentation can be performed by perturbing the second component of an image in PCA space. Preliminary visual comparison of transformed images showed that a multiplication with a factor $f \in [1 - 0.01x, 1 + 0.01x]$, with x being the augmentation strength results in realistically augmented images.

2.4 Experimental setup

For the evaluation, the set of normally stained images (NI) is divided into six subsets. In six-fold cross-validation, we first train a network on four training and one validation set. Evaluation is performed separately on the held out test set as well as on OS1 and OS2. For augmentation, we evaluate augmentation strengths from $x \in [1, 9]$.

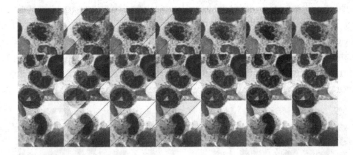

Fig. 2. Augmentation and normalization for three sample cells (normal stain classification dataset). From left to right: original, Macenko augmentation, HSV augmentation, PCA augmentation, Macenko normalization, grayscale normalization, LAB normalization. For the augmentation methods, the largest change in each direction is shown (top left and bottom right of each image, both augmentation strength 9), with a medium augmentation in the middle (augmentation strength 4).

For detection, we employ a U-Net [4] of depth five on random patches of size $512 \times 512\,\mathrm{px}^2$ followed by Watershed [5] segmentation. This model showed excellent results in previous comparisons to other state-of-the-art architectures. Training takes at most 100 epochs with early stop after ten epochs without improvement. The matching of prediction and ground truth is performed using centroid distance. For classification, we employ a Dense-121 [6] architecture with cross entropy loss. Training takes at most 300 epochs with early stop after 50 epochs without improvement. In both cases, we additionally perform data augmentation with random rotation, mirroring and random crop.

3   Results

Fig. 3 shows the results for detection and classification. In general, augmentation methods yield better results than normalization methods. However, in both cases results frequently decrease compared to the baseline without normalization or augmentation. Notable exception is the HSV augmentation method: while the absolute score stays mostly unchanged on NI with a slight increase in variance between folds, results for the stained images of OS1 (for both detection and classification) and OS2 (only for detection) improve. It is further noteworthy that for classification, the PCA augmentation method has decreasing scores with increasing augmentation strength, which is not the case for detection.

4   Discussion

The results show that most standard augmentation and normalization methods commonly used in digital histopathology do not yield improved results on heavily stained hematology data and even decrease classification and detection scores in most cases. Only the HSV augmentation methods mostly improves results: particularly the dataset OS1 benefits from the additional variance in the training data. While methods based on color deconvolution yield good results on histopathological image data, no improvement is observed for hematological images. The varying density of a large number of very different objects (cells) might make computation of accurate stain and concentration matrices more challenging. The poor results of the PCA augmentation methods are unexpected as their color transformation is based on a large data basis containing patches from all three staining types.

It stands to reason that these common data-augmentation methods are not able to sufficiently capture the color distribution of the staining variabilities in hematological image data. In future work, we will further look into generative models that are able to learn more accurately from training data.

It needs to be further noted that the datasets OS1 and OS2 in this work constitute extreme cases, which are already difficult to analyze for human experts. While it might be an option to exclude such images from training or in application, researching the limitations of a neural network is important for translation into clinical practice.

Fig. 3. Top: results for detection in terms of Average Precision (AP). Bottom: results for classification in terms of macro f1-Score. Horizontal lines denote the reference results, colors denote the test set (black for NI, red for OS1, blue for OS2). Each column shows results from all six folds (brighter markers) as well as the result over all folds.

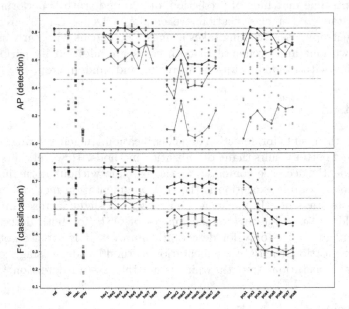

Acknowledgement. The authors would like thank Xinyi Gao for his support in improving the data transformation pipeline. This study was supported by the following grants: DFG: SFB/TRR57, SFB/TRR219, BO3755/6-1, BMBF: STOP-FSGS-01GM1901A, BMWi: EMPAIA project to PB.

References

1. Tellez D, Litjens G, Bandi P, et al. Quantifying the effects of data augmentation and stain color normalization in convolutional neural networks for computational pathology. arXiv preprint arXiv:190206543. 2019;.
2. Reinhard E, Adhikhmin M, Gooch B, et al. Color transfer between images. IEEE Comput Graph Appl. 2001;21(5):34–41.
3. Macenko M, Niethammer M, Marron JS, et al.; IEEE. A method for normalizing histology slides for quantitative analysis. 2009 IEEE International Symposium on Biomedical Imaging: From Nano to Macro. 2009; p. 1107–1110.
4. Ronneberger O, Fischer P, Brox T; Springer. U-net: Convolutional networks for biomedical image segmentation. MICCAI. 2015; p. 234–241.
5. Beucher S, Meyer F. The morphological approach to segmentation: the watershed transformation. Mathematical morphology in image processing. 1993;34:433–481.
6. Huang G, Liu Z, Van Der Maaten L, et al. Densely connected convolutional networks. Proc IEEE CVPR. 2017; p. 4700–4708.

Cell Detection for Asthma on Partially Annotated Whole Slide Images
Learning to be EXACT

Christian Marzahl[1,2], Christof A. Bertram[3], Frauke Wilm[1], Jörn Voigt[2],
Ann K. Barton[4], Robert Klopfleisch[3], Katharina Breininger[1], Andreas Maier[1],
Marc Aubreville[5]

[1]Pattern Recognition Lab, Department of Computer Science,
Friedrich-Alexander-Universität Erlangen-Nürnberg (FAU), Germany
[2]R & D Projects, EUROIMMUN Medizinische Labordiagnostika AG
[3]Institute of Veterinary Pathology, Freie Universität Berlin, Germany
[4]Equine Clinic, Freie Universität Berlin, Berlin, Germany
[5]Technische Hochschule Ingolstadt, Ingolstadt, Germany
c.marzahl@euroimmun.de

Abstract. Asthma is a chronic inflammatory disorder of the lower respiratory tract and naturally occurs in humans and animals including horses. The annotation of an asthma microscopy whole slide image (WSI) is an extremely labour-intensive task due to the hundreds of thousands of cells per WSI. To overcome the limitation of annotating WSI incompletely, we developed a training pipeline which can train a deep learning-based object detection model with partially annotated WSIs and compensate class imbalances on the fly. With this approach we can freely sample from annotated WSIs areas and are not restricted to fully annotated extracted sub-images of the WSI as with classical approaches. We evaluated our pipeline in a cross-validation setup with a fixed training set using a dataset of six equine WSIs of which four are partially annotated and used for training, and two fully annotated WSI are used for validation and testing. Our WSI-based training approach outperformed classical sub-image-based training methods by up to 15% mAP and yielded human-like performance when compared to the annotations of ten trained pathologists.

1 Introduction

Asthma is a chronic inflammatory disorder of the lower respiratory tract and can occur in multiple species. While asthma can affect humans, horses can also suffer from asthma and are often used as models for human disease [1] due to their similar symptoms and pathogenesis. The gold standard for diagnosis of equine and human asthma is to collect bronchoalveolar lavage fluid (BALF) and to examine the sample under a microscope or on digitised whole slide images

(WSIs). Asthma and other pulmonary disorders are diagnosed based on the relative proportion of different cell types including eosinophils, mast cells, neutrophils, macrophages and lymphocytes. This typically requires manual counting of 300-500 cells and is therefore time-consuming and strenuous for the pathologist [2]. Therefore, automatic solutions that support this task are of high interest. Although asthma is a common disease in horses and humans, to the author's knowledge there is no trained model or method published analysing asthma on WSI automatically. For the development of machine learning algorithms, huge annotated datasets are generally required. A particular challenge for the annotation process of asthma is the large number of cells per WSI, which can easily reach hundreds of thousands. This makes the annotation process very labour-intensive and time-consuming. In order to increase the efficiency of the annotation process, expert-algorithm collaboration can be used where experts enhance pre-computed annotations of a trained model. Marzahl et al.[2] showed this for mitotic figures or pulmonary haemorrhage. An alternative option is to annotate multiple WSIs only partially to capture the domain variability between WSIs, and train a network to complete the annotation. On the one hand, training deep learning-based methods on partially annotated WSIs faces some additional challenges regarding tracking annotated WSI areas and leads to higher demands on the coordination and synchronisation between the participating institutes. On the other hand, training on partially annotated data simplifies training pipelines in terms of data augmentation and live patch sampling in contrast to extracted sub-image-based approaches. Nevertheless, sub-image-based approaches, where patches from the WSI have to be extracted before the training, are the only supported method for the most prominent object detection frameworks [3] and are used in multiple WSI-based detection applications [4, 5].

As the main contribution to the field of deep learning-based cytological WSI analysis, we propose a training pipeline to train object detection models with live sampling on partially annotated WSIs. Additionally, we create a baseline with a state-of-the-art deep learning-based object detection model for detecting five types of cells on WSIs. All code to train, evaluate, test our models and to reproduce our results for public is accessible at GitHub [1]. Furthermore, the WSIs can be accessed at reasonable request from the corresponding author.

2   Material and methods

The dataset consists of six cytological samples (Tab. 1) of equine BALF which were cytocentrifugated and stained using May-Grunwald Giemsa stain. Afterwards, the glass slides were digitized using a linear scanner (Aperio ScanScope CS2, Leica Biosystems, Germany) at a magnification of 400× with a resolution of 0.25 $\frac{\mu m}{px}$. Finally, two slides were completely annotated and the remaining four partially annotated by a veterinary pathologist. Twenty patches from the same six WSI have been used in a recent study [2] to investigate the annotation accuracy from ten trained pathologist. We exclude these twenty patches

---

[1] https://github.com/ChristianMarzahl/Asthma_WSI

Table 1. Overview of the dataset including the file id, the number of cells per type and the screened sample area. The top two rows represent the completely annotated validation and test slides for the cross validation with a fixed train set.

ID	eosinophils	mast cells	neutrophils	macrophages	lymphocytes	total	screened
1	21	511	3301	3934	14846	22613	100%
2	47	762	951	16748	10342	28850	100%
3	10	69	1321	3081	15666	20147	8%
4	20	37	2467	729	2144	5397	28%
5	8	116	4491	1639	3077	9331	43%
6	2	40	26	370	323	761	1%
	108	1535	12557	26501	46398	87099	46%

from training to compare the accuracy of human experts with our algorithmic approach.

2.1 Label generation and training pipeline

The dataset containing only six WSIs appears to be comparably small. However, the cells in the WSIs are annotated by experts and subdivided into five classes using SlideRunner [6], rendering it one of the largest manually annotated cytology datasets to date. The dataset displays an extreme class imbalance, with the rarest class of eosinophils representing only 0.12% of all annotations. A particular challenge for training neuronal networks emerges from the sparse annotation of four WSIs, as shown in the column "screened" in table 1. To

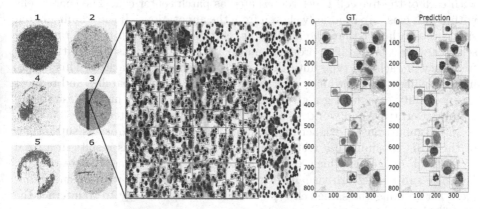

Fig. 1. Left: visualisation of the annotated regions/cells of the included slides. Center: visualisation of the 16 traditional fully annotated sub-images for sampling in green and 624 cell-based sampling positions for our live sampling approach within the red area. To prevent sampling from unannotated WSI areas, the red area is restricted to half of the patch size to the annotation border. Right: The ground truth (GT) and the deep learning based predictions; neutrophils (red), eosinophils (green), lymphocytes (blue), macrophages (yellow), mast cells (purple).

meet this challenge of partially annotated WSIs, we apply an online training approach using the open-source online annotation platform EXACT [7]. EX-ACT supports a persistent screening mode that allows experts to screen WSIs in a self-determined resolution. By reusing the information this screening mode provides, we are able to track exactly which areas of the slide have already been annotated by the expert and can download them into the training process via the provided REST-API.

We propose the following online training pipeline for equine asthma. As a first step, screened areas of the slides and associated annotations are downloaded from the EXACT server via the REST-API. The training pipeline is then initialised with the downloaded information, the network architecture and the loss function. During training, new patches are sampled live from the WSI according to the patch selection and sampling strategy described in the following sections and are restricted by information about the screened area provided by EXACT. The trained models can be applied to new data and the results can be synchronised with the server for expert review.

2.2 Live patch selection and sampling strategy

To counteract the described class imbalance and partial annotations, we propose the following sampling strategy which uses annotated cells as seeds for training patches: Each training patch has a cell that was manually annotated by an expert in its center. Consequently, only cells that have at least a distance of half of the patch size to the border of the annotated region can be used as patch centers (red area in Fig. 1). Each training batch contains at least five patches with each of the five cell types represented as patch center cell. The center cells within each class are randomly chosen from the annotations. If the training batch size is chosen larger than the number of cell types, a new cell type is randomly selected with a probability proportional to $1 - p_k$ where p_k is the relative class frequency of each cell type until the required batch size is reached. This results in a sampling strategy which can freely choose the sampled patches and reduces the possibility of sampling a given region repeatedly. This is highly desirable to counter overfitting and works as an advanced augmentation technique.

For comparison we extract all available fully annotated areas as sub-images of the WSIs to simulate a traditional training pipeline. This results in a total of 1862 sub-images of which 851 belong to the two fully annotated test WSIs. Example sub-images are visualised in Figure 1 on the right with green rectangles. For training the same cell type-based sampling strategy to counteract the described class imbalance is applied.

2.3 Object detection methods

Since the training strategy itself is the main contribution of this work, we use a publicly available and for cytology optimised implementation [8] of the successful RetinaNet [9] architecture. Different ResNet-variants [10] (ResNet-18, -34,

Table 2. The mean average precision for the five types of cells in respect to the number of layers used for the ResNet backbone network (BB) and batch size (BS). The modes represent our method working on partially annotated WSIs and a classical approach with extracted sub-images.

Mode	BB	BS	eosinophils	mast cell	neutrophils	macrophages	lymphocytes	∅
ours	18	16	0.93	0.85	0.88	0.89	0.81	0.87
sub-image	18	16	0.69	0.72	0.68	0.80	0.71	0.72
ours	34	16	0.91	0.86	0.90	0.89	0.78	0.87
sub-image	34	16	0.70	0.71	0.68	0.80	0.72	0.72
ours	50	6	0.92	0.80	0.90	0.89	0.81	0.86
sub-image	50	6	0.72	0.69	0.68	0.81	0.75	0.73

-50) pretrained on ImageNetare applied as backbone networks with appropriate mini-batch sizes. The networks are trained using the sub-images-based and the proposed live sampling-based approach with a patch size of 1024×1024 px. Each of the two fully annotated WSIs (Tab. 1) are used once as the validation set and once as the test set while keeping the training set static to allow for a form of cross-validation given the limited amount of cases. During training, data augmentation (rotation between zero and 90 degrees, horizontal and vertical flips, random increase or decrease of intensity in the range of -20 to +20%) is applied and the networks are trained until convergence on the validation set. The initial learning rate is set to 1e-3 and reduced to 1e-4 and 1e-5 if the validation loss doesn't decrease for three epochs. One epoch consists of 500 training patches regardless of the WSI-based sampling mode or the extracted sub-images. The object detection accuracy is measured as mean Average Precision (mAP) according to the 2007 PASCAL VOC challenge.

3   Results

Independent of the backbone model or batch size, the accuracy of our WSI-based sampling approach converge at an mAP of 0.87 (min=0.86, max=0.87, IoU=0.5, epochs=73), outperforming the model trained on sub-images (mAP=0.72, min = 0.72, max=0.73, IoU=0.5, epochs=23) as shown in Table 2. After 23 epochs the sub-images-based training is terminated due to overfitting. The backbone network of the model has no effect on the accuracy. The live sampling approaches show the lowest performance for the lymphocytes, which are the smallest and most clustered type of cells. The sub-images-based approach scores lowest on the rare classes of eosinophils and mast cells due to overfitting.

When applying the trained solution with a ResNet-18 as a backbone on the image patches and ground-truth published in [blinded for peer review], we reach a mean mAP across images of 0.76 with the proposed method and 0.63 with the sub-images-based approach compared to the experts reaching a published mean concordance of μ=0.73 mAP (min=0.56, max=0.82,σ=0.08).

4   Discussion and outlook

We demonstrated the creation of an object detection training pipeline which is able to use partially annotated WSIs efficiently and is superior to a simple sub-image-based approach. Our proposed approach allows for better sampling strategies and data augmentation for rare classes which massively reduces the chance to sample the same patch repeatedly and therefore mitigate overfitting, as apparent in the considerable difference in performance for eosinophils in the evaluation. This resulted in a object detection model with human like performance on a small set of example patches. However, this work has the limitation that only six images have been partially annotated by one expert, which needs to be addressed in further research. This work can be used as a baseline for further enhancements, like increasing the detection performance of small cells, optimising the non-maximum suppression algorithm for high quantities of cells but also to create new annotations in an expert-algorithm based manner on the remaining WSIs.

Acknowledgement. CAB gratefully acknowledges financial support received from the Dres. Jutta & Georg Bruns-Stiftung für innovative Veterinärmedizin.

References

1. Bullone M, Lavoie JP. Asthma "of horses and men"—how can equine heaves help us better understand human asthma immunopathology and its functional consequences? Mol Immunol. 2015;66(1):97–105.
2. Marzahl C, Bertram CA, Aubreville M, et al. Are fast labeling methods reliable? A case study of computer-aided expert annotations on microscopy slides. Proc MICCAI. 2020; p. 24–32.
3. Huang J, Rathod V, Sun C, et al. Speed/accuracy trade-offs for modern convolutional object detectors. Proc CVPR. 2017; p. 7310–7311.
4. Kawazoe Y, Shimamoto K, Yamaguchi R, et al. Faster r-cnn-based glomerular detection in multistained human whole slide images. Imaging. 2018;4(7):91.
5. Yang F, Yu H, Silamut K, et al. Parasite detection in thick blood smears based on customized Faster-RCNN on smartphones; 2019. p. 1–4.
6. Aubreville M, Bertram C, Klopfleisch R, et al. SlideRunner. In: Bildverarbeitung für die Medizin 2018. Springer; 2018. p. 309–314.
7. Marzahl C, Aubreville M, Bertram CA, et al. EXACT: a collaboration toolset for algorithm-aided annotation of almost everything. arXiv preprint arXiv:200414595. 2020;.
8. Marzahl C, Aubreville M, Bertram CA, et al. Deep learning-based quantification of pulmonary hemosiderophages in cytology slides. Sci Rep. 2020;10(1):1–10.
9. Lin TY, Goyal P, Girshick R, et al. Focal loss for dense object detection. Proc IEEE ICCV. 2017; p. 2980–2988.
10. He K, Zhang X, Ren S, et al. Deep residual learning for image recognition; 2016. p. 770–778.

Combining Reconstruction and Edge Detection in Computed Tomography

Jürgen Frikel[1], Simon Göppel[2], Markus Haltmeier[2]

[1]Department of Computer Science and Mathematics, OTH Regensburg
[2]Department of Mathematics, University of Innsbruck
juergen.frikel@oth-regensburg.de

Abstract. We present two methods that combine image reconstruction and edge detection in computed tomography (CT) scans. Our first method is as an extension of the prominent filtered backprojection algorithm. In our second method we employ ℓ^1-regularization for stable calculation of the gradient. As opposed to the first method, we show that this approach is able to compensate for undersampled CT data.

1 Introduction

Detection of edges in computed tomography (CT) scans is a challenging task because the underlying image reconstruction problem is ill-posed and, hence, even small errors in the x-ray measurements may lead to huge reconstruction errors that have to be compensated by the edge detection algorithms [1]. This task becomes even more challenging, when the CT scans are generated from a small number of x-ray measurements, as it is the case, e.g., in digital breast tomosynthesis or dental CT, where the x-ray measurements can be taken only from a small number of views in a limited angular range. In such situations, classical reconstruction algorithms may generate characteristic reconstruction artifacts (in addition to noise amplification) and, thus, substantially degrade the image quality [2]. Performing edge detection after image reconstruction, can therefore lead to unreliable edge maps. In this article, we present two methods that allow for a stable reconstruction of edges directly from CT data and, thus, stabilizes edge detection in CT images. In particular, we focus on a stable reconstruction of the gradient of a CT scan, because it is the main ingredient in most prominent edge detection algorithms, such as the Canny algorithm [3].

In what follows, we model CT scans as functions $f : \mathbb{R}^2 \to \mathbb{R}$ and the corresponding CT data by the Radon transform of f, which is defined as [1]

$$\mathcal{R}f(\phi, s) := \int_{\mathbb{R}} f(s\theta(\phi) + t\theta^{\perp}(\phi)) \mathrm{d}t \tag{1}$$

where $\theta(\phi) = (\cos(\phi), \sin(\phi))^{\top}$ and $\theta^{\perp}(\phi) = (-\sin(\phi), \cos(\phi))^{\top}$. Here, the value $\mathcal{R}f(\phi, s)$ represents one x-ray measurement along the x-ray path that is given

Springer Fachmedien Wiesbaden GmbH, ein Teil von Springer Nature 2021
C. Palm et al. (Hrsg.), *Bildverarbeitung für die Medizin 2021*,
Informatik aktuell, https://doi.org/10.1007/978-3-658-33198-6_37

by the line $L(\phi, s) = \{s\theta(\phi)) + t\theta^{\perp}(\phi) : t \in \mathbb{R}\} = \{x \in \mathbb{R}^2 : \langle x, \theta(\phi)\rangle = s\}$, where $\phi \in [0, \pi)$ and $s \in \mathbb{R}$.

We will present two methods for stable reconstruction of the gradient of the smooth function $f_\epsilon := f * g_\epsilon$, where

$$g_\epsilon(x) := \frac{1}{2\pi\epsilon^2} \exp\left(-\frac{\|x\|^2}{2\epsilon^2}\right), \quad \epsilon > 0 \tag{2}$$

First, we derive a method that is of the same type as the famous filtered back-projection algorithm (FBP). This method follows the spirit of [4] and yields good results whenever the CT data is well sampled (for exact conditions for a proper sampling of the Radon transform see, e.g., [5]). In our second approach, we employ ideas from compressed sensing and propose to use sparse regularization for the reconstruction of the image gradient. We show that this method leads to a more robust edge detection, especially when the data is not sampled properly.

2   Materials and methods

2.1   Method 1: An FBP-type approach for calculating the gradient

In order to calculate the smoothed partial derivatives derivatives

$$\frac{\partial f_\epsilon}{\partial x_j} = \frac{\partial}{\partial x_j}(f * g_\epsilon) = f * \frac{\partial g_\epsilon}{\partial x_j} \tag{3}$$

directly form CT data, we use the well-known relations between the Radon transform, convolutions and derivatives [1] and obtain the following result.

Lemma 1. *Let the Gaussian g_ϵ be defined by (2). Then, we have for $j \in \{1, 2\}$:*

$$\mathcal{R}\left[f * \frac{\partial g_\epsilon}{\partial x_j}\right](\phi, s) = [\mathcal{R}f *_s G_{\epsilon,j}](\phi, s) \tag{4}$$

where $*_s$ denotes the convolution with respect to the second variable s, and

$$G_{\epsilon,j}(\phi, s) := -\frac{\theta_j(\phi)}{\epsilon^3 \sqrt{2\pi}} \cdot s \cdot \exp\left(-\frac{s^2}{2\epsilon^2}\right) \tag{5}$$

with $(\phi, s) \in [0, \pi) \times \mathbb{R}$ and $\theta_1(\phi) := \cos(\phi)$, $\theta_2(\phi) := \sin(\phi)$

Lemma 1 shows that the partial derivatives (3) can be obtained by applying the inverse Radon transform $\mathcal{R}^{-1}$ to the preprocessed data (4), that is

$$\frac{\partial f_\epsilon}{\partial x_j} = \mathcal{R}^{-1}[\mathcal{R}f *_s G_{\epsilon,j}] \tag{6}$$

Since the FBP algorithm is a regularized implementation of $\mathcal{R}^{-1}$ [1], a standard toolbox implementation could be used in practice to obtain ∇f_ϵ.

Moreover, it is well-known that the inverse Radon transform is given by $\mathcal{R}^{-1} = \mathcal{B} \circ P$, where P is a filtering (convolution) operator and $\mathcal{B}$ is the so-called backprojection operator [1]. Therefore, the filter used in the FBP algorithm, given by the operator P, can be combined with the filtering in (6). In this way, we obtain a reconstruction formula of FBP-type for the derivatives (6), that is stated in the following theorem.

Theorem 1. *Let $W_{\epsilon,j}$ be the function of two variables (ϕ, s) which is defined in the Fourier domain by*

$$\widehat{W}_{\epsilon,j}(\phi, \omega) := \frac{1}{4\pi} \cdot \theta_j(\phi) \cdot i \cdot \omega \cdot |\omega| \cdot \exp\left(\frac{-\epsilon^2 \omega^2}{2}\right) \tag{7}$$

where $\widehat{W}_{\epsilon,j}$ denotes the 1D-Fourier transform of $W_{\epsilon,j}$ with respect to the s-variable and $i \in \mathbb{C}$ is the imaginary unit. Then

$$\frac{\partial f_\epsilon}{\partial x_j} = \mathcal{B}(\mathcal{R}f *_s W_{\epsilon,j}) \tag{8}$$

where $\mathcal{B}$ is the backprojection operator for the Radon transform [1].

The proof of Theorem 1 follows from (4) together with the convolution theorem for the Fourier transform and Theorem II.2.1 in [1]. It shows that the derivatives (3) can be calculated using a FBP-algorithm with angle-dependent filters that are given by (7).

Remark 1. The accuracy of the presented method (given by (6) and (8)) will strongly depend on the sampling of the Radon transform [1]. If the CT data does not satisfy the sampling requirements, e.g., when the angles are sampled rather sparsely, the algorithm will produce artifacts which can substantially degrade the performance of edge detection.

2.2   Method 2: gradient calculation using sparse regularization

In order to account for the negative effects of (possible) undersampling of CT data, we propose to replace $\mathcal{R}^{-1}$ in (6) by a regularization method for $\mathcal{R}^{-1}$ that is able to deal with undersampled data. From the theory of compressed sensing it is well known that sparsity can help to overcome the classical Shannon sampling paradigm [6]. As we are interested in the recovery of gradients of images which have large values only around edges, we aim at enforcing sparsity of image gradients. Thus, we calculate the derivatives (3) approximately via [6]

$$\mathbf{f}_{\lambda,\epsilon}^{(j)} = \underset{\mathbf{f}}{\operatorname{argmin}} \|\mathbf{R}\mathbf{f} - \mathbf{y} * G_{\epsilon,j}\|_2^2 + \lambda \|\mathbf{f}\|_1 \tag{9}$$

where $\lambda > 0$ is regularization parameter. Note that in (9) the bold face symbols denote the discretized versions of the corresponding continuous objects.

3   Results

We implemented the methods 1 and 2 in Matlab and tested them on the x-ray CT data of a lotus root [7]. In our experiments we converted the fan-beam data to a parallel-beam data using Matlab function `fan2para` and downsampled this data in order to simulate angular undersampling. Thereby, we used 738 equispaced samples in the s-variable and 36 evenly distributed angles in $[0, \pi)$. For our implementations, we used the Matlab functions `radon` and `iradon` as numerical realizations of the Radon transform, the inverse Radon transform and the backprojection operator. For the minimization of the ℓ^1-functional (9), we implemented the iterative soft thresholding algorithm [8].

The CT data and the corresponding FBP reconstruction are shown in Fig. 1(a) and 1(d). It can be clearly observed that the FBP reconstruction contains many undersampling artifacts (streaks) that could complicate the detection of edges in that image. Hence, we calculated the gradient directly from CT data using the methods 1 and 2, where we chose the parameters based on visual inspection of edge detection results. These parameters are presented in the captions of Fig. 1.

In Fig. 1(b) and 1(e) one can see that the Gaussian smoothing cannot compensate for the undersampling artifacts and, thus, many edges in the edge map are not coming from actual image features. However, the ℓ^1-regularization suc-

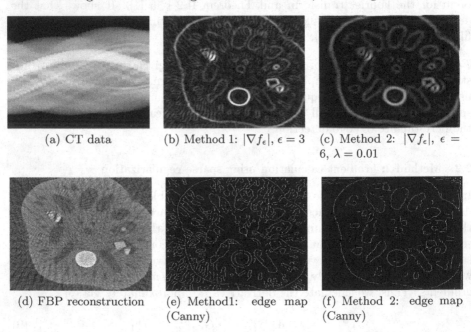

(a) CT data   (b) Method 1: $|\nabla f_\epsilon|$, $\epsilon = 3$ (c) Method 2: $|\nabla f_\epsilon|$, $\epsilon = 6$, $\lambda = 0.01$

(d) FBP reconstruction   (e) Method1:   edge map   (f) Method 2:   edge map
                         (Canny)   (Canny)

Fig. 1. Rebinned CT data of a lotus root (a) and the corresponding FBP reconstruction (d) from an angular range given by $[0, \pi)$ and 36 evenly distributed angles [7]. The images of the gradient magnitude $|\nabla f_\epsilon|$ are shown in (b) and (c), and the corresponding edge detection results using the Canny algorithm are presented in (e) and (f).

cessfully reduces the number of artifacts and detects the edges more reliably, as can be seen in Fig. 1(c) and 1(f).

In other experiments that are not presented here, we also observed that the method 2 outperforms the method 1 whenever the CT data was not sampled properly. However, in the case that the CT data was sampled densely, we found that both methods produce similar edge detection results.

4 Discussion

We presented two methods for calculating the gradient of a CT scan directly from CT data. As our first method, we introduced a variant of the filtered backprojection algorithm and explained two different ways for its implementation. As our second approach, we introduced a sparsity based gradient recovery from CT data and showed in numerical experiments that this method is able to account for data undersampling and to provide more reliable edge detection results. Moreover, the second approach provides more flexibility and can be more easily applied to different scanning geometries.

Acknowledgement. The contribution by S. G. is part of a project that has received funding from the European Union's Horizon 2020 research and innovation programme under the Marie Skłodowska-Curie grant agreement No 847476. The views and opinions expressed herein do not necessarily reflect those of the European Commission.

References

1. Natterer F. The mathematics of computerized tomography. Stuttgart: B. G. Teubner; 1986.
2. Frikel J, Quinto ET. Characterization and reduction of artifacts in limited angle tomography. Inverse Probl. 2013;29(12):125007.
3. Canny J. A computational approach to edge detection. IEEE Trans Pattern Anal Mach Intell. 1986;PAMI-8(6):679–698.
4. Louis AK. Combining image reconstruction and image analysis with an application to two-dimensional tomography. SIAM J Imaging Sci. 2008;1:188–208.
5. Natterer F, Wübbeling F. Mathematical methods in image reconstruction. SIAM Monographs on Mathematical Modeling and Computation. Philadelphia, PA: Society for Industrial and Applied Mathematics (SIAM); 2001.
6. Candès EJ, Romberg JK, Tao T. Stable signal recovery from incomplete and inaccurate measurements. Comm Pure Appl Math. 2006;59(8):1207–1223.
7. Bubba TA, Hauptmann A, Huotari S, et al. Tomographic X-ray data of a lotus root filled with attenuating objects. 2016; p. 1–11. arXiv:1609.07299 [physics.data-an].
8. Daubechies I, Defrise M, De Mol C. An iterative thresholding algorithm for linear inverse problems with a sparsity constraint. Comm Pure Appl Math. 2004;57(11):1413–1457.

2D Respiration Navigation Framework for 3D Continuous Cardiac Magnetic Resonance Imaging

Elisabeth Hoppe[1], Jens Wetzl[2], Philipp Roser[1], Lina Felsner[1],
Alexander Preuhs[1], Andreas Maier[1]

[1]Pattern Recognition Lab, Friedrich-Alexander-Universität Erlangen-Nürnberg,
Germany
[2]Magnetic Resonance, Siemens Healthineers, Erlangen, Germany
elisabeth.hoppe@fau.de

Abstract. Continuous protocols for cardiac magnetic resonance imaging enable sampling of the cardiac anatomy simultaneously resolved into cardiac phases. To avoid respiration artifacts, associated motion during the scan has to be compensated for during reconstruction. In this paper, we propose a sampling adaption to acquire 2D respiration information during a continuous scan. Further, we develop a pipeline to extract the different respiration states from the acquired signals, which are used to reconstruct data from one respiration phase. Our results show the benefit of the proposed workflow on the image quality compared to no respiration compensation, as well as a previous 1D respiration navigation approach.

1 Introduction

Cardiac magnetic resonance imaging (MRI) is an established tool for the diagnosis of various cardiomyopathies [1, 2]. For a comprehensive diagnosis, two factors are essential: First, the anatomy of the heart has to be imaged for the evaluation of different cardiac structures. Second, dynamic imaging, i.e., the resolution into different cardiac phases, is needed for the evaluation of the cardiac function. Recent 3D protocols were proposed for the sampling of dynamic cardiac 3D volumes [3, 4, 5]. Most protocols sample data continuously during free-breathing and multiple cardiac cycles, often combined with incoherent subsampling [4, 5]. However, the permanent respiration motion during scanning can have a substantial influence on the image quality, yielding severe artifacts. This can be improved by reconstructing data from only one respiration state. Recent approaches for respiration extraction use either additional navigation readouts [6] (which prolong the scan times), or 1D self-navigation, where central k-space lines (mainly orientated in the superior-inferior (SI) direction) are processed with, e.g., principal component analysis (PCA) [5, 7]. However, only 1D central k-space lines might be insufficient for the extraction of respiration, as it mainly comprises anterior-posterior (AP) as well as SI motion. Consequently,

Springer Fachmedien Wiesbaden GmbH, ein Teil von Springer Nature 2021
C. Palm et al. (Hrsg.), *Bildverarbeitung für die Medizin 2021*,
Informatik aktuell, https://doi.org/10.1007/978-3-658-33198-6_38

this motion is not properly encoded in the 1D central k-space lines. In this work, we propose an adapted sampling and navigation framework for extracting 2D respiration motion from continuous cardiac sequences to reduce the influence of respiration-induced artifacts. We show the superior performance of our 2D navigation on the image quality compared to no respiration navigation and previous 1D navigation.

2 Method

Our proposed framework uses 2D navigation signals from the adapted sampling scheme (Sec. 2.1, Fig. 1) for extracting the different respiration states (Sec. 2.2, Fig. 2). Readouts from one particular respiration state are jointly reconstructed, reducing respiration-induced artifacts.

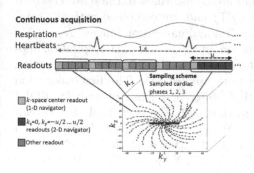

Fig. 1. Adaption of the sampling pattern (figure adopted from [8]). Samples on the phase-encoding plane are collected continuously on pseudo-spiral spokes, every $t = 1\,s$ the navigation signals are sampled on the $k_z = 0$, $k_y = -u/2, ..., 0, ..., u/2$ line.

2.1 Sampling pattern

We extended a previously proposed prototypical method for 3D free-breathing, continuous, cardiac MRI [5]. Data is collected during multiple cardiac and respiration phases. The Cartesian phase encoding (PE) plane is incoherently undersampled with samples on pseudo-spiral spokes, each starting in the k-space

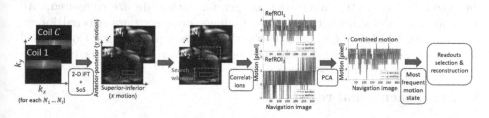

Fig. 2. Respiration motion extraction pipeline. Raw navigation signals from single coils are reconstructed with the 2D inverse Fourier transform (iFT) and sum-of-squares (SoS) coil combination. For motion extraction, correlations between different ROIs on navigation images are computed. PCA extracts the main motion values. The cluster with the highest amount of readouts corresponding to one particular motion state is used for image reconstruction.

center (Fig. 1). We adapted this scheme to sample 2D respiration motion information: Every $t = 1\,s$, data is sampled on the $k_z = 0$, $k_y = -u/2, ..., 0, ..., u/2$ line, where u is number of samples on one pseudo-spiral spoke. This leads to a fully sampled k-space center with size $u \times v$, where v is the length of the k_x-line, the remaining positions are zero-filled. The 2D navigation signals are planes within the imaged 3D volume, mainly orientated in the AP and SI direction. These readouts are simultaneously used for navigation and reconstruction of the 3D dynamic volumes, avoiding additional scan time for navigation. All acquired readouts after a navigation signal i and prior to the next navigation signal $i + 1$ are considered to have the same motion state as the navigation signal i.

2.2 Navigation motion extraction pipeline

All 2D navigation signals from single coils are transformed to the spatial domain with the 2D inverse Fourier transform (iFT) and are combined with the sum-of-squares (SoS) resulting in final low-resolutional navigation images, $N_1, ..., N_I$, where I is the total number of navigation images. The 2D respiration motion in AP and SI direction can be observed there (Fig. 3). For the selection of one respiration state, following steps are applied: (1) The first navigation image is selected as reference N_{ref} with R different regions of interest (ROIs) $N_{\text{refROI}_1}, ..., N_{\text{refROI}_R}$ with observable motion. (2) For each ROI the correlation coefficients CC between $N_{\text{refROI}_1}, ..., N_{\text{refROI}_R}$ and $N_{\text{ROI}_1}, ..., N_{\text{ROI}_R}$ in each $N_2, ..., N_I$ are calculated, while moving the ROI within a selected search window on $N_2, ..., N_I$. The spatial positions of $N_{\text{ROI}_1}, ..., N_{\text{ROI}_R}$ in $N_2, ..., N_I$ with the highest CC result in the x and y shifts for the two motion directions compared to the $N_{\text{refROI}_1}, ..., N_{\text{refROI}_R}$, yielding the current motion vector $\boldsymbol{m_{ir}} = (\hat{x}_{ir}, \hat{y}_{ir})^\top$ for each $N_2, ..., N_I$ and each $N_{\text{ROI}_1}, ..., N_{\text{ROI}_R}$. (3) We assume that each ROI will mainly contain one direction of motion (e.g., a ROI on the chest wall will contain mainly AP motion). PCA is applied on all motion vectors from step (2) to select the dominant 1D shifts from each ROI, resulting in a combined $\boldsymbol{m_{comb}} = (\hat{x}_{ir_{\max}}, \hat{y}_{ir_{\max}})^\top$ for each $N_2, ..., N_I$, where $r_{\max}$ is the selected ROI for one particular motion direction (x or y). (4) Different motion states and the amount of respective navigation images for each state are computed. All readouts from the state with the most frequent occurence are selected for reconstruction, which is based on a previously proposed prototypical Compressed Sensing framework combined with spatiotemporal Wavelet regularization [8].

3 Experiments and results

3.1 Experimental setup

We acquired a 3D free-breathing, continuous in-vivo scan from one volunteer (female, 55 years) after written consent was obtained. Data was acquired with the proposed prototypical sequence in short-axis orientation and balanced steady-state free precession readouts on a $1.5\,T$ scanner (MAGNETOM Aera, Siemens

Healthcare, Erlangen, Germany) with these parameters: Field-of-view: $310 \times 310 \times 86\,mm$, spatial resolution: $1.8^3\,mm$, flip angle: $46\,°$, echo time: $1.7\,ms$, repetition time: $3.3\,ms$, scan time: $5.3\,min$. Cardiac signal from an external ECG device was used to bin the data into cardiac phases [5]. We selected $R = 2$ navigation ROIs, which correspond mainly to AP (green ROI in Fig. 3) and SI motion (red ROI in Fig. 3). A search window of ± 25 pixels in x, y directions on $N_2, ..., N_I$ was used. The m_{comb} was selected with $\hat{x} = 2$ (from green ROI with a principal component coeffiecent of 0.99) and $\hat{y} = 1$ (from red ROI with a principal component coeffiecent of 0.99) with 39.9 % of all data (108/339 navigation images). We compared three different reconstructions: (1) Without respiration compensation (No Nav), (2) with 1D navigation (1D Nav), with respiration motion extracted from central 1D k-space lines [5] (Fig. 3) and (3) with our proposed 2D navigation (2D Nav). For the quantitative evaluation, three commonly used image quality metrics in motion compensation [9] were applied (Tab. 1): (1) Histogram entropy H, (2) total variation TV and (3) wavelet-based estimation of the standard deviation of Gaussian noise distribution σ_{Noise} [10].

3.2   Results

Figure 4 shows one slice resolved into different cardiac phases from 3D volumes reconstructed with different approaches. Our 2D based navigation shows a visually sharper image quality compared to the other reconstructions, especially in the cardiac region (marked with orange box for cardiac phase 2). For all quantitative metrics shown in Tab. 1, the 2D based navigation approach yields superior results. The Student's t-test results confirm that the differences in the image quality between the approaches are statistically significant (p-value < 0.05).

4   Discussion and conclusion

No respiration compensation yields artifact-corrupted images, which are of limited diagnostic utility: The myocardial structure (marked with orange box for cardiac phase 2) is heavily disturbed by the permanent chest wall motion (especially in cardiac phases 2, 14), that manifests as folding artifacts. The reconstruction based on the 1D navigation also results in artifact-corrupted images.

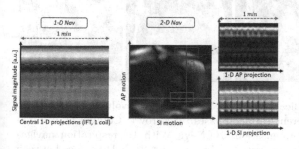

Fig. 3. Examples of 1D lines for extracting 1D motion from central k-space lines (left, readouts corresponding to different states are marked with the black and white line, respectively), and navigation images (right) for extracting 2D motion from our proposed 2D navigation, which result in 1D projections over time, mainly orientated in AP and SI directions.

162   Hoppe et al.

Table 1. Quantitative image quality metrics for different reconstructions, each given as $\mu \pm \sigma$ for the 3D dataset (48 slices, 20 cardiac phases). No Nav: Without respiration compensation, 1D Nav: With 1D navigation [5], 2D Nav: With the proposed 2D navigation, H: Histogram entropy (lower is better), TV: Total variation (lower is better), σ_{Noise}: Standard deviation of Gaussian noise distribution (lower is better).

Method	Metric ($\mu \pm \sigma$), [95 % confidence intervals]		
	Histogram entropy	Total variation	σ_{Noise}
No Nav	3.80 ± 0.11 [3.79, 3.80]	90868 ± 790 [90817, 90918]	6.17 ± 1.00 [6.11, 6.24]
1D Nav	3.77 ± 0.12 [3.77, 3.78]	90575 ± 856 [90521, 90629]	5.41 ± 0.95 [5.35, 5.47]
2D Nav	$\mathbf{3.68 \pm 0.11}$ [3.67, 3.68]	$\mathbf{86197 \pm 1831}$ [86081, 86313]	$\mathbf{4.36 \pm 0.69}$ [4.31, 4.39]

Even if 1D motion is visible in the central 1D k-space lines (Fig. 3), it can only represent one motion direction, which is insufficient for respiration. For our subject, the image quality could only be slightly improved with the 1D navigation. Our proposed 2D navigation yields the visually sharpest image quality. Even if

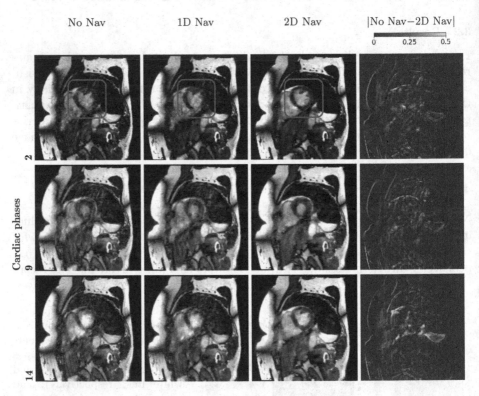

Fig. 4. Qualitative results. One slice from the reconstructed 3D volume (48 slices, 20 cardiac phases) is shown for different cardiac phases (each row). Column by column: No Nav: Without respiration compensation, 1D Nav: With 1D respiration navigation, 2D Nav: With 2D respiration navigation, |No Nav−2D Nav|: Difference between reconstructions without navigation and 2D respiration navigation.

the subsampling is increased with the 2D navigation by removing parts of data for the reconstruction (up to a factor 11.5, compared to max. 4.1 without respiration compensation), the image quality can be greatly improved with data from only one stable respiration state. This is confirmed by our quantitative analysis, where the 2D navigation has significantly superior results in all metrics.

To summarize, we proposed a sampling pattern adaption and a 2D respiration navigation pipeline that improves image quality compared to previously proposed 1D navigation. Using our adapted continuous sampling, the same data can be used for 2D navigation and 3D reconstruction, without introducing the need for sampling navigation data only. Our approach can be potentially combined with a data-driven cardiac navigation, e.g., [11] without further adaptions on the sampling, yielding an ECG-free workflow. Future work will deal with the automatic detection of ROIs for the motion computation, as well as the application to other protocols, such as multi-contrast sampling [5].

References

1. Al-Mallah MH, Shareef MN. The role of cardiac magnetic resonance imaging in the assessment of non-ischemic cardiomyopathy. Heart Fail Rev. 2011;16(4):369–380.
2. Florian A, Jurcut R, Ginghina C, et al. Cardiac magnetic resonance imaging in ischemic heart disease: a clinical review. J Med Life. 2011;4(4):330.
3. Wetzl J, Schmidt M, Pontana F, et al. Single-breath-hold 3-D cine imaging of the left ventricle using cartesian sampling. MAGMA. 2018;31(1):19–31.
4. Feng L, Coppo S, Piccinni D, et al. 5D whole-heart sparse mri. Magn Reson Med. 2018;79(2):826–838.
5. Hoppe E, Wetzl J, Forman C, et al. Free-breathing, self-navigated and dynamic 3-D multi-contrast cardiac cine imaging using cartesian sampling and compressed sensing. In: Proc Int Soc Magn Reson Med Sci Meet Exhib; 2019. p. 1608.
6. Shaw JL, Yang Q, Zhou Z, et al. Free-breathing, non-ecg, continuous myocardial t1 mapping with cardiovascular magnetic resonance multitasking. Magn Reson Med. 2019;81(4):2450–2463.
7. Di Sopra L, Piccini D, Coppo S, et al. An automated approach to fully self-gated free-running cardiac and respiratory motion-resolved 5D whole-heart mri. Magn Reson Med. 2019;82(6):2118–2132.
8. Wetzl J, Lugauer F, Schmidt M, et al. Free-breathing, self-navigated isotropic 3-D CINE imaging of the whole heart using cartesian sampling. In: Proc Int Soc Magn Reson Med Sci Meet Exhib; 2016. p. 411.
9. Preuhs A, Manhart M, Roser P, et al. Appearance learning for image-based motion estimation in tomography. IEEE Trans Med Imaging. 2020;.
10. Donoho DL, Johnstone JM. Ideal spatial adaptation by wavelet shrinkage. biometrika. 1994;81(3):425–455.
11. Hoppe E, Wetzl J, Yoon S, et al. DeepECG: towards 3-D continuous cardiac mri without ecg-gating - deep learning-based r-wave classification for automated cardiac phase binning. In: Proc Int Soc Magn Reson Med Sci Meet Exhib; 2020. p. 2129.

Residual Neural Network for Filter Kernel Design in Filtered Back-projection for CT Image Reconstruction

Jintian Xu[1], Chengjin Sun[1], Yixing Huang[2], Xiaolin Huang[1]

[1]Institute of Image Processing and Pattern Recognition, Shanghai Jiao Tong University, Shanghai, China
[2]Pattern Recognition Lab, Friedrich-Alexander-University Erlangen-Nuremberg
xiaolinhuang@sjtu.edu.cn

Abstract. Filtered back-projection (FBP) has been widely applied for computed tomography (CT) image reconstruction as a fundamental algorithm. Most of the filter kernels used in FBP are designed by analytic methods. Recently, the precision learning-based ramp filter (PL-Ramp) has been proposed to formulate FBP to directly learn the reconstruction filter. However, it is difficult to introduce regularization terms in this method, which essentially provides a massive solution space. Therefore, in this paper, we propose a neural network based on residual learning for filter kernel design in FBP, named resFBP. With such a neural network, it is possible for us to limit the solution space by introducing various regularization terms or methods to achieve better reconstruction quality on the test set. The experiment results demonstrate that both quality and reconstruction error of the proposed method has great superiority over FBP and also outperforms PL-Ramp when projection data are polluted by Poisson noise or Gaussian noise.

1 Introduction

Computed tomography (CT) is a technology to obtain internal information of an unknown object and has been extensively used in many areas, such as medical imaging and electron microscopy in materials science. Filtered back-projection (FBP), one of the most popular methods for CT image reconstruction, requires a large number of noise-free projections to yield accurate reconstructions. It is applied widely for its low computational cost and ease of implementation. However, in practice, noisy projections and projection discretization can make the image reconstructed by FBP suffer from severe artifacts. To suppress artifacts, the filter kernel designs for specific cases have been proposed to improve the quality of reconstruction images.

The methods for filter kernel design can be divided into two categories: (i) analytic design, (ii) data-driven learning. For analytic design, Ram-Lak filter [1] is mathematically optimized from the ramp filter for the discrete image and projection. Shepp-Logan filter [2], imposing a different noise assumption, is one common filter for FBP. To derive new filters, Wei et al. [3] propose a filter design methodology in the real space, and apply this methodology to deduce new filters as well as classic filters. New filters have been demonstrated to produce equivalent image quality in comparison to classic filters.

For data-driven methods, a novel scheme is proposed by Shi et al. [4] to design the reconstruction filters to replace the ramp filter. The reconstruction filters are optimized to drive the reconstruction matrix approach δ-matrix as close as possible with constraints. Wang et al. [5] propose an end-to-end network FBP-Net, combining the FBP algorithm with a denoiser neural network, to directly reconstruct positron emission tomography (PET) images from sinograms. The frequency filter is adaptively learned in the FBP part. Syben et al. [6] propose the precision learning-based ramp filter (denoted as PL-Ramp) to optimize discrete filter kernels by back-propagation, which solves the problem of manually designing filters. Experiments have proved that the initialized ramp filter can automatically approximate the hand-crafted Ram-Lak filter by training, and it greatly reduces the burden of manual design and allows the filter to be trained to adapt to more noise conditions.

Although PL-Ramp has been proved to have the ability to learn a discrete optimal reconstruction filter from the ramp filter, its performance on training noisy data is not as good as expected according to our experiments. Moreover, PL-Ramp does not have any regularization term to avoid over-fitting. To solve the problems mentioned above, in this paper, we propose a residual neural network to learn the filter in FBP, named resFBP. In detail, resFBP includes a residual fully connected neural network and a residual convolution neural network. Experiments on Poisson noise and Gaussian noise data demonstrate that our proposed method can better suppress the artifacts and has lower reconstruction root-mean-squared error (RMSE) than PL-Ramp.

2   Materials and methods

2.1   resFBP

The architecture of the proposed resFBP is illustrated in Fig. 1. The whole procedure can be described as following: the projection data first undergo Fourier transform F, and then are filtered in the frequency domain with the learned

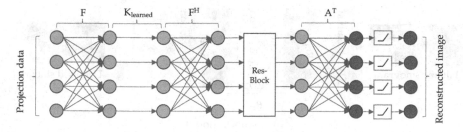

Fig. 1. The general architecture of resFBP.

filter K_{learned} before undergoing inverse Fourier transform F^H. Next, the result is refined through the resBlock, and finally is back-projected to get the reconstructed image with rectified linear unit (ReLU) activation. In Fig. 1, the light blue circle and the dark blue circle represent data in the projection domain and in the image domain, respectively.

Mathematically, the objective function of resFBP can be described as the following function

$$f(\theta_1, \theta_2) = \frac{1}{2} \left\| A^\top K_2(\theta_2) F^H K_1(\theta_1) F p - x \right\|_2^2 + R(\theta_1) \tag{1}$$

in which p denotes the projection data; x denotes the image to be reconstructed; F and F^H denote Fourier transform and inverse Fourier transform respectively; θ_1 denotes the weights and biases of all layers in the kernel-learning module; θ_2 denotes the kernel values of convolution layers and scale variables of batch normalization in the resBlock module; $K_1(\theta_1)$ and $K_2(\theta_2)$ denote effects of kernel-learning module and resBlock module on projection data; $f(\theta_1, \theta_2)$ denotes the loss function; A^T denotes the transpose of the projection operator A; $R(\theta_1)$ denotes the l_2-norm regularization term of weights in the kernel-learning module. In the training stage, θ_1 and θ_2 are simultaneously updated by the corresponding gradients of the objective function.

The biggest difference from the existing work[6] lies in two modules, the kernel-learning module and the resBlock module, which are described in detail in the following. Fig. 2 (a) illustrates the kernel-learning module, in which K_{learned} is the summation of the Ramp filter kernel K and its residual part that goes through a two-layer fully connected neural network. The first layer has only 10 neurons and the second layer has 400 neurons, which equals the number of

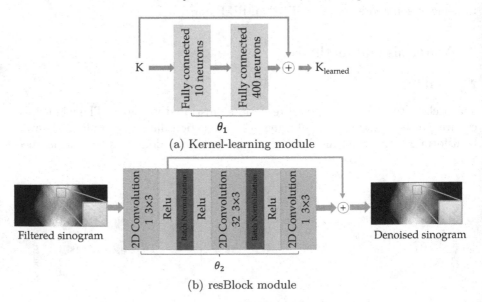

(a) Kernel-learning module

(b) resBlock module

Fig. 2. Two modules designed for filter kernel learning.

detector pixels. The width (from 10 neurons to 400 neurons) and depth (from 1 layer to 3 layers) of the fully connected network are optimized by minimizing reconstruction error on the validation set. This configuration achieves state-of-the-art performance while requiring the least training parameters. This residual module brings two advantages. On the one hand, it can be adapted to noise projection data while maintaining a similar performance as the Ramp filter in noise-free cases. On the other hand, it is possible to introduce a regularization term, such as a l_2-norm on weights, in training to avoid over-fitting.

The resBlock module is shown in Fig. 2 (b), where a typical ResNetV2 [7] structure is used. This structure has been proved to make information propagation smooth. The resBlock can further denoise the data in the projection domain, improving the quality of the reconstructed image. With batch normalization, it need not add any regularization term. The number (ranging from 1 to 3) of ResNetV2 and the number (ranging from 8 to 64) of convolution kernels of the resBlock module are optimized by grid search on the validation set.

2.2 Experimental setup

In this paper, the resFBP is implemented with PY-RONN [8], which is an open-source platform for applying deep learning to medical image reconstruction. Experiments are conducted on medical images, provided by American Association Physicists Medicine (AAPM, [9]). In the dataset, AAPM provides 5936 CT slice images from 10 patients for 4 kinds of scanning settings. The training set, validation set and test set contain 4795, 823, and 318 CT slice images respectively. In this paper, we use the CT slice images reconstructed by the full dose projection and 1.0 mm image pixel and reshape them to 256×256. The projection data are simulated from the AAPM volumes by parallel-beam scanning, which has 400 1.0 mm detector pixels collecting projection data from 180 uniformly distributed positions at a range of 180°.

The value of the pixel in the original image is a positive integer, which represents the attenuation rate in the Hounsfield unit (HU) with an offset of 1000 HU. In this paper, the value is normalized to [0,1] for training. To simulate noise in the process of reconstruction, Gaussian noise and Poisson noise are added to the projection data. The mean and variance of Gaussian noise are 0 and 0.5, while Poisson noise is simulated by assuming each detector pixel is exposed to 10^5 photons before attenuation. The RMSE between ground truths and reconstructed CT images is employed as the evaluation metric.

The parameters of the fully connected neural network in the kernel-learning module and convolution layer in the resBlock module are initialized with truncated normal distribution with small-variance and zero-mean. The loss function consists of a data fidelity term and a regularization term of weights in the kernel-learning module. The training batch size is 50 and the model is trained for 1000 epochs with the Adam optimizer using a 0.01 learning rate.

To validate the advantages of resFBP, we train PL-Ramp and resFBP using two kinds of training datasets, which are polluted by Poisson noise or Gaussian

Table 1. The reconstruction RMSE (HU) comparison of PL-Ramp and resFBP in Poisson noise and Gaussian noise under two kinds of training data.

Training dataset	Test on Poisson noise			Test on Gaussian noise		
	FBP	PL-Ramp	resFBP	FBP	PL-Ramp	resFBP
None	133.9±1153.2	–	–	90.3±0.689	–	–
Poisson noise	–	90.7±12.7	80.0±8.8	–	88.6±20.9	77.4±14.6
Gaussian noise	–	96.1±16.5	84.2±15.6	–	94.5±23.6	83.1±21.6

noise. Then, we compare the reconstruction RMSE of FBP and the trained models with projection data polluted by Poisson noise and Gaussian noise.

3 Results

Table 1 displays the reconstruction RMSE (mean±std) (HU) of FBP, RL-Ramp and resFBP under Poisson noise and Gaussian noise training dataset. It can be observed that regardless of the training dataset used, resFBP achieves lower RMSE mean and RMSE standard deviation than PL-Ramp and has great superiority over FBP under the same condition. For those two filter learning methods, the models trained with Poisson noise have better performance than those trained with Gaussian noise when tested on Gaussian noise data.

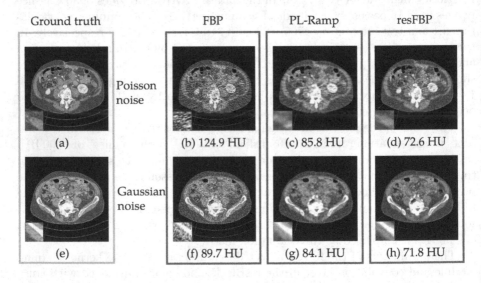

Fig. 3. Reconstruction results of two sample slices from the test patient, in the window of [-300,300] HU. The RMSE value of each reconstruction result is displayed. (a)(e) are ground truths. (b)(c)(d) are tested with Poisson noise data, and (f)(g)(h) are tested with Gaussian noise data. (a), (b), (e) and (f) use FBP with Ram-Lak filter. (c) and (g) use PL-Ramp. (d) and (h) use resFBP.

The reconstruction results of two sample slices from the test patient are visualized in the window of [-300,300] HU (Fig. 3). The images are reconstructed from Poisson noise data (the first row) and Gaussian noise data (the second row). Ground truths from original CT slice images are shown in Fig. 3 (a) and (e) for reference. Fig. 3 (b) and (f) show the results of FBP, which produced severe artifacts due to the high-pass filter designed in FBP. Fig. 3(c) and (g) show the results of PL-ramp, while Fig. 3(d) and (h) show the results of resFBP. The images reconstructed by PL-Ramp are much better than that by FBP due to its capability of learning from data, however, resFBP reconstructs images with sharper boundaries and lower reconstruction error. Therefore, resFBP is less sensitive to noise.

4 Discussion

With the help of the residual neural network, resFBP can achieve lower reconstruction error with sharper boundaries compared to PL-Ramp on Poisson noise data and Gaussian noise data. Due to regularization terms, resFBP is more robust than PL-Ramp and less likely to suffer from over-fitting. In consideration of the complexity of designing, this method is better than the analytical filter kernel design method. Meanwhile, it can still provide a good filter by learning in a noisy situation, where it is difficult to design analytic filters. In addition, the reconstruction by resFBP can serve as a better prior for deep learning-based post-processing methods. Robustness against noise on real datasets and the contribution of different modules remain to be further studied.

References

1. Ramachandran, G, N, et al. Three-dimensional reconstruction from radiographs and electron micrographs: application of convolutions instead of Fourier transforms. Proc Natl Acad Sci U S A. 1971;68(9):2236–2240.
2. Shepp LA, Logan BF. The fourier reconstruction of a head section. IEEE Trans Nucl Sci. 1974;NS21(3):21–43.
3. Wei Y, Bonse U, Wang G, et al. CT reconstruction filter design in the real space. Proc SPIE. 2004;5535:628–635.
4. Shi H, Luo S. A novel scheme to design the filter for CT reconstruction using FBP algorithm. Biomed Eng Online. 2013;12(1):50–50.
5. Wang B, Liu H. FBP-Net for direct reconstruction of dynamic PET images. Phys Med Biol. 2020;.
6. Syben C, Stimpel B, Breininger K, et al. Precision learning: reconstruction filter kernel discretization. arXiv preprint arXiv:171006287. 2017;.
7. He K, Zhang X, Ren S, et al. Identity mappings in deep residual networks. European Conference on Computer Vision. 2016; p. 630–645.
8. Syben C, Michen M, Stimpel B, et al. Technical note: PYRO-NN: python reconstruction operators in neural networks. Med Phys. 2019;46(11):5110–5115.
9. Mccollough CH, Bartley AC, Carter RE, et al. Low-dose CT for the detection and classification of metastatic liver lesions: results of the 2016 low dose CT grand challenge. Med Phys. 2017;44(10).

Abstract: Automatic Plane Adjustment in Surgical Cone Beam CT-volumes

Celia Martín Vicario[1], Florian Kordon[1,2,3], Felix Denzinger[1,2],
Markus Weiten[2], Sarina Thomas[5], Lisa Kausch[5], Jochen Franke[6], Holger Keil[7],
Andreas Maier[1,3,4], Holger Kunze[2,1]

[1]Pattern Recognition Lab, Universität Erlangen-Nürnberg (FAU), Erlangen
[2]Siemens Healthcare GmbH, Forchheim
[3]Erlangen Graduate School in Advanced Optical Technologies (SAOT), Universität Erlangen-Nürnberg (FAU), Erlangen
[4]Machine Intelligence, Universität Erlangen-Nürnberg (FAU), Erlangen
[5]Division of Medical Image Computing, German Cancer Research Center, Heidelberg
[6]Department for Trauma and Orthopaedic Surgery, BG Trauma Center Ludwigshafen, Ludwigshafen
[7]Department of Trauma and Orthopedic Surgery, University Hospital Erlangen, Universität Erlangen-Nürnberg (FAU), Erlangen
Celia.Martin@fau.de

Cone beam computed tomography (CBCT) is used intra-operatively to assess the result of surgery. Due to limitations of patient positioning and the operating theater in general, the acquisition usually cannot be performed such that the axis-aligned multiplanar reconstructions (MPR) of the volume match the anatomically oriented MPRs. This needs to be corrected manually, which is a time-consuming and complex task and requires the surgeon to interact with non-sterile equipment. To this end, this study investigates a fully-automatic solution to directly regress the standard plane parameters from a CBCT volume of the calcaneus and ankle regions. A PoseNet convolutional neural network (CNN) is adapted and trained, comparing a 6D-, Euler angle- and quaternion-based approach to represent the plane rotation [1]. In addition, a cost function is optimized to incorporate orientation constraints. The best-performing CNN – which uses the 6D representation – estimates the plane normal with a median accuracy of $5°$, the in-plane rotation with a median accuracy of $6°$, and the position with a median accuracy of 6 mm. The inference time is less than 0.05 s.

References

1. Martin Vicario C, Kordon F, Denzinger F, et al. Automatic plane adjustment of orthopedic intraoperative flat panel detector CT-volumes. Proc MICCAI. 2020; p. 486–495.

© Der/die Autor(en), exklusiv lizenziert durch
Springer Fachmedien Wiesbaden GmbH, ein Teil von Springer Nature 2021
C. Palm et al. (Hrsg.), *Bildverarbeitung für die Medizin 2021*,
Informatik aktuell, https://doi.org/10.1007/978-3-658-33198-6_40

Abstract: Towards Automatic C-arm Positioning for Standard Projections in Orthopedic Surgery

Lisa Kausch[1], Sarina Thomas[1], Holger Kunze[2], Maxim Privalov[3], Sven Vetter[3], Jochen Franke[3], Andreas H. Mahnken[4], Lena Maier-Hein[1], Klaus Maier-Hein[1]

[1]German Cancer Research Center, Heidelberg
[2]Imaging and Therapy Systems Division, Siemens Healthineers, Erlangen
[3]Division of Medical Imaging and Navigation in Trauma and Orthopedic Surgery, BG Unfallklinik Ludwigshafen
[4]Division of Diagnostic and Interventional Radiology, Universitätsklinikum Marburg
l.kausch@dkfz-heidelberg.de

Guidance and quality control in orthopedic surgery increasingly relies on intra-operative fluoroscopy using a mobile C-arm. The accurate acquisition of standardized and anatomy-specific projections is essential in this process. The corresponding iterative positioning of the C-arm is error-prone and involves repeated manual acquisitions or even continuous fluoroscopy. To reduce time and radiation exposure for patients and clinical staff, and to avoid errors in fracture reduction or implant placement, we aim at guiding - and in the long run automating - this procedure. In contrast to the state of the art, we tackle this inherently ill-posed problem without requiring patient-individual prior information like pre-operative computed tomography scans, and without requiring additional technical equipment besides the projection images themselves. We propose learning the necessary anatomical hints for efficient C-arm positioning from in silico simulations, leveraging masses of 3D CTs. Specifically, we propose a convolutional neural network regression model that predicts 5 degrees of freedom pose updates directly from 2D projections. Quantitative and qualitative validation was performed for two clinical applications involving two highly dissimilar anatomies, namely the lumbar spine and the proximal femur. Starting from one initial projection, the mean absolute pose error to the desired standard pose is iteratively reduced across different anatomy-specific standard projections. Acquisitions of both hip joints on 4 cadavers allowed for an evaluation on clinical data, demonstrating that the approach generalizes without re-training. Overall, the results suggest the feasibility of an efficient deep learning-based 2-step automated positioning procedure, which is trained on simulations. This work was first presented at IPCAI 2020 [1].

References

1. Kausch L, Thomas S, Kunze H, et al. Towards automatic C-arm positioning for standard projections in orthopedic surgery. IJCARS. 2020;15:1095–1105.

Open-Science Gefäßphantom für neurovaskuläre Interventionen

Lena Stevanovic[1], Benjamin J. Mittmann[2,3], Florian Pfiz[1], Michael Braun[4],
Bernd Schmitz[4], Alfred M. Franz[2]

[1]Institut für Medizintechnik und Mechatronik, Technische Hochschule Ulm
[2]Institut für Informatik, Technische Hochschule Ulm
[3]Medizinische Fakultät, Universität Heidelberg
[4]Sektion Neuroradiologie, Bezirkskrankenhaus Günzburg
`alfred.franz@thu.de`

Zusammenfassung. Computerassistenzsysteme könnten Ärzten in neurovaskulären Interventionen eine Hilfestellung bei bestehenden Schwierigkeiten, wie der Positionierung der eingesetzten Instrumente bieten, indem sie deren Lage im Gefäßbaum des Patienten anzeigen. Zur Evaluierung derartiger Systeme stellen wir ein Gefäßphantom der hirnversorgenden Arterien für die Simulation neurovaskulärer Interventionen vor.
Das Phantom wurde durch Segmentierung des Gefäßbaums der computertomographischen Angiographie-Aufnahme (CTA) eines Patienten erstellt, nachbearbeitet und anschließend als flexibler 3D-Druck gefertigt.
Die Methodik zur Phantom-Erstellung wurde beschrieben, um im Sinne des open-science-Gedankens die eigenständige Fertigung individueller
Phantome zu ermöglichen. Anhand einer CTA des gefertigten Phantoms
konnte eine weitgehende Übereinstimmung mit dem Gefäßbaum des Patienten gezeigt werden. Die Einsatzfähigkeit des Phantoms wurde zudem
durch das Einbringen neurovaskulärer Instrumente untersucht. Darüber
hinaus konnte das Phantom erfolgreich in einer Beispielanwendung von
Comupterassistenzsystemen eingesetzt werden. Alle für die Herstellung
des Phantoms relevanten Dateien wurden zusammen mit den Versuchs-
ergebnissen unter https://osf.io/yg95d/ zur Verfügung gestellt.

1 Einleitung

Neurovaskuläre Interventionen sind minimalinvasive Verfahren zur Behandlung
intrakranieller, vaskulärer Erkrankungen, wie Aneurysmen oder Stenosen. Ver-
glichen mit offenen Gefäßoperationen bieten sie mitunter Vorteile, wie kürzere
Heilungs- und Rehabilitationszeiten. Bei der Thrombektomie, einem Verfahren
zur katheterbasierten Bergung von Thromben beim akuten ischämischen Schlag-
anfall, konnte beispielsweise eine bessere Prognose bezüglich neurologischer Aus-
fälle und der Mortalität im Vergleich zur medikamentösen Therapie erzielt werden [1]. Insbesondere bei stark gewundenen Gefäßverläufen ist die korrekte Positionierung der Katheter zur Bergung der Thromben erschwert [2], wodurch

C. Palm et al. (Hrsg.), *Bildverarbeitung für die Medizin 2021*,
Informatik aktuell, https://doi.org/10.1007/978-3-658-33198-6_42

die Prognose des Patienten tendenziell schlechter ausfällt [3]. Im Rahmen von
Image-Guided-Therapy(IGT)-Projekten entwickelte Computerassistenzsysteme
könnten die Lage der Katheter zum Gefäßsystem visualisieren und damit die
Navigation der Katheter zum betroffenen Gefäß erleichtern. Zur Erforschung
derartiger Systeme wird ein Gefäßphantom der hirnversorgenden Arterien benötigt, das die realitätsnahe Simulation neurovaskulärer Interventionen ermöglicht.

Kommerzielle Gefäßphantome können bei den Herstellern „United Biolo-
gics Inc." (Santa Ana, Kalifornien) und „Elastrat Sàrl" (Genf, Schweiz) erworben werden und basieren auf einer Zusammensetzung verschiedener Patienten-
daten. Wird ein Phantom hingegen anhand eines medizinischen Datensatzes
eines einzelnen Patienten erstellt, ergeben sich Vorteile, wie die Möglichkeit
zur Registrierung des Phantoms zum klinischen Datensatz und die Erstellung
patienten-spezifischer Phantome. Solche Phantome können bei Unternehmen wie
der „HumanX GmbH" (Wildau, Deutschland) erworben werden und wurden beispielsweise in einer verwandten Arbeit für Aortenphantome genutzt [4]. Eine
weitere Arbeit zur Erstellung eines Aorten-Phantoms zeigt auf, dass sich die
Anforderungen von denen eines neurovaskulären Phantoms unterscheiden [5].
Unseres Wissens existiert bisher keine Arbeit zur Erstellung eines Gefäßphantoms für neurovaskuläre Interventionen mit open-source Mitteln. Im Sinne des
open-science Gedankens [6] beschreiben wir in dieser Arbeit die Methodik zur
Herstellung eines neurovaskulären Phantoms auf Basis frei zugänglicher, medizinischer Bilddaten und veröffentlichen für die Herstellung benötigte Konstruktionsdaten, um den Nachbau des Phantoms sowie die Übertragbarkeit der Methodik auf andere Gefäßanatomien zu ermöglichen.

Vom gefertigten Phantom wurde eine computertomographischen Angiographie-Aufnahme (CTA) erstellt. Zudem wurde es durch Einbringen neurovaskulärer Instrumente und durch den Einsatz in einer IGT-Beispielanwendung erprobt.

2 Material und Methoden

Zur Herstellung des Phantoms ist in fünf Teilprozesse gegliedert. Die Evaluation
erfolgt durch Simulation einer neurovaskulären Intervention.

2.1 Herstellungsprozess

I Die Erstellung des Gefäßphantoms erfolgte auf Basis frei zugänglicher, ra-
diologischer Daten des University College London Hospitals [7]. Als Aus-
gangsdatensatz diente eine CTA des Patienten 17 mit einer Voxelgröße von
0,5 x 0,5 x 0,3 mm, bei dem die Blutgefäße einen Graustufenbereich von 110
- 390 HU umfassen.

II Die kontrastierten Blutgefäße wurden aufgrund des geringen Durchmessers
und der erforderlichen Präzision mittels des „The Medical Imaging Interaction Toolkit" (MITK) manuell segmentiert. Dabei wurden die Gefäße beider Körperhälften beginnend von der *Arteria carotis communis* (ACC) und
der *Arteria vertebralis* (AV) bis zur *Arteria cerebri posterior* (ACP) sowie

der *Arteria cerebri anterior* (ACA) und der *Arteria cerebri media* (ACM, Segmente: rechts M2, links M3) schichtweise in der axialen Ansicht segmentiert, wobei jede zweite bis dritte Schicht interpoliert wurde. Die Segmentierung wurde in der sagittalen und coronalen Ansicht korrigiert. Da die Grenze zwischen der dünnen Gefäßwand und dem Gefäß-Inneren in der CTA nicht erkennbar war, wurden die Gefäße als ausgefüllte Struktur inklusive der Gefäßwand segmentiert. Aus dem segmentierten Gefäßbaum wurde eine Stereolithographie-Datei erstellt und exportiert.

III Da die Segmentierung anhand eines diskret aufgelösten Datensatzes erfolgt war, zeigte die Oberfläche des Gefäßbaums Unebenheiten. Zur Erstellung eines kontinuierlichen Modells wurde der Gefäßbaum geglättet. Um Interventionen im Inneren des Phantoms zu ermöglichen ohne den Innendurchmesser der Gefäße zu verkleinern, wurde ein Offset der Außenfläche des Gefäßbaums im Abstand von 1,5 mm erzeugt, der den ursprünglichen Gefäßbaum umschloss. Aus dem entstandenen Raum zwischen der Außenfläche des Gefäßbaums und der Offset-Fläche konnte ein Volumenkörper erstellt werden, dessen hohler Innenraum mit dem Gefäßbaum des Patienten übereinstimmt. Die Gefäßwandstärke wurde entsprechend der Möglichkeiten des Fertigungsverfahrens auf 1,5 mm gesetzt. Für den Zugang zu den Gefäßen wurden deren Enden abgetrennt und geöffnet. Im letzten, optionalen Schritt wurde ein Grundgestell zur Stabilisierung um den digitalen Gefäßbaum herum konstruiert. Die Nachbearbeitung wurde zunächst mit den Programmen „MeshLab" und „Siemens NX" getestet. Die einzelnen Schritte der Nachbearbeitung konnten daraufhin auch mit ausschließlich freier Software unter Verwendung der Programme „Meshmixer" (Glätten, Aushöhlen, Abtrennen) und „FreeCAD" (Volumenkörper, Grundgestell) durchgeführt werden.

IV Das digitale Modell wurde schließlich im Polyjet - Verfahren 3D-gedruckt. Um den Gefäßbaum hohl, flexibel und dennoch robust zu gestalten, wurde das Druckmaterial „Agilus30" (Stratasys Ltd., Eden Prairie, Minnesota) und wasserlösliches Stützmaterial eingesetzt. Das Grundgestell wurde im selben Druckvorgang aus dem starren Material „VeroClear" von Stratasys an den Gefäßbaum angrenzend gedruckt.

V Durch die Ergänzung von Kunststoffschläuchen über Silikon-Klebestellen wurde das Phantom mithilfe von Reduzierstücken sowie 3D-gedruckten Verbindungsstücken zu einem Kreislauf verbunden. Zur Stabilisierung wurde das Phantom zuletzt auf einer Grundplatte fixiert (Abb. 1).

2.2 Evaluierung des Phantoms

Zur Evaluierung der Einsatzfähigkeit des Phantoms wurde zunächst eine CTA des Phantom durch die Befüllung mit einem Jod-Wasser-Gemisch (20 mg Jod/ml, Imeron 400 MCT, Bracco S.p.A., Mailand, Italien) angefertigt. Daraufhin wurde der Gefäßbaum der Phantom-CTA entsprechend dem oben beschriebenen Vorgehen segmentiert und geglättet. Die Segmentierung wurde über anatomische Landmarken (ACC rechts, Arteria carotis externa (ACE) links,

ACA mittig, Arteria basilaris) zur ursprünglichen Patienten-Segmentierung registriert, um die Übereinstimmung der Gefäßbäume zu prüfen. Da in neurovaskulären Interventionen Katheter entlang eines Führungsdrahts in die Gefäße des Patienten eingebracht werden, wurde die Erreichbarkeit vordefinierter Stellen im Phantom (rechts: ACA, ACP, ACM-M3; links: ACA, ACP, ACM-M1) mit einem 0,018 inch großen Führungsdraht (Terumo Corporation, Tokio, Japan) je zwei Mal von drei Laien geprüft. Das Phantom wurde zudem in MITK mithilfe des Aurora Tracking-Systems mit Tabletop Feldgenerator (Northern Digital, Inc., Waterloo, Kanada) über vier CT-Marker auf der Grundplatte des Phantoms zur Phantom-CTA registriert. Ein trackbarer Prototyp eines Führungsdrahts wurde durch die Verbindung des Führungsdrahts mit einem NDI Aurora 5 DOF Sensordraht durch einen Latex-Überzug erstellt. Der Prototyp wurde beidseitig je vier Mal in die Arteria carotis interna (ACI) und die ACE des Phantoms vorgeschoben, um seine Position in der Phantom-CTA aufzuzeichnen.

3 Ergebnisse

In der Arbeit wurde ein flexibles, neurovaskuläres Gefäßphantom 3D-gedruckt und für seinen Einsatzzweck zur Simulation neurovaskulärer Interventionen erweitert. Folgende Dateien wurden unter https://osf.io/yg95d/ im Open Science Framework veröffentlicht: Segmentierungen, Konstruktionsdaten der Nachbearbeitung, Anleitung zur Erstellung des Phantoms sowie Daten der Registrierungsversuche. Das Vorschieben eines Führungsdrahts zu definierten Stellen im Phantom gelang in acht von zwölf Versuchen, wohingegen vier Versuche scheiterten. Dabei handelte es sich um die distalen Gefäße ACP, ACA, ACM-M3. Es konnte eine CTA des Phantoms erstellt werden, in der die Gefäße stark kontrastiert (bis zu 900 HU) dargestellt wurden. Die rechte ACM wurde ab dem M2-Segment nicht mehr durchgängig dargestellt und daher nicht segmentiert. Die Co-Registrierung der segmentierten Gefäßbäume aus Phantom-CTA und Patienten-CTA zeigte hinsichtlich des Gefäßverlaufs eine weitgehende Übereinstimmung (Abb. 2a) und einen Fiducial Registration Error von 2,4 mm. Abweichungen konnten vor allem im distalen Phantombereich durch eine Absenkung der Gefäße zur Grundplatte hin beobachtet werden, die im Bereich der ACP am größten ausfiel (2 cm). Um

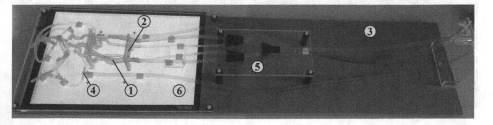

Abb. 1. Gedrucktes Gefäßphantom (1) mit Grundgestell (2) auf stabilisierender Grundplatte (3). Ergänzungen durch Schläuche mit Reduzierstücken (4), 3D-gedruckte Verbindungsstücke (5) und LED-Panel (6) zur besseren Sichtbarkeit des Führungsdrahts.

176   Stevanovic et al.

die Größenordnung der Abweichungen abschätzen zu können, wurde der Abstand der Gefäßmittelpunkte beider Gefäßbaume an folgenden Referenzpunkten gemessen: links: ACE (0,9 mm), ACI (2,2 mm), AV-V4 (4,7 mm); rechts: ACC (0,4 mm), ACA (1,7 mm) und AV-V3 (0,1 mm).

Bei der Lokalisierung des trackbaren Führungsdrahts wurde dessen Position bis auf einzelne Ausreißer (ca. 1,5%) auch bei mehrfacher Wiederholung des Versuchs innerhalb des Gefäßbaums angezeigt (Abb. 2b).

4 Diskussion

Die besonderen Anforderungen eines neurovaskulären Phantoms wie die geringen Durchmesser (1,5 - 8 mm) und starken Windungen der Gefäße konnten in dieser Arbeit über den flexiblen 3D-Druck realisiert werden. Die überwiegende Übereinstimmung der Gefäßbaum-Segmentierungen von Phantom und Patient im proximalen Bereich zeigt, dass der Gefäßverlauf des Patienten weitestgehend im Phantom wiedergegeben wird. Abweichungen durch die Absenkung der Gefäße sind vor allem im distalen Phantombereich zu beobachten und der Flexibilität des Materials geschuldet. Ein starrer 3D-Druck des Gefäßbaums kann die Patientenanatomie potentiell genauer abbilden, jedoch konnten Führungsdraht und Katheter bei Testdrucken aus starrem Material nur mühsam ins Phantom vorgeschoben werden. Um realitätsnahe Bedingungen für die Beschaffenheit der Gefäße und das Handling der Instrumente zu schaffen, wurde das Phantom aus flexiblem Material gefertigt. Die Absenkung der Phantom-Gefäße könnte durch weitere Stützstrukturen oder die Imitation des umliegenden Gewebes vermindert werden. Ein weiterer möglicher Grund für die Abweichung zwischen den Gefäßbäumen sind Registrierungsfehler, bedingt durch die Schwierigkeit, die anatomischen Landmarken bei der Co-Registrierung manuell präzise anzuwählen.

Die erfolgreiche Positionsanzeige des trackbaren Führungsdrahts bildet eine vielversprechende Basis für weitere Untersuchungen der Einsatzfähigkeit des

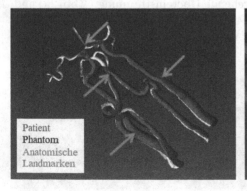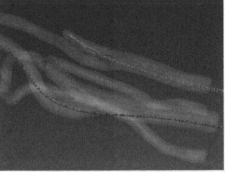

Abb. 2. Ergebnisse der Registrierungsversuche zur Untersuchung der Einsatzfähigkeit des Phantoms. Links: Co-Registrierung der Segmentierung von Patienten-CTA und Phantom-CTA. Rechts: Positionsanzeige des getrackten Führungsdrahts innerhalb des Gefäßbaums.

Phantoms zur Evaluierung von Computerassistenzsystemen. Diese soll künftig unter klinischen Bedingungen näher geprüft werden. Die einzelnen, außerhalb der Gefäße liegenden Positionswerte sind vermutlich Trackingfehlern zuzuschreiben.

Die Unterbrechung des M2-Segments in der Phantom-CTA ist wahrscheinlich durch Luftblasen innerhalb des Phantoms entstanden, weshalb es vor der Erstellung medizinischer Bilddaten gründlich darauf untersucht werden sollte.

In der Versuchsreihe zum Erreichen definierter Gefäße mit dem Führungsdraht lagen die nicht erreichten Stellen ausschließlich in distalen Gefäßen, die auch am Patienten eine Herausforderung darstellen. Die Versuche wurden von Laien durchgeführt, die Schwierigkeiten im Handling der Instrumente hatten. Die Annahme, dass erfahrene Neuroradiologen größere Erfolgsquoten erreichen würden, konnte bisher aufgrund der Pandemie noch nicht überprüft werden.

Die zur Ergänzung des Kreislaufes angebrachten Klebestellen erwiesen sich bei häufigem Gebrauch als Schwachstellen hinsichtlich der Wasserundurchlässigkeit und könnten durch 3D-gedruckte Verbindungsstücke ersetzt werden.

Zusammenfassend wurde in der Arbeit ein neurovaskuläres Phantom zur Simulation katheterbasierter Interventionen erstellt und evaluiert. Die open-science Vorgehensweise ermöglicht sowohl die Reproduktion des vorgestellten Phantoms als auch die Übertragbarkeit auf andere Gefäßanatomien.

Danksagung. Diese Arbeit wird vom BMBF gefördert (ZF4640301GR8). Wir danken Herrn Michael Moroch (Alphacam GmbH), Herrn Prof. Dr.-Ing. Rainer Brucher (Technische Hochschule Ulm), Herrn Thomas Szimeth (Technische Hochschule Ulm) und Herrn Daniel Gröner (Universitätsklinikum Frankfurt) für die Unterstützung.

Literatur

1. Goyal M, et al. Endovascular thrombectomy after large-vessel ischaemic stroke: a meta-analysis of individual patient data from five randomised trials. Lancet. 2016;.
2. Yoo AJ, Andersson T. Thrombectomy in acute ischemic stroke: challenges to procedural success. J Stroke. 2017;.
3. Saver JL. Time is brain — quantified. Stroke. 2005; p. 263–266.
4. Jäckle S, et al. Three-dimensional guidance including shape sensing of a stentgraft system for endovascular aneurysm repair. Int J Comput Assist Radiol Surg. 2020; p. 1033–1042.
5. Heidemanns S. Konzeption, Entwicklung und Evaluation eines kostengünstigen reproduzierbaren Gefäßmodells für die Simulation und das Training endovaskulärer interventioneller Prozeduren an der Aorta anhand anatomischer Vorlagen eines realen Patienten. Dissertation: LMU München; 2015.
6. Darrel IC, Hatton L, Graham-Cumming J. The case for open computer programs. nature. 2012; p. 485–488.
7. Goren N, et al. UCLH stroke EIT dataset radiology data [data set]. zenodo. http://doi.org/10.5281/zenodo.1199398: University College London Hospital; 2017.

Abstract: Semi-supervised Segmentation Based on Error-correcting Supervision

Robert Mendel[1], Luis Antonio de Souza Jr[2], David Rauber[1],
João Paulo Papa[3], Christoph Palm[1]

[1]Ostbayerische Technische Hochschule Regensburg, Regensburg, Germany
[2]Federal University of São Carlos, São Carlos, Brazil
[3]São Paulo State University, Bauru, Brazil
robert1.mendel@oth-regensburg.de

Pixel-level classification is an essential part of computer vision. For learning from labeled data, many powerful deep learning models have been developed recently. In this work, we augment such supervised segmentation models by allowing them to learn from unlabeled data. Our semi-supervised approach, termed Error-Correcting Supervision, leverages a collaborative strategy. Apart from the supervised training on the labeled data, the segmentation network is judged by an additional network. The secondary correction network learns on the labeled data to optimally spot correct predictions, as well as to amend incorrect ones.As auxiliary regularization term, the corrector directly influences the supervised training of the segmentation network. On unlabeled data, the output of the correction network is essential to create a proxy for the unknown truth. The corrector's output is combined with the segmentation network's prediction to form the new target. We propose a loss function that incorporates both the pseudo-labels as well as the predictive certainty of the correction network. Our approach can easily be added to supervised segmentation models. We show consistent improvements over a supervised baseline on experiments on both the Pascal VOC 2012 and the Cityscapes datasets with varying amounts of labeled data. This work was was presented at the European Conference on Computer Vision 2020 [1].Semi-supervised learning is especially important in domains where labeled data is sparse. Although this work did not specifically focus on medical imaging, we believe that the proposed method can be valuable for the community, and applications in the medical image segmentation setting should be considered.

References

1. Mendel R, de Souza LA, Rauber D, et al. Semi-supervised segmentation based on error-correcting supervision. Proc ECCV. 2020; p. 141–157.

Abstract: Efficient Biomedical Image Segmentation on EdgeTPUs

Andreas M. Kist[1], Michael Döllinger[1]

[1] Division for Phoniatrics and Pediatric Audiology, Department of
Otorhinolaryngology, Head and Neck Surgery, University Hospital Erlangen,
Friedrich-Alexander-University Erlangen-Nürnberg
andreas.kist@uk-erlangen.de

The U-Net architecture [1] is a state-of-the-art neural network for semantic image segmentation that is widely used in biomedical research. It is based on an encoder-decoder framework and its vanilla version shows already high performance in terms of segmentation quality. Due to its large parameter space, however, it has high computational costs on both, CPUs and GPUs. In a research setting, inference time is relevant, but not crucial for the results. However, especially in mobile, clinical applications a light and fast variant would allow deep-learning assisted, objective diagnosis at the point of care. In this work, we suggest an optimized, tiny-weight U-Net for an inexpensive hardware accelerator. We first mined the U-Net architecture to reduce computational complexity to increase runtime performance by simultaneously keeping the accuracy on a high level. Using an open, biomedical dataset for high-speed videoendoscopy (BAGLS, [2]), we show that we can dramatically reduce the parameter space and computations by over 99.8% while keeping the segmentation performance at 95% of our baseline. Using a custom upscaling routine, we further successfully deployed our optimized U-Net to an EdgeTPU hardware accelerator to gain cost-effective speed improvements on conventional computers and to showcase the applicability of EdgeTPUs for biomedical imaging processing of large images on portable devices. Combining the optimized architecture and the EdgeTPU, we gain a speedup of >79-times compared to our initial baseline while keeping high accuracy. This combination allows to provide immediate results to the clinician, especially in constrained computational environments, and an objective diagnosis at the point of care. This work has been previously published [3].

References

1. Ronneberger O, Fischer P, Brox T. U-net: convolutional networks for biomedical image segmentation. Proc MICCAI. 2015; p. 234–241.
2. Gómez P, Kist AM, Schlegel P, et al. BAGLS, a multihospital benchmark for automatic glottis segmentation. Scientific data. 2020;7(1):1–12.
3. Kist AM, Döllinger M. Efficient biomedical image segmentation on edgeTPUs at point of care. IEEE Access. 2020;8:139356–139366.

© Der/die Autor(en), exklusiv lizenziert durch
Springer Fachmedien Wiesbaden GmbH, ein Teil von Springer Nature 2021
C. Palm et al. (Hrsg.), *Bildverarbeitung für die Medizin 2021*,
Informatik aktuell, https://doi.org/10.1007/978-3-658-33198-6_44

Human Axon Radii Estimation at MRI Scale

Deep Learning Combined with Large-scale Light Microscopy

Laurin Mordhorst[1], Maria Morozova[2,3], Sebastian Papazoglou[1], Björn Fricke[1],
Jan M. Oeschger[1], Henriette Rusch[3], Carsten Jäger[2], Markus Morawski[2,3],
Nikolaus Weiskopf[2,4], Siawoosh Mohammadi[1,2]

[1]Institute of Systems Neuroscience, University Medical Center Hamburg-Eppendorf
[2]Department of Neurophysics, Max Planck Institute for Human Cognitive and Brain
Sciences
[3]Paul Flechsig Institute of Brain Research, University of Leipzig
[4]Felix Bloch Institute for Solid State Physics, University of Leipzig
l.mordhorst@uke.de

Abstract. Non-invasive assessment of axon radii via MRI is of increasing interest in human brain research. Its validation requires representative reference data that covers the spatial extent of an MRI voxel (e.g., $1\,mm^2$). Due to its small field of view, the commonly used manually labeled electron microscopy (mlEM) can not representatively capture sparsely occurring, large axons, which are the main contributors to the effective mean axon radius (r_{eff}) measured with MRI. To overcome this limitation, we investigated the feasibility of generating representative reference data from large-scale light microscopy (lsLM) using automated segmentation methods including a convolutional neural network (CNN). We determined large, mis-/undetected axons as the main error source for the estimation of r_{eff} ($\approx 10\,\%$). Our results suggest that the proposed pipeline can be used to generate reference data for the MRI-visible r_{eff} and even bears the potential to map spatial, anatomical variation of r_{eff}.

1 Introduction

In vivo axon radius assessment in human brain using MRI-based models [1] is of neuroscientific relevance [2]. Often, these models have been compared to manually labeled electron microscopy (mlEM) images with a very small field of view containing up to 10^3 or less axons [3, 4] whereas MRI voxels of $1\,mm^3$ contain two to three orders of magnitude more axons. While mlEM is commonly used to report the arithmetic mean axon radii (r_{arith}) in histology studies [3, 4], it can largely underestimate the axon radius indices measured with MRI such as the effective mean axon radius (r_{eff}) [1]. r_{eff} based on mlEM is often underestimated because sparsely occurring, large axons, which are the main contributors to r_{eff}, are underrepresented in the mlEM based axon distribution [5]. Here, we assessed the potential of large-scale light microscopy (lsLM) and automated segmentation

Springer Fachmedien Wiesbaden GmbH, ein Teil von Springer Nature 2021
C. Palm et al. (Hrsg.), *Bildverarbeitung für die Medizin 2021*,
Informatik aktuell, https://doi.org/10.1007/978-3-658-33198-6_45

methods including a convolutional neural network (CNN) to generate representative reference data for axon radii distributions in typical MRI voxels. We evaluated the error and bias of both r_{eff} and r_{arith} on six lsLM sections across a human corpus callosum sample including a cross-microscopy comparison to their mlEM-based counterparts.

2   Materials and methods

2.1   Ensemble mean axon radii

The MRI-visible, effective mean radius [1] of an ensemble of N axons can be defined as $r_{\text{eff}} = \sqrt[4]{(\sum_{i=1}^{N} r_i^6)/(\sum_{i=1}^{N} r_i^2)}$, where r_i is the i-th radius. It deviates from the arithmetic mean radius $r_{\text{arith}} = \frac{1}{N} \sum_{i=1}^{N} r_i$ and is weighted towards the tail of its distribution rather than its bulk.

2.2   Normalized root-mean-square deviation and mean bias

To measure the residuals between observed (y) and estimated ($\hat{y}$) values (e.g., mean axon radii) over multiple observations, we used the normalized root-mean-square deviation NRMSD $= (\sqrt{\frac{1}{N} \sum_{i=1}^{N} (\hat{y}_i - y_i)^2})/(\frac{1}{N} \sum_{i=1}^{N} y_i)$ and the relative mean bias $\bar{b}_r = (\sum_{i=1}^{N} \hat{y}_i - y_i)/(\sum_{i=1}^{N} y_i)$, where y_i and $\hat{y}_i$ are the i-th observation and estimation.

2.3   Dataset

A human optic chiasm (OC), a corticospinal tract (CST) and a corpus callosum (CC) sample were scanned at autopsy. The entire procedure of case recruitment, acquisition of the patient's personal data, the protocols and the informed consent forms, performing the autopsy and handling the autopsy material have been approved by the responsible authorities (Approval #205/17-ek). We acquired lsLM images of semi-thin (500 nm) sections using a Zeiss AxioScan Z1 (resolution: 0.112 µm/px; resolution limit: 0.3 µm) and EM images of consecutively cut, ultra-thin (50 nm) sections using a Zeiss EM 912 Omega (resolution: 0.0043 µm/px).

From the total of 20 lsLM sections (18 CC, 1 CST, 1 OC), we annotated 17 subsections (11 CC, 3 CST, 3 OC; size: $\sim 100 \times 100\,\mu\text{m}^2$) as background, axon or myelin for training and validation. For testing, we reserved six regions (no overlap with training/validation regions) of the CC sample (Fig. 1) and annotated EM sections and subsections of their corresponding lsLM sections at different granularity: EM subsections (one per region; size: $\sim 50 \times 50\,\mu\text{m}^2$) and small lsLM subsections were annotated entirely (five per region; size: $\sim 28 \times 28\,\mu\text{m}^2$), whereas larger subsections (two of size $\sim 110 \times 110\,\mu\text{m}^2$ per region to evaluate the segmentation performance; one per region of size $\sim 550 \times 550\,\mu\text{m}^2$ to evaluate the estimation of r_{eff}) were annotated selectively for MRI-relevant, large axons with $r >= 1.6\,\mu\text{m}$. The threshold was determined so that r_{eff} was halved when axons with radii above this threshold were removed.

Fig. 1. Schematic of the human corpus callosum sample. LsLM and consecutively cut EM sections were investigated for six regions of interest: anterior genu (G1, G2), posterior genu (PG2), midbody (M3), isthmus (I2) and splenium (S3).

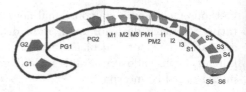

2.4 Axon radius estimation pipeline

Axon radius estimation was split up into three parts (Fig. 2): pixel-wise classifications were obtained using a U-Net [6] (Fig. 2a; details below) in a sliding window manner (patch size 512×512 px). After identification of axon instances (Fig. 2b) through connected-component labeling, axon radii were extracted (Fig. 2c) as circular area equivalent radii from the segmented instance areas.

We used a U-Net [6] implemented in PyTorch [7] and employed transfer learning, i.e., we used pretrained (on the ImageNet dataset) ResNet18 [8] encoders and adapted all weights during training.

The training process was split into pseudo-epochs of 75 random patches, matching the number of available patches. Augmentations were employed on-the-fly: geometric, brightness and saturation transformations, Gaussian blurring and stain augmentation [9]. Patches were standardized with respect to the ImageNet dataset. We used Adam [10] with a learning rate of 10^{-3} and a learning rate decay of $\gamma = 0.75$ every 25 epochs to minimize a cross-entropy loss with classes weighted inversely proportional to their occurrences. Hyperparameter optimization was carried out in a 4-fold cross-validation split at the level of entire lsLM subsections. The model with the best hyperparameters was determined in terms of the averaged dice score for axon and myelin and trained for 250 epochs.

2.5 Experiment 1: Segmentation performance

We assessed the general segmentation quality on small, entirely labeled subsections as well as the MRI-relevant, large-axon specific segmentation quality on large, selectively labeled subsections in terms of accuracy, dice, precision and recall for the binary classification between axon and background.

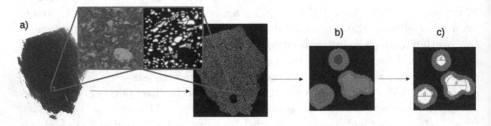

Fig. 2. The axon radius estimation pipeline. Radius estimation was performed in three steps: semantic segmentation (a), instance segmentation (b) and radius extraction (c).

2.6   Experiment 2: Accuracy of mean axon radii estimation

1. *Cross-microscopy comparison with mlEM:* The estimation of r_{arith} from lsLM sections was compared to its counterpart obtained from consecutively cut mlEM subsections with $(r \geq 0.3\,\mu m)$ and without $(r \geq 0.0\,\mu m)$ rejection of small axons irresolvable due to the lsLM resolution limit.

2. *Spatial variance of r_{arith}/r_{eff} and their correlation with lsLM image intensity:* To assess the spatial variance, r_{arith} and r_{eff} were computed for randomly positioned subsections (size: $0.12\,mm^2$) of each lsLM sample and the average of overlapping subsections was computed locally, resulting in spatially smoothed axon radii maps. To investigate the influence of lsLM image intensity on the spatial variance of the axon radii maps, we first estimated the r_{arith} and r_{eff} maps on an equally spaced grid (pixel area: $0.12\,mm^2$) and resampled the corresponding original lsLM images to the same size. Then, we estimated the correlation between image intensity and mapped axon radii across all pixels in the grid and all sections with similar axon radii distributions (i.e., G1, G2, PG2, M3 and I2).

3. *Error propagation of small axons into r_{eff}:* To measure the error in the axon radii range irresolvable in lsLM $(r < 0.3\,\mu m)$, we compared r_{eff} obtained from lsLM with $(r >= 0.3\,\mu m)$ and without $(r >= 0.0\,\mu m)$ rejection of small axons to a mlEM-informed reference. To generate the mlEM-informed reference, we added small axon radii drawn from the mlEM distribution to its lsLM equivalent, so that the ratio between small $(r < 0.3\,\mu m)$ and remaining $(r >= 0.3\,\mu m)$ axons equaled the ratio observed in mlEM.

4. *Error propagation of large, false negative/positive axons into r_{eff}:* To assess the error introduced by large, false negative (fn) and false positive (fp) axons, we compared the estimated r_{eff} to a manually corrected r_{eff}. The latter was generated by manually correcting large axons in the aforementioned subsections (Sec. 2.3). As false negative, we determined a matching predicted axon for each labeled axon in terms of the highest pairwise dice score and defined labeled axons with no matching predicted axon or a dice score < 0.75. As false positive, we determined predicted axons with no matching labeled axon and $r \geq 1.6\,\mu m$. Small axons $(r < 0.3\,\mu m)$ irresolvable in lsLM were rejected for both estimated and manually corrected r_{eff}.

3   Results

3.1   Experiment 1: Segmentation performance

The segmentation metrics are given as (mean for all axons/mean for large axons): accuracy was (0.92/0.98), axon dice was (0.74/0.84), axon precision was (0.77/0.83) and axon recall was (0.72/0.86).

3.2   Experiment 2: Accuracy of mean axon radii estimation

1. r_{arith} was overestimated by $5\,\%$ to $7\,\%$. The rejection of small axons decreased the NRMSD from $10\,\%$ to $8\,\%$.

Table 1. Mean axon radii estimation results. The errors of r_{arith} and r_{eff} (Sec. 2.6) are given as normalized root-mean-square deviations and relative mean biases $\bar{b}_r$ (Sec. 2.2) over six corpus callosum regions with ($r >= 0.3\,\mu\text{m}$) and without ($r >= 0.0\,\mu\text{m}$) rejection of small axons irresolvable in lsLM.

Measure	Experiment	$r >= 0.0\,\mu\text{m}$		$r >= 0.3\,\mu\text{m}$	
		NRMSD [%]	$\bar{b}_r$ [%]	NRMSD [%]	$\bar{b}_r$ [%]
r_{arith}	Cross-microscopy comparison	10.1	4.5	8.4	6.7
r_{eff}	Error prop. of small axons	0.3	0.2	1.7	1.6
	Error prop. of large fn/fp axons			9.6	-6.1

2. r_{eff}, estimated with or without inclusion of small axons, had a high local heterogeneity (Fig. 3a, bottom) and no correlation with the image intensity (Fig. 3c). The smooth spatial pattern across the sample visible in r_{arith} (Fig. 3a, top) roughly coincided with the lsLM image intensity (Fig. 3b). The visual correspondence was supported by the significant correlation between r_{arith} and the image intensity (Fig. 3c). Removing smaller axons, reduced the correlation coefficient for r_{arith} (without small axons: $\rho = 0.67, p < 10^{-5}$; with small axons: $\rho = 0.83, p < 10^{-5}$).
3. The rejection of small axons ($r < 0.3\,\mu\text{m}$) increased the bias from 0.2 % to 1.6 % and the error from 0.3 % to 1.7 % (Tab. 1).
4. The comparison between manually corrected r_{eff} and predicted r_{eff} (Tab. 1) revealed an underestimation of 6 % and an error of 10 %.

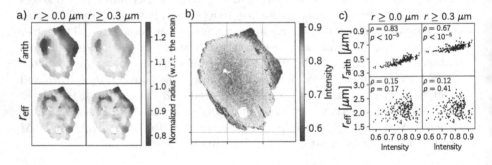

Fig. 3. Spatial variance of $r_{\text{arith}}/r_{\text{eff}}$ and their correlation with lsLM image intensity. Depicted are: (a) spatially smoothed r_{arith} and r_{eff} maps, (b) lsLM image of section PG2 (a) adjusted to illustrate the correlation with r_{arith} map in (a), and scatter plots between $r_{\text{arith}}/r_{\text{eff}}$ maps and lsLM image intensities (c). The r_{arith} and r_{eff} maps in (a) and (c) were generated with ($r >= 0.3\,\mu\text{m}$) and without ($r >= 0.0\,\mu\text{m}$) rejection of small axons. The correlation plots in (c) pools across 5 sections, its p-value has been multiplied by the number of regions, to correct for multiple comparisons (ρ is the correlation coefficient). The grid overlaid in (b) illustrates a typical MRI voxel ($1\,\text{mm}^2$ resolution).

4 Discussion

We demonstrated that our pipeline employing a CNN on large-scale light microscopy (lsLM) data is more suitable to estimate the MRI-visible effective mean radius r_{eff} than the arithmetic mean radius r_{arith}. Albeit r_{arith} had comparable bias (r_{eff}: -6.1 % and r_{arith}: 4.5 %) and error (r_{eff}: 9.6 % and r_{arith}: 10.1 %), the significant correlation with the image/staining intensity proved our pipeline incapable to capture the spatial, anatomical variation. The correlation was particularly high when small axons (i.e., axons below the lsLM resolution limit: $r < 0.3\,\mu\text{m}$) were included, which was reflected in consistently lower segmentation performance for small axons. For r_{eff}, the error and bias was dominated by false negative and positive predicted large axons ($r \geq 1.6\,\mu\text{m}$). Consequently, the presented pipeline is potentially suited to map anatomical, spatial variation at MRI voxel resolution, but requires further quantification of errors in the large axon range, e.g., systematic under-/overestimation to qualify it as a robust reference for the validation of MRI-based axon diameter models.

References

1. Veraart J, Nunes D, Rudrapatna U, et al. Noninvasive quantification of axon radii using diffusion MRI. elife. 2020;9:e49855.
2. Schmidt H, Knösche TR. Action potential propagation and synchronisation in myelinated axons. PLoS Comput Biol. 2019;15:e1007004.
3. Aboitiz F, Scheibel AB, Fisher RS, et al. Fiber composition of the human corpus callosum. Brain Res. 1992;598(1):143–153.
4. Caminiti R, Ghaziri H, Galuske R, et al. Evolution amplified processing with temporally dispersed slow neuronal connectivity in primates. PNAS USA. 2009;106(46):19551–19556.
5. Mordhorst L, Morozova M, Papazoglou S, et al.. Towards a representative estimation of the MRI-visible axon-radius distribution using large-scale light microscopy images. ESMRMB; 2020.
6. Ronneberger O, Fischer P, Brox T. U-Net: convolutional networks for biomedical image segmentation. MICCAI. 2015; p. 234–241.
7. Paszke A, Gross S, Massa F, et al.. PyTorch: an imperative style, high-performance deep learning library; 2019.
8. He K, Zhang X, Ren S, et al. Deep residual learning for image recognition. Proc IEEE Comput Soc Conf Comput Vis Pattern Recognit. 2016; p. 770–778.
9. Macenko M, Niethammer M, Marron JS, et al. A method for normalizing histology slides for quantitative analysis. ISBI. 2009; p. 1107–1110.
10. Kingma DP, Ba J. Adam: a method for stochastic optimization; 2017.

Age Estimation on Panoramic Dental X-ray Images using Deep Learning

Sarah Wallraff[1], Sulaiman Vesal[1], Christopher Syben[1], Rainer Lutz[2], Andreas Maier[1]

[1]Pattern Recognition Lab, Friedrich-Alexander-University Erlangen-Nürnberg, Germany,
[2]Department of Oral and Maxillofacial Surgery, Friedrich-Alexander-University Erlangen-Nürnberg, Germany
sarah.wallraff@web.de

Abstract. Dental panoramic X-ray images provide important information about an adolescent's age because the sequential development process of teeth is one of the longest in the human body. Such dental panoramic projections can be used to assess the age of a person. However, the existing manual methods for age estimation suffer from a low accuracy rate. In this study, we propose a supervised regression-based deep learning method for automatic age estimation of adolescents aged 11 to 20 years to reduce this estimation error. To evaluate the model performance, we used a new dental panoramic X-ray data set with 14,000 images of patients in the considered age range. In an early investigation, our proposed method achieved a mean absolute error (MAE) of 1.08 years and error-rate (ER) of 17.52% on the test data set, which clearly outperformed the dental experts' estimation.

1 Introduction

Milk and permanent teeth breakthrough with such regularity that there is a close correlation with the patient's chronological age (CA). Furthermore, tooth development is only minimally affected by environmental and nutritional influences compared to skeletal growth. Since the dentition is usually very well preserved after death, its analysis is particularly suitable for determining the age and identity of deceased persons. A forensic examination of the teeth is also carried out to estimate whether a person has already reached the age of majority if no birth certificate is available [1, 2]. Several manual methods have been developed to assess the CA of adolescents as a function of the degree of calcification of their milk and permanent teeth, such as the London Atlas [3] and Demirjian's [4] method. These methods are based on the evaluation of dental X-rays. However, already after the breakthrough of the second molars at the age of about 13 years, the age determination becomes increasingly less accurate, as the changes in dentition are more irregular than in childhood [2]. The results of manual estimation methods differ from the actual CA by about ±1 year for adolescents on average. In up to 40% of the examined persons, the absolute deviation is even more than two years [5].

In 2017 Stern et al. [6] presented a deep learning based approach to determine the CA of adolescents. A deep convolutional neural network (DCNN) was trained with MRI images of the left hand, upper thorax, and jaw. Before training cropping of age-relevant structures was performed such that the regression is applicable for a relatively small data set. Therefore from the dental MRI data, only the four wisdom teeth were extracted. The approach was trained and evaluated on a data set of 3D MRI data of 103 male Caucasian volunteers in the age range of 13.01 to 24.89 years. The regression-based solution achieved a mean absolute error (MAE) of 1.3 ± 1.13 years.

Kahaki et al. [7] developed a DCNN for roughly classifying adolescent's age only based on their dental X-ray images. First, the images have been segmented using fuzzy c-means, and afterward, convolutional filtering was used to extract the molar teeth. Then a DCNN was trained with those cropped teeth images captured of 356 Malaysian children aged between 1 and 17 years. The age categories were defined as 1-4, 5-7, 8-10, 11-13, and 14-17 years. On average the accuracy achieved was about 81.83% for this five-class problem.

In this paper, we investigate the feasibility of an extensive data set of 14,000 dental panoramic X-ray images for regression-based automatic age estimation on non-cropped panoramic X-rays to reduce the estimation error. To the best of our knowledge, no such extensive data set has yet been used for an automated age estimation on medical data. Compared to the mentioned related works, no pre-processing and cropping of images is necessary.

2   Material and methods

2.1   Data

We use a clinical image data set with 110,595 dental panoramic X-rays. As teeth develop in a predictable sequence for the first 20 years of life [2], only images of patients aged 11 to 20 years were used for our approach, which leads to 14,000 images in total. Projections of the first ten years of life were omitted because there were relatively few images available from this age range, which would have resulted in a highly unbalanced data set. The age distribution is shown in Table 1. All images are labeled with the age of the patients in days, their sex and a patient identification number (PID). With regard to the patients' sex, the data set is almost equally distributed. Our data set includes various types of clinical images such as low contrast X-rays and images of denture deviating from regular dentition caused by accidents, diseases and jaw malpositions. The data set was provided by our clinical partners[2]. 244 images were split off as unique test data set. The age of the patients in this test data set was manually estimated by an senior physician for oral and maxillofacial surgery and three dental students specially trained in age estimation.

Table 1. Age distribution of the data set for patients in the age range of 11 to 20 years.

Age in years	11	12	13	14	15	16	17	18	19	20	Total
Number of images	975	1103	1362	1432	1621	1621	1653	1537	1501	1599	14019

2.2 Network architecture

For our regression-based approach, we used the original ResNet18 [8] architecture. The fully-connected block at the end of the network architecture was adapted to have one node as output and consists of three fully-connected layers. Since a patient's sex influences the development of teeth [2], two architectures were compared: A uni-sex architecture and a sex-specific architecture, which receives the sex of the patients in the last fully-connected layer as additional information. In initial tests, similarly promising results were achieved with other architectures from the ResNet, VGG and DenseNet families.

As loss function, the Huber-Loss with $\delta = 1$ was chosen. Stochastic Gradient Decent (SGD) with a learning rate of 0.001 was used as optimizer. To make use of the capacities of our large data set, the architecture was pre-trained for regression with the images that do not fall into the age group considered and whose PID does not appear in the training, validation and test data set.

2.2.1 Training. 5-fold cross-validation was used to obtain more stable results. Per fold, approximately 10,000 images were used for training, 2,500 for validation and 244 for testing. Thereby we ensured a unique data split, which ensures that images from one and the same patient are only used for (pre-)training, validation or testing. To compensate for the high variability of patient positioning for the data acquisition, we augment the training images by random flipping, rotating by +/- 5 degrees, slight cropping along the y-axis, and variations in brightness and contrast. Since the X-ray images vary in height and width, all images were resized with interpolation to 1024 × 1024 pixels.

2.2.2 Metrics. Different metrics were used to assess the accuracy of the estimation. First, MAE, standard deviation (std) and mean error (ME) were analyzed. Since an exact daily estimation is not necessary for our approach, the metrics accuracy and error rate are introduced. The accuracy rate describes the percentage of estimates that differ from the actual age by less than ± 1 year, while the error rate describes the percentage of estimates that differ from the actual age by more than ± 2 years.

3 Results

The performance of the trained uni-sex network on the test data set is shown in Figure 1 depending on the patient's sex. The linear regression line for male patients runs almost parallel to the line for optimal estimation. Male patients are generally estimated slightly too young. Female patients' age is overestimated until the age of 16 years and underestimated after that. This is inline with the earlier tooth development of females reported in [2]. With a ME of -0.174 and a MAE of 1.122 years are predictions worse for female than for male patients with a ME of -0.191 and a MAE of 0.951 years.

Using the sex-specific architecture, the accuracy for female patients could be improved from 50.67% to 54.24% and the error rate was reduced from 19.12% to 15.75% but leads on the other hand to an even worse ME of -0.309 and a MAE of 1.180 years. For male patients, the sex-specific training did not lead to an improvement in performance with an accuracy of 55.08% instead of 55.75% and an error rate of 14.97% instead of 15.58%.

For a better understanding of the considered image features, the trained uni-sex architecture was analyzed with Grad-CAM++ [9]. Figure 2 presents two examples of accurate estimates and Figure 3 inaccurate estimates. The focused regions are colored as a heat-map. It is noticeable that those regions do not differ between accurate and inaccurate estimates. In both cases, the area of teeth is mainly focused. The image description also shows the mean of the clinical expert's estimates (CE), in comparison to the automatic estimation (AE). After careful evaluation of the results, it was observed that images of patients whose age was strongly misjudged do not share common characteristics such as poor image quality or conspicuous disease- and patient-specific features. It is particularly noticeable for the inaccurate estimates that the experts similarly

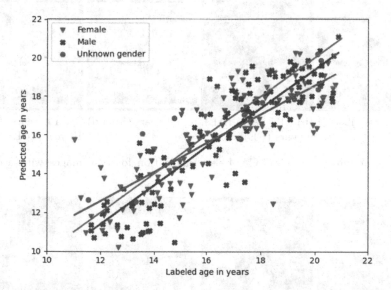

Fig. 1. Accuracy of age estimation on the test data set of the uni-sex regression-based approach depending on sex of the patients. Grey line: linear locations of perfect estimation, blue line: linear regression of estimation for male patients, red line: linear regression of estimation for female patients.

Table 2. Performance comparison between our uni-sex regression-based approach and the clinical evaluation in years on the test data set.

Methods	ME	std	MAE	Accuracy	Error rate
Automatic estimation (uni-sex)	-0.30	±1.41	1.08	54.61%	17.52%
Automatic estimation (sex-specific)	-0.24	±1.39	1.12	54.59%	15.13%
Clinical estimation	0.04	±1.85	1.50	36.17%	30.14%

misjudged the age. Furthermore, they confirmed that forensic experts would also evaluate the areas highlighted by Grad-CAM++ primarily.

Compared to the age estimation by the clinical experts, our uni-sex and sex-specific approaches achieve better results on the test data set as shown in Table 2. A lower MAE, std and error rate were achieved as well as a higher accuracy rate. Our approaches tend to underestimate or overestimate mean age, respectively.

4   Discussion

In this paper, we have shown that regression-based deep learning for CA estimation of adolescents on dental panoramic X-rays achieves better results than

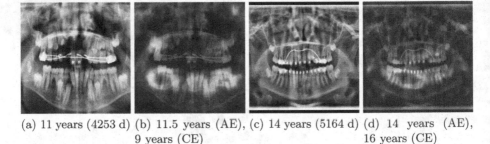

(a) 11 years (4253 d) (b) 11.5 years (AE), (c) 14 years (5164 d) (d) 14 years (AE),
9 years (CE)   16 years (CE)

Fig. 2. Input image and Grad-CAM++ visualization for two images with accurate estimates.

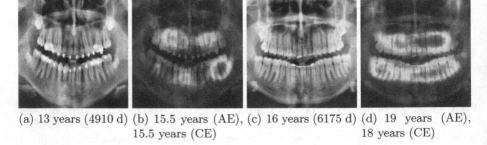

(a) 13 years (4910 d) (b) 15.5 years (AE), (c) 16 years (6175 d) (d) 19 years (AE),
15.5 years (CE)   18 years (CE)

Fig. 3. Input image and Grad-CAM++ visualization for two images with inaccurate estimates.

manual estimation methods conducted by clinical experts. The proportion of severe misjudgments can be reduced by using an architecture that takes the patient's sex as additional input.

The available extensive data set allows training an architecture capable of learning age-specific features without first cropping to relevant areas. This is advantageous compared to related deep learning approaches [6, 7].

The achieved MAE of 1.1 years in the age range of 11 to 20 years is similar to the a MAE of 1.3 years of the multi-factorial approach based on MRI data by Stern et al. [6] considering patients in the age from 13 to 24 years although only the images of one body region were used.

Kahaki et al. [7] introduced a classification algorithm based on X-rays cropped to the molar regions for the age classes 1-4, 5-7, 8-10, 11-13, and 14-17 years with an accuracy of 81.83%. This is outperformed by the error rate of 15.13% of the proposed sex-specific approach which describes the percentage of estimates that differ from the actual age by more than ±2 years. This shows that consideration of the entire dentition and a higher number of images allows age estimation even for older patients, who are therefore more difficult to estimate [2].

The available data set provides extensive data for the age range from 11 to 20 years while the range from 0 to 11 is underrepresented. In future, a representative data set from 0 to 20 years would be desirable to train the network.

References

1. AlQahtani SJ, Hector MP, Liversidge HM. Accuracy of dental age estimation charts: Schour and massler, ubelaker, and the london atlas. Am J Phys Anthropol. 2014;154(1):70–78.
2. Müller N. Zur Altersbestimmung beim Menschen unter besonderer Berücksichtigung der Weisheitszähne. Universität Erlangen-Nürnberg: Dissertation; 1990.
3. AlQahtani SJ, Hector MP, Liversidge HM. The london atlas of human tooth development and eruption. Am J Phys Anthropol. 2010;142(3):481–490.
4. Demirjian A, Goldstein H, Tanner JM. A new system of dental age assessment. Hum Biol. 1973;45(2):211–227.
5. Khorate MM, Dinkar AD, Ahmed J. Accuracy of age estimation methods from orthopantomograph in forensic odontology: A comparative study. Forensic Sci Int. 2013;184.
6. Stern D, Kainz P, et al. Multi-factorial age estimation from skeletal and dental MRI volumes. In: Machine Learning in Med Im. Cham: Springer International; 2017. p. 61–69.
7. Kahaki SMM, Nordin J, et al. Deep convolutional neural network designed for age assessment based on orthopantomography data. In: Neural Computing and Applications. vol. 32. Springer; 2019. p. 9357–9368.
8. He K, Zhang X, Ren S, et al. Deep residual learning for image recognition. Proc IEEE Comput Soc Conf Comput Vis Pattern Recognit. 2015; p. 770–778.
9. Chattopadhyay A, Sarkar A, et al. Grad-CAM++: Improved visual explanations for deep convolutional networks. Proc IEEE Workshop Appl Comput Vis. 2018; p. 839–847.

Multi-modal Unsupervised Domain Adaptation for Deformable Registration Based on Maximum Classifier Discrepancy

Christian N. Kruse[1], Lasse Hansen[1], Mattias P. Heinrich[1]

[1]Institute of Medical Informatics, Lübeck University
christian.kruse@uni-luebeck.de

Abstract. The scarce availability of labeled data makes multi-modal domain adaptation an interesting approach in medical image analysis. Deep learning-based registration methods, however, still struggle to outperform their non-trained counterparts. Supervised domain adaptation also requires labeled- or other ground truth data. Hence, unsupervised domain adaptation is a valuable goal, that has so far mainly shown success in classification tasks. We are the first to report unsupervised domain adaptation for discrete displacement registration using classifier discrepancy in medical imaging. We train our model with mono-modal registration supervision. For cross-modal registration no supervision is required, instead we use the discrepancy between two classifiers as training loss. We also present a new projected Earth Mover's distance for measuring classifier discrepancy. By projecting the 2D distributions to 1D histograms, the EMD L1 distance can be computed using their cumulative sums.

1 Introduction

Labeled 3D medical images in particular for multi-modal scans are rare due to the necessity of expert knowledge and the large time consumption for labeling. However, datasets containing either a large number of landmarks [1] or anatomical labels [2] are required for training deep learning models for automatic image analysis. Unsupervised domain adaptation for multi-modal or multi-domain images allows using labeled data of one domain to be used on other domains thereby reducing the need for expensive expert-labeled data. In computer-vision, classifier discrepancy for unsupervised domain adaptation has been successfully used for classification and segmentation tasks [3]. This approach requires a metric for comparing the output of two classifiers [4]. Different approaches exist for this discrepancy measures, for example, the Earth Mover's distance (EMD) [5] for 1D cases and adaptations for 2D histograms [6]. These approaches are, however, computationally expensive and based on sensitive hyper-parameters.

1.1 Contribution

We are the first to employ unsupervised domain adaptation for medical image registration using a discrete displacement setting. We train our model for mono-modal registration with strong supervision from pre-computed displacement fields. In a next step we use the discrepancy between two classifiers as a training loss to first maximise the discrepancy by updating the classifier weights and then minimising the discrepancy by updating the feature extractor weights. We further improve over the sliced Wasserstein metric [3] using a novel 2D histogram projected Earth Mover's distance. An early proof-of-concept abstract of this approach on only synthetic MR T1/T2 patches and without instance optimization was published in [7].

1.2 Related work

For supervised multi-modal image registration some recent methods include using a Twin CNN-architecture to predict similarity of patches using aligned multi-modal training data [8] and U-Net like registration with anatomical segmentations [2, 9]. In [9] the latter method is extended using a normalized gradient metric. Discrete displacement labeling in deep learning-based registration was proposed in [10] to capture large deformations. In [11] Cycle-GANs were used for unpaired multi-modal segmentation via knowledge distillation. Recently, promising methods for domain adaptation for image classification and multi-modal segmentation have been published in [12].

2 Materials and methods

In this work, we formulate medical image registration as a discrete labelling task to exploit the strengths of domain adaptation for classification tasks. We apply our approach to 2D CT to MR registration using a 21x21 displacement vector resulting in a 441-class classification task.

The training is supervised with pre-computed CT $\rightarrow$ CT and MR $\rightarrow$ MR displacement fields. This pseudo-ground truth was computed using the pdd-net [10]. For the task of registering CT to MR images no supervision is provided.

Our domain adaptation model is shown in Fig. 1: The two input images (240x260 resolution) for registration (fixed and moving image) are first passed to a feature extractor. The feature extractor produces 120x130 feature maps with 24 channels. We then sample a multidimensional tensor from the feature map of the moving image using an identity grid (interpreted as 1D-column vector per image dimension) to which the relative displacement search offsets (interpreted as 1D row vector per image dimension) are added. This yields a resampled feature tensor of size 24x3900x441, where 24 is the number of feature channels, 3900 the number of (downsampled) pixels (quarter resolution: 60x65) and 441 the size of the displacement vector (spatial region of 21×21). This 24x3900x441 feature tensor is then concatenated with the feature map of the fixed image, which is repeated 441 times, and then passed to the classifiers. These classifiers are set up equally except for their random initialization. The classifiers then calculate a smooth metric of both tensors. Each training epoch consists of three steps:

1. train the feature extractor and both classifiers to register CT → CT or MR → MR (in alternating training epochs) with displacement supervision
2. maximise the discrepancy for cross-modal registration between both classifiers while minimising the classification loss for mono-modal registration by only updating the classifier weights.
3. minimise the classifier discrepancy by updating the feature extractor weights

For feature extraction we employ an OBELISK net [13] with 105k weights. The OBELISK net takes a 240x260 pixel input image (CT or MR) and produces a 120x130 (later down-sampled to 60x65) feature map with 24 channels. For discrete displacement labeling we use two classifiers with 5 blocks of Conv2d, InstanceNorm and PReLU with 33k weights per classifier. The classifiers take two 24x3900x441 feature maps and compute a smooth metric of both inputs. We train the model for 3000 epochs with a learning rate of 0.005 for both the feature net optimizer and the classifier optimizer.

The sliced Wasserstein metric [3] is not invariant to histogram bin/ displacement class permutations and, therefore, not ideally suited for measuring the classifier discrepancy in our approach. In our case we can convert the displacement prediction into 2D spatial probability maps for the x- and y-displacements.

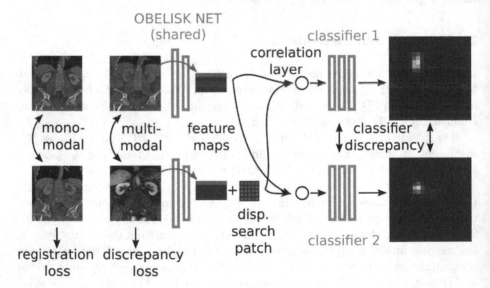

Fig. 1. Domain adaptation approach presented in this work: The model consists of one feature extractor, an OBELISK net, shown in green and two classifiers, shown in red and blue, which yield discrete displacement vectors.

Table 1. Dice scores calculated from 6 labels for different training setups on VISCERAL data. Avg. is the average across all labels. L, S, K and P are the labels for liver, spleen, kidneys and psoas major muscles, respectively, where the two labels each for K and P are averaged.

	CT → CT	MR → MR	CT → MR				
	avg.	avg.	avg.	L	S	K	P
No registration	55.4%	58.4%	50.1%	55.6%	39.6%	48.7%	54.0%
Classifier only	77.9%	75.4%	57.4%	76.1%	57.1%	55.7%	50.1%
Domain adaptation	76.8%	74.6%	62.3%	77.2%	60.4%	61.5%	56.6%

Hence, we propose the new projected Earth Mover's distance (p-EMD) as a discrepancy measure for our approach. The EMD for 1D histograms with linear complexity can be exactly solved [5]. Based on the 2D-histogram displacements being close to mono-modal Gaussians we approximate the optimal transport problem by projecting the normalized histograms to 16 lines rotated between 0 and 90 degrees with bi-linear interpolation. The L1 distance of the different projections then yields the p-EMD, which matches computationally expensive full EMD calculations almost perfectly and is, at least for our experiments, much more stable than the 2D diffusion distance in [6]. As a post-processing step we perform instance optimization using semi-global matching [14] to improve the alignment.

3 Results and discussion

We test our approach on 2D coronal CT and MR slices from the VISCERAL dataset [15]. We have a total of 9 CT and 9 MR unpaired image slices with six labels for the liver, spleen, kidneys and psoas major muscles. We use all data for training and later also test the cross-modal registration from all 9 CT slices to all 9 MR slices. We employ our training method with supervision on CT and MR in alternating training epochs. We set up the displacement vector to cover displacements of up to 40% of the image width. We test our trained

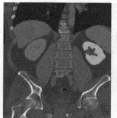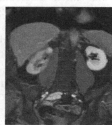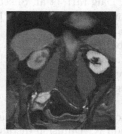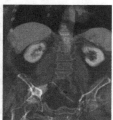

Fig. 2. From left to right: CT image (fixed) with labels for liver (red), spleen (pink), left and right kidney (blue and teal) and left and right psoas major muscle (green and orange), MR image (moving) with CT labels, warped MR image with CT labels and overlay of CT and warped MR image.

model on mono-modal (CT → CT, MR → MR) and multi-modal (CT → MR) registration and compare the resulting label Dice scores (averaged over all labels) with the initial alignment and the registration with the same model setup but trained without any domain adaptation. The results are shown in table 1. We see that both models improve over initial alignment for mono-modal registration and increase Dice scores from about 55% and 58% to about 77% and 75% for CT and MR, respectively. The Dice scores for the individual labels for mono-modal registration were also very similar for both training methods and are therefore not shown here. For the cross-modal registration of 81 pairs we see an improved alignment even for the model trained without domain adaption with an increase from 50.1% to 57.4% in Dice score. Our proposed domain adaption approach increases the Dice score by an additional 4.9% points to 62.3%. The label specific Dice scores for multi-modal registration are also shown in table 1. We see that the liver Dice score is only about 1% higher with domain adaptation. The spleen, kidneys and psoas major muscles however benefit stronger from the domain adaptation with a Dice score increase from 3.3% up to 6.5% This shows the benefit of domain adaptation with maximum classifier discrepancy and projected Earth Mover's distance. Future work will focus on an extension to 3D and applying our approach to other multi-modal registration tasks.

Acknowledgement. This work was in part supported by the German ministry of Education and Research (BMBF) within the project Multi-Task Deep Learning for Large-Scale Multimodal Biomed- ical Image Analysis (MDLMA) FKZ 031L0202B.

References

1. Xiao Y, Rivaz H, Chabanas M, et al. Evaluation of MRI to ultrasound registration methods for brain shift correction: the CuRIOUS2018 challenge. IEEE Trans Med Imaging. 2020 mar;39(3):777–786.
2. Hu Y, Modat M, Gibson E, et al. Weakly-supervised convolutional neural networks for multimodal image registration. Med Image Anal. 2018;49:1–13. Available from: http://www.sciencedirect.com/science/article/pii/S1361841518301051.
3. Lee CY, Batra T, Baig MH, et al. Sliced wasserstein discrepancy for unsupervised domain adaptation. Procs IEEE CVPR. 2019; p. 10277–10287. Available from: http://arxiv.org/abs/1903.04064.
4. Saito K, Watanabe K, Ushiku Y, et al. Maximum classifier discrepancy for unsupervised domain adaptation. Procs IEEE CVPR. 2018; p. 3723–3732. Available from: http://arxiv.org/abs/1712.02560.
5. Werman M, Peleg S, Rosenfeld A. A distance metric for multidimensional histograms. Comp Vis Graph Image Proc. 1985;32(3):328–336. Available from: http://www.sciencedirect.com/science/article/pii/0734189X85900556.
6. Haibin Ling, Okada K. Diffusion distance for histogram comparison. Procs IEEE CVPR. 2006 jun;1:246–253.
7. Heinrich MP, Hansen L. Unsupervised learning of multimodal image registration using domain adaptation with projected earth move's discrepancies. Medical Imaging with Deep Learning. 2020 may;Available from: http://arxiv.org/abs/2005.14107.

8. Simonovsky M, Gutiérrez-Becker B, Mateus D, et al. A deep metric for multimodal registration. Proc MICCAI. 2016; p. 10–18.

9. Hering A, Kuckertz S, Heldmann S, et al. Memory-efficient 2.5D convolutional transformer networks for multi-modal deformable registration with weak label supervision applied to whole-heart CT and MRI scans. Int J Comput Assist Radiol Surg. 2019;14(11):1901–1912. Available from: https://doi.org/10.1007/s11548-019-02068-z.

10. Heinrich MP. Closing the gap between deep and conventional image registration using probabilistic dense displacement networks. Lect Notes Comp Scie. 2019;11769:50–58. Available from: http://arxiv.org/abs/1907.10931.

11. Wolterink JM, Dinkla AM, Savenije MHF, et al. Deep MR to CT synthesis using unpaired data. In: Tsaftaris SA, Gooya A, Frangi AF, et al., editors. Simulation and Synthesis in Medical Imaging. Cham: Springer International Publishing; 2017. p. 14–23.

12. Dou Q, Liu Q, Heng PA, et al. Unpaired multi-modal segmentation via knowledge distillation. IEEE Trans Med Imaging. 2020;39(7):2415–2425.

13. Heinrich MP, Oktay O, Bouteldja N. OBELISK – one kernel to solve nearly everything: unified 3D binary convolutions for image analysis. In: MidlProceedings of the Conference on Medical Imaging with Deep Learning (MIDL). Amsterdam; 2018. p. 9.

14. Hirschmuller H. Accurate and efficient stereo processing by semi-global matching and mutual information. Proc IEEE CVPR. 2005; p. 807–814.

15. Jimenez-del Toro O, Müller H, Krenn M, et al. Cloud-based evaluation of anatomical structure segmentation and landmark detection algorithms: VISCERAL anatomy benchmarks. IEEE Trans Med Imaging. 2016 nov;35(11):2459–2475.

Abstract: A Completely Annotated Whole Slide Image Dataset of Canine Breast Cancer to Aid Human Breast Cancer Research

Marc Aubreville[1,2], Christof A. Bertram[3], Taryn A. Donovan[4],
Christian Marzahl[2], Andreas Maier[2], Robert Klopfleisch[3]

[1]Technische Hochschule Ingolstadt, Ingolstadt, Germany
[2]Pattern Recognition Lab, Friedrich-Alexander-Universität Erlangen-Nürnberg, Germany
[3]Institute of Veterinary Pathology, Freie Universität Berlin, Germany
[4]Department of Anatomic Pathology, Animal Medical Center, New York, USA
marc.aubreville@thi.de

Canine mammary carcinoma (CMC) has been used as a model to investigate the tumorigenesis of human breast cancer and the same histological grading scheme is commonly used to estimate patient outcome for both. One key component of this grading scheme is the density of cells undergoing cell division (mitotic figures, MF). Current publicly available datasets on human breast cancer only provide annotations for small subsets of whole slide images (WSIs). We present a novel dataset[1] of 21 WSIs of CMC completely annotated for MF. For this, a pathologist screened all WSIs for potential MF and structures with a similar appearance. A second expert blindly assigned labels, and for non-matching labels, a third expert assigned the final labels. Additionally, we used machine learning to identify previously undetected MF. Finally, we performed representation learning and two-dimensional projection to further increase the consistency of the annotations. Our dataset consists of 13,907 MF and 36,379 hard negatives. We achieved a mean F1-score of 0.791 on the test set. Testing our algorithms without any further adaptation on a human breast cancer dataset (AMIDA13) yielded a mean F1-score of 0.635. The F1-score increased to 0.696 when using threshold optimization and model selection, and to 0.733 using transfer learning, both on the human tissue training set.

References

1. Aubreville M, Bertram CA, Donovan TA, et al. A completely annotated whole slide image dataset of canine breast cancer to aid human breast cancer research. Scientific Data. 2020;7(417).

Acquisition Parameter-conditioned Magnetic Resonance Image-to-image Translation

Jonas Denck[1,2,3], Jens Guehring[2], Andreas Maier[2], Eva Rothgang[3]

[1]Pattern Recognition Lab, FAU Erlangen-Nürnberg, Erlangen, Germany
[2]Siemens Healthcare GmbH, Erlangen, Germany
[3]Department of Industrial Engineering and Health, Ostbayerische Technische
Hochschule Amberg-Weiden, Weiden, Germany
jonas.denck@fau.de

Abstract. A Magnetic Resonance Imaging (MRI) exam typically consists
of several sequences that yield different image contrasts. Each sequence
is parameterized through a multitude of acquisition parameters that influence image contrast, signal-to-noise ratio, scan time and/or resolution.
Depending on the clinical indication, different contrasts are required by
the radiologist to make a diagnosis. As the acquisition of MR sequences
is time consuming, and acquired images may be corrupted due to motion,
a method to synthesize MR images with fine-tuned contrast settings is
required. We therefore trained an image-to-image generative adversarial
network conditioned on the MR acquisition parameters repetition and
echo time. Our approach is able to synthesize missing MR images with
adjustable MR image contrast and yields a mean absolute error of 0.05,
a peak signal-to-noise ratio of 23.23 dB and structural similarity of 0.78.

1 Introduction

Magnetic Resonance Imaging (MRI) is an important but complex imaging
modality in radiology. An MRI exam typically consists of several MR image
acquisition steps to obtain a set of MR sequences that yield different image
contrasts. The sequence configurations are parameterized through a multitude
of acquisition parameters that influence image contrast, signal-to-noise ratio,
scan time and/or resolution. Depending on the clinical indication, different
contrasts are required by the radiologist to make a reliable diagnosis. Besides
the given clinical indication and imaged body part, the parameterization of
an MR sequence depends on various factors, such as available hardware (1.5T
vs. 3T), clinical guidelines, scan time constraints, and radiologists' preferences.
This leads to large variations in MR sequence configurations across radiology
sites, but also within a single site.

An MRI scan is time consuming, prone to premature scan termination due
to claustrophia of the patient [1] or re-scanning due to motion artefacts [2].
Therefore, methods to shorten scan time or synthesize missing contrasts can
add significant value to MRI.

One possible approach to achieve this is to use artificial intelligence (AI) to synthesize missing contrasts from existing ones. Different approaches for medical image synthesis using generative adversarial networks [3] have already been proposed [4, 5, 6, 7, 8]. However, these approaches are only trained on different categories of MR contrasts (e.g. T1-, T2- or PD-weighted) and cannot synthesize MR images with fine-tuned image contrast. Acquisition parameters influencing the image contrast are e.g. the repetition time (TR) and echo time (TE).

In order to address the variability of sequence parameterizations, we trained an MR image-to-image GAN conditioned on the acquisition parameters TR and TE to enable fine-tuned contrast synthesis for a given MR image.

2   Materials and methods

Our model consists of three networks (Fig. 1): a generator that translates an MR image to a target image contrast, defined by the acquisition parameters TR and TE, a discriminator that learns to distinguish between synthetic and real MR images as well as an auxiliary classifier that is trained to determine the acquisition parameters TR and TE from the image itself.

The generator is based on a U-Net architecture [9] with residual blocks [10]. The acquisition parameters of the source and target contrast are normalized to values between 0 and 1 and injected into the generator through an adaptive instance normalization layer (AdaIN) [11]. The discriminator learns to distin-

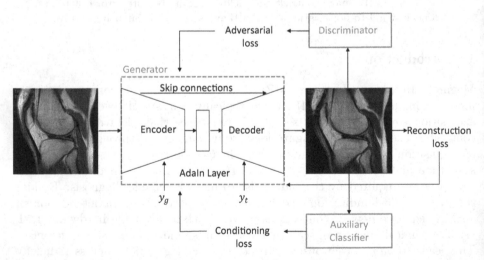

Fig. 1. Training procedure of our approach: The generator receives a real input image (left image), including its acquisition parameters TR and TE (y_g) as well as the target acquisition parameters (y_t) and translates the image to the synthesized target contrast (right image). The discriminator learns to distinguish between real and synthetic MR images, and the auxiliary classifier is pre-trained to determine the acquisition parameters from the image.

guish between real and synthetic MR images only, while the auxiliary classifier is pre-trained to determine the acquisition parameters from the image.

We use a non-saturating adversarial loss with R1 regularization [12], combined with a reconstruction and conditioning loss to train the GAN. The reconstruction loss is given by the L1-loss of the predicted and target image, if a target image is available, and by the cycle consistency loss [13], if no target image is available. The mean squared error between predicted and target acquisition parameters is used as conditioning loss.

For training and validation, we used the clinical part of the fastMRI dataset [14] containing knee MR images from different MR scanners with different sequence parameterizations. We used the DICOM images from the image series without fat saturation from 1.5 T Siemens scanners (Siemens Healthcare, Erlangen, Germany). After applying several data filters, this results in a dataset of 67,956 MR images (2,114 paired and 65,842 unpaired images) of which 60 unique DICOM studies (1,022 images) are used for testing and the rest for training (66,934 images).

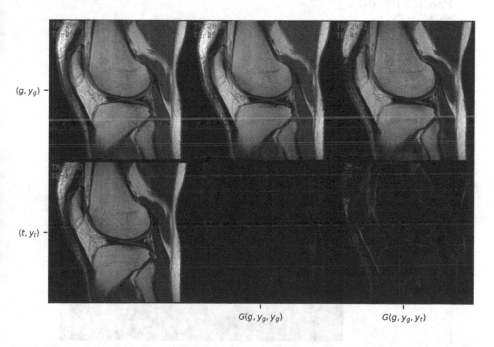

Fig. 2. Example of two paired MR images with different acquisition parameters including their synthesized images. The first column shows the real image g with acquisition parameters y_g (top) and the real target image pair t with acquisition parameters y_t (bottom). The second column shows the result and the absolute error map, when synthesizing image g with the generator G, and the third column shows the result of the image synthesis of image t. The image annotations show the real (first column) and predicted TR and TE values.

3   Results

The auxiliary classifier reached a mean absolute error of 247 ms for the determination of TR and 1.8 ms for TE on the test set, respectively. Thus, it is able
to reliably guide the training of the generator to produce MR images with the
correct image contrast.

Besides visual assessment (Fig. 2 and 3), we computed the mean absolute
error (MAE), peak signal-to-noise ratio (PSNR), and the structural similarity
(SSIM) index [15] to measure both pixel-wise intensity differences and structural
similarities between reconstructed and reference images.

The performance metrics were computed on the test set with cyclic reconstruction and randomly selected acquisition parameters, since slice pairs were
not available for all test images. Our approach reached the following MAE,
PSNR and SSIM values:

- MAE: 0.05
- PSNR: 23.23 dB
- SSIM: 0.78

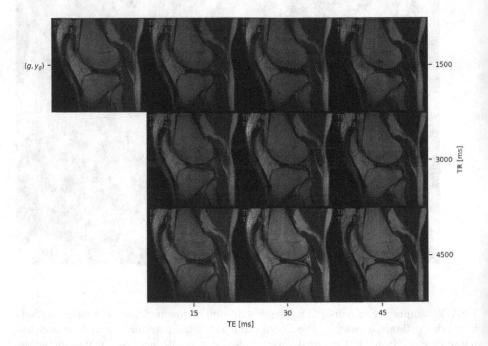

Fig. 3. Example of acquisition parameter interpolation for a given real image g with
acquisition parameters y_g (first column). The image grid shows the synthesized images
with varying acquisition parameters in the TE intervals [15, 30, 45] ms and TR intervals
[1500, 3000, 4500] ms including their predicted TR and TE values.

4 Discussion

The generator is able to produce realistic and sharp MR images that also show fine anatomical structures within the image. Although several approaches have already been published that apply image-to-image GANs to synthesize MR image contrasts, these results are difficult to compare due to the fact that our presented approach is the first to condition the contrast translation of MR images on acquisition parameters and not only on different categories of contrasts. Moreover, a different dataset (including body regions trained on) was used in our work, since the recently published fastMRI dataset offers the required image contrast variations. However, the reported performance metrics are comparable to reference literature [4, 5, 6, 7], demonstrating the potential of our presented approach.

One limitation of the dataset is that it only contains different parameterizations of PD-weighted MR images. Consequently, the network is not able to translate an existing image into a T1- or T2-weighted MR image as it has not been trained on such. However, it is anticipated that the approach is transferable to a wider range of acquisition parameters given a proper dataset. A limitation of the cycle consistency loss is that it may hallucinate features in the generated images [16]. Consequently, a reader study must evaluate the diagnostic value of the synthesized MR images.

This work has the potential to synthesize missing or replace corrupted contrasts and therefore is anticipated to reduce the duration of an MRI exam.

In future work, we aim at extending the capabilities of the network on additional acquisition parameters (e.g. scan options such as fat-saturation) and evaluate the work on data with additional body regions.

Acknowledgement. This work is supported by the Bavarian Academic Forum (BayWISS)—Doctoral Consortium "Health Research", funded by the Bavarian State Ministry of Science and the Arts.

References

1. Munn Z, Moola S, Lisy K, et al. Claustrophobia in magnetic resonance imaging: a systematic review and meta-analysis. Radiography. 2015 May;21(2):e59–e63.
2. Andre JB, Bresnahan BW, Mossa-Basha M, et al. Toward quantifying the prevalence, severity, and cost associated with patient motion during clinical MR examinations. J Am Coll Radiol. 2015 Jul;12(7):689–695.
3. Goodfellow I, Pouget-Abadie J, Mirza M, et al. Generative adversarial nets. In: Adv Neural Inf Process Syst; 2014. p. 2672–2680.
4. Yu B, Zhou L, Wang L, et al. Ea-GANs: Edge-aware generative adversarial networks for cross-modality MR image synthesis. IEEE Trans Med Imaging. 2019 Jul;38(7):1750–1762.
5. Sharma A, Hamarneh G. Missing MRI pulse sequence synthesis using multi-modal generative adversarial network. IEEE Trans Med Imaging. 2020 Apr;39(4):1170–1183.

6. Zhou T, Fu H, Chen G, et al. Hi-Net: hybrid-fusion network for multi-modal MR image synthesis. IEEE Trans Med Imaging. 2020 Sep;39(9):2772–2781.
7. Wang G, Gong E, Banerjee S, et al. Synthesize high-quality multi-contrast magnetic resonance imaging from multi-echo acquisition using multi-task deep generative model. IEEE Trans Med Imaging. 2020 Oct;39(10):3089–3099.
8. Stimpel B, Syben C, Würfl T, et al. Projection-to-projection translation for hybrid X-ray and magnetic resonance imaging. Sci Rep. 2019 Dec;9(1).
9. Ronneberger O, Fischer P, Brox T. U-net: convolutional networks for biomedical image segmentation. MICCAI. 2015; p. 234–241.
10. He K, Zhang X, Ren S, et al. Deep residual learning for image recognition. In: Proc IEEE CVPR; 2016. p. 770–778.
11. Huang X, Belongie S. Arbitrary style transfer in real-time with adaptive instance normalization. In: Proc IEEE ICCV. IEEE; 2017. p. 1501–1510.
12. Lucic M, Kurach K, Michalski M, et al. Are GANs created equal? A large-scale study. In: Adv Neural Inf Process Syst. NIPS'18. Red Hook, NY, USA: Curran Associates Inc; 2018. p. 698–707.
13. Zhu JY, Park T, Isola P, et al. Unpaired image-to-image translation using cycle-consistent adversarial networks. Proc IEEE ICCV. 2017; p. 2223–2232.
14. Zbontar J, Knoll F, Sriram A, et al. fastMRI: an open dataset and benchmarks for accelerated MRI. arXiv preprint arXiv:181108839. 2018;.
15. Wang Z, Bovik AC, Sheikh HR, et al. Image quality assessment: from error visibility to structural similarity. IEEE Trans Image Process. 2004 Apr;13(4):600–612.
16. Cohen JP, Luck M, Honari S. Distribution matching losses can hallucinate features in medical image translation. MICCAI. 2015; p. 234–241.

Fine-tuning Generative Adversarial Networks using Metaheuristics

A Case Study on Barrett's Esophagus Identification

Luis A. Souza[1,2], Leandro A. Passos[3], Robert Mendel[2], Alanna Ebigbo[4],
Andreas Probst[4], Helmut Messmann[4], Christoph Palm[2,5], João P. Papa[3]

[1]Department of Computing, São Carlos Federal University - UFSCar, Brazil
[2]Regensburg Medical Image Computing (ReMIC), Ostbayerische Technische
Hochschule Regensburg (OTH Regensburg) - Germany
[3]Department of Computing, São Paulo State University - UNESP, Brazil
[4]Department of Gastroenterology, University Hospital Augsburg - Germany
[5]Regensburg Center of Health Sciences and Technology (RCHST), OTH Regensburg
- Germany
luis.souza@dc.ufscar.br

Abstract. Barrett's esophagus denotes a disorder in the digestive system
that affects the esophagus' mucosal cells, causing reflux, and showing
potential convergence to esophageal adenocarcinoma if not treated in
initial stages. Thus, fast and reliable computer-aided diagnosis becomes
considerably welcome. Nevertheless, such approaches usually suffer from
imbalanced datasets, which can be addressed through Generative Adversarial Networks (GANs). Such techniques generate realistic images based
on observed samples, even though at the cost of a proper selection of its
hyperparameters. Many works employed a class of nature-inspired algorithms called metaheuristics to tackle the problem considering distinct
deep learning approaches. Therefore, this paper's main contribution is to
introduce metaheuristic techniques to fine-tune GANs in the context of
Barrett's esophagus identification, as well as to investigate the feasibility of generating high-quality synthetic images for early-cancer assisted
identification.

1 Introduction

Barrett's esophagus (BE) is a dangerous condition in which the mucosal cells of
the lower part of the esophagus changes due to chronic gastrointestinal reflux,
and may progress into esophageal adenocarcinoma [1]. Computer-aided analysis of Barrett's esophagus and adenocarcinoma has been subjected to intensive
research in the past years using both handcrafted features from endoscopic images, as well as the application of Convolutional Neural Networks (CNN) for
automatic identification. Some examples can be observed in recent works of
Souza Jr. et al. [1], van der Sommen [2] and Passos et al. [3].

© Der/die Autor(en), exklusiv lizenziert durch
Springer Fachmedien Wiesbaden GmbH, ein Teil von Springer Nature 2021
C. Palm et al. (Hrsg.), *Bildverarbeitung für die Medizin 2021*,
Informatik aktuell, https://doi.org/10.1007/978-3-658-33198-6_50

A usual drawback, the limited amount of data, restricts the development and validation of more effective methods to detect early-stage illness in medical applications. Recently, such a bottleneck has been coped through data augmentation (DA) techniques. In this context, Generative Adversarial Networks (GAN) [4] have presented significant improvements in image generation, with highlights for medical imaging [5, 6]. GAN's primary idea is to train a generator and a discriminator simultaneously, aiming to generate convincing and high-quality synthetic images.

One of the main hindrances regarding GANs and most modern deep learning approaches concerns a proper selection of their hyperparameters since they pose a significant influence in the model's final output. Several works addressed a similar problem through metaheuristic optimization techniques [3]. Metaheuristic approaches refer to stochastic nature-inspired methods that mimic some natural behavior observed in groups of animals, social conduct, among others, to solve complex problems. The paradigm obtained notorious popularity due to positive results in a wide variety of applications.

As far as we know, there is no work addressing the use of metaheuristic techniques to optimize the GAN hyperparameters itself. Therefore, the main contributions of this work are three-fold: (i) to introduce metaheuristic optimization algorithms in the context of GAN hyperparameter optimization; (ii) to investigate the feasibility of using GAN parameter optimization to generate high-quality synthetic images for further assisting the identification of Barrett's esophagus and adenocarcinoma; and (iii) to evaluate whether it makes sense to perform such parameter optimization of image generation for further data augmentation and classification purposes.

2   Materials and methods

The GAN training procedure demands the user an appropriate selection of the network hyperparameters, which poses a far from straightforward task due to the context-dependence and the sensitivity related to the selected values. To cope with such an issue, this work proposes employing nature-inspired metaheuristic optimization techniques to fine-tune a set of five main hyperparameters $\theta = \{\eta, \beta_1, ngf, ndf, batch\ size\}$ considering a pre-defined range, described as follows: the learning rate $\eta \in [0.0001, 0.001]$, the Adam optimizer decay control $\beta_1 \in [0.002, 0.5]$, the $ngf \in [1, 128]$ and the $ndf \in [1, 128]$, which are related to the generator and discriminator feature map depths, respectively, and the $batch\ size \in [1, 128]$.

The main idea behind metaheuristic optimization techniques consists of stochastically initializing a set of random solutions, and iteratively evolving towards the solution whose decision variables best fit a target objective, i.e., minimizing the quadratic difference between generator and discriminator losses. The pipeline employed to perform GAN hyperparameter fine-tuning is depicted in Fig. 1. In a nutshell, the optimization technique selects the set of hyperparameters that minimize the loss function over the training set considering an augmented dataset composed of endoscopy images and synthetic images generated during the process.

The following metaheuristic techniques from [3] are considered:

- BSA: Backtracking Search Optimization is an evolutionary algorithm that combines stored memories with crossover and mutation operations to generate new individuals.
- BSO: Brain Storm Optimization is a swarm-based optimization technique inspired by the creative human brainstorming process.
- FA: Firefly Algorithm tries to mimic the fireflies' behavior while searching for mating partners and preys.
- FPA: Flower Pollination Algorithm is a swarm-based optimization method that mimics the pollination process of flowering plants.
- JADE [3]: a differential evolution-based algorithm that implements the "DE/current-to-p-best" mutation strategy.

3 Results

This section briefly describes the datasets used in this work and the setup employed during the experiments.

3.1 Datasets

Two white-light endoscopic datasets were used for an in-depth analysis concerning the robustness of the proposed approach. The first one, provided at the "MICCAI 2015 EndoVis Challenge (MICCAI), comprises 100 lower esophagus endoscopic images captured from 39 individuals, 22 of them being diagnosed with Barrett's esophagus (BE), and 17 showing early-stage signs of esophageal adenocarcinoma (AD). Five different experts have individually delineated suspicious regions observed in the cancerous images.

The second dataset used for the experiments was provided by the Augsburg Hospital University and it is composed of 76 endoscopic images captured from different patients with BE (42 samples) and early AD (34 samples). The cancerous images were manually annotated by one expert. The annotations provided

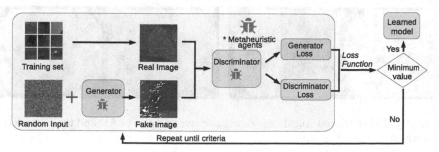

Fig. 1. Proposed approach to encode the decision variables of each optimization agent.

by the experts were considered for the patch label definition for both datasets. Fig. 2 (a) and (b) depicts some positive samples of the MICCAI and the Augsburg datasets.

3.2 Experimental setup

Regarding the pre-processing step, the images were split into patches [1]. The idea is to cover the entire image with a sliding window of 200 × 200 pixels and overlapping of 50 pixels in horizontal and vertical directions. The label of each patch was based on the expert annotations of the full-images.

To obtain the best parameters for each dataset and class, the metaheuristic techniques were run for 40 epochs. For the data augmentation evaluation, experiments were conducted over 12,000 epochs, generating 525 synthetic samples at every 2,000 iterations, for each sample class (AD and BE) using the best parameters obtained in the metaheuristic experimental design. The output sample amount was related to computational limitations. We employed two different strategies to sample the synthetic images: (i) the last batch during learning, and (ii) the five last batches. The statical analysis was conducted using the Wilcoxon signed-rank test with confidence level of 5% [7].

After performing data augmentation, 80% of the new dataset was randomly selected for training purposes, and the remaining 20% was used for the testing. Such a partitioning was conducted over 20 runs for more robust evaluation. For the classification step, we employed two CNN architectures pre-trained with the ImageNet dataset: LeNet-5 and AlexNet, also running for 12,000 epochs.

3.3 Optimization results

The metaheuristic results for the hyperparameters fine-tuning can be observed in Tab. 1. The best results for MICCAI dataset (closest to 0) were obtained using BSA and FA, for AD and BE diagnosed patches, respectively, with values of 0.0033 and 0.0010. Regarding the Augsburg metaheuristic fine-tuning, best results were achieved, respectively, for AD and BE, using FA and BSA, with values of 0.0025 and 0.0011. Fine-tuned synthetic samples can be observed in Figure 3.

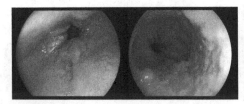 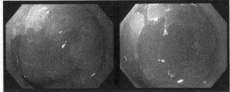

Fig. 2. MICCAI (left) and Augsburg (right) positive samples to AD and their respective delineations.

Table 1. Mean loss value and time consumption considering MICCAI and Augsburg datasets.

Dataset	Diagnosis	Metric	BSA	BSO	FA	FPA	JADE	RANDOM
MICCAI	AD	Loss	0.0033	0.0056	0.0046	0.0037	0.0057	0.0310
		Time(h)	2.9238	2.7872	3.7210	3.7254	3.4264	1.0706
	BE	Loss	0.0045	0.0029	0.0010	0.0011	0.0018	0.0034
		Time(h)	13.6447	15.1997	16.1333	14.6826	10.8849	4.8940
Augsburg	AD	Loss	0.0049	0.0074	0.0025	0.0140	0.0053	0.0129
		Time(h)	2.8345	2.5835	2.1745	4.0850	2.4363	0.6976
	BE	Loss	0.0011	0.0045	0.0036	0.0057	0.0105	0.0051
		Time(h)	8.6632	8.7128	8.7699	9.9796	9.3854	2.6029

3.4 Classification results

Regarding the classification performed after the data augmentation step, one can observe the results in Table 2. Concerning MICCAI dataset, the best classification rates were obtained using BSA and FA data augmentation for AD and BE patches, respectively, with a value of 0.93 using LeNet-5 architecture and "5-last" augmentation protocol. For the Augsburg dataset classification, the best results were achieved, respectively, for AD and BE, using FA and BSA parameters, with an accuracy of 0.90 also using LeNet-5 and "5-last" augmentation protocol. The Wilcoxon test revealed statistical simmilarity for MICCAI classification results for both LeNet-5 and AlexNet architectures. The augmented dataset results using fine-tuned GAN outperformed the other experimental delineations.

4 Discussion

This paper dealt with computer-assisted Barrett's esophagus and adenocarcinoma identification through GAN-fine-tuned data augmentation and CNNs as feature extractors. The GAN hyperparameter fine-tuning showed promising

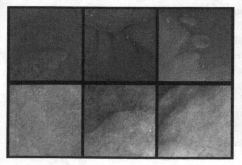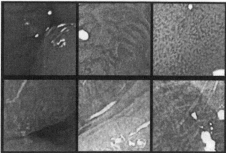

Fig. 3. MICCAI (left) and Augsburg (right) dataset experiments using patches: original (top) and synthetic (bottom) images.

210   Souza et al.

Table 2. Accuracy results considering MICCAI and Augsburg datasets taking different kinds of augmentation into account.

Dataset	AD param.	BE param.	No aug.		Standard Aug.		Last GAN-aug.		5-last GAN-aug.	
			Le-5	Alex	Le-5	Alex	Le-5	Alex	Le-5	Alex
MICCAI	BSA	FA	0.81	0.82	0.83	0.83	0.89	0.88	⋆ **0.93**	**0.91**
Augsburg	FA	BSA	0.73	0.73	0.75	0.83	0.88	0.87	0.90	0.86

classification results after the data augmentation step, outperforming the classification rates of original and standard augmented datasets. Regarding the fine-tuning process, FA and BSA provided the best results for both datasets, suggesting the best performance for BE and adenocarcinoma high-quality and trustworthy sample generation for classification purposes. Such procedures provided improvements compared to previous works, suggesting the importance of enough data and CNN generalization ability to deal with BE and adenocarcinoma distinction problem. In regard of future works, we intend to evaluate fine-tuned GAN to generate full-image samples, aiming to reinforce the impact of the best hyperparameter selection in the synthetic image generation quality.

Acknowledgement. The authors thank Capes/Alexander von Humboldt Foundation grant number BEX 0581-16-0, CNPq grants 306166/2014-3 and 307066/2017-7, as well as FAPESP grants 2013/07375-0, 2014/12236-1, and 2016/19403-6, 2017/04847-9 and 2019/08605-5.

References

1. Souza Jr LA, Palm C, Mendel R, et al. A survey on Barrett's esophagus analysis using machine learning. Comput Biol Med. 2018;96:203 – 213.
2. van der Sommen F, Zinger S, Curvers WL, et al. Computer-aided detection of early neoplastic lesions in Barret's esophagus. Endoscopy. 2016;68:617–624.
3. Passos LA, Souza Jr LA, Mendel R, et al. Barrett's esophagus analysis using infinity restricted Boltzmann machines. J Vis Commun Image Represent. 2019;59:475 – 485.
4. Goodfellow I, Pouget-Abadie J, Mirza M, et al. Generative adversarial nets. In: Ghahramani Z, Welling M, Cortes C, et al., editors. Advances in Neural Information Processing Systems 27. Curran Associates, Inc.; 2014. p. 2672–2680.
5. Souza Jr LA, Passos LA, Mendel R, et al. Assisting Barrett's esophagus identification using endoscopic data augmentation based on generative adversarial networks. Comput Biol Med. 2020; p. 104029.
6. Han C, Murao K, Satoh S, et al. Learning more with less: GAN-based medical image augmentation. CoRR. 2019;abs/1904.00838.
7. Wilcoxon F. Individual comparisons by ranking methods. Biometrics Bulletin. 1945;1(6):80–83.

Neural Networks with Fixed Binary Random Projections Improve Accuracy in Classifying Noisy Data

Zijin Yang[1], Achim Schilling[2], Andreas Maier[1], Patrick Krauss[2]

[1]Pattern Recognition Lab, FAU Erlangen-Nürnberg
[2]Neuroscience Lab, University Hospital Erlangen
michael.yang@fau.de

Abstract. The trend of Artificial Neural Networks becoming "bigger" and "deeper" persists. Training these networks using back-propagation is considered biologically implausible and a time-consuming task. Hence, we investigate how far we can go with fixed binary random projections (BRPs), an approach which reduces the number of trainable parameters using localized receptive fields and binary weights. Evaluating this approach on the MNIST dataset we discovered that contrary to models with fully-trained dense weights, models using fixed localized sparse BRPs yield equally good performance in terms of accuracy, saving 98% computations when generating the hidden representation for the input. Furthermore, we discovered that using BRPs leads to a more robust performance – up to 56% better compared to dense models – in terms of classifying noisy inputs.

1 Introduction

In recent years, algorithms of artificial intelligence (AI) and machine learning (ML) have undergone significant improvements, enabling machines to automatically perform tasks such as semantic analysis of images or language patterns with high accuracy and reliability. To increase the performance of artificial neural networks (ANN), which are a major part of this development, the model architecture tends to become more complex by using a large number of parameters and hidden layers [1]. These "deep" architectures allow for a broad spectrum of different network topologies with various numbers of hidden neurons, hidden layers, parameters configurations, or optimization strategies. As a result, it is increasingly hard to train these networks and to find a suitable hyper-parameter configuration for the task at hand.

As we all have experienced, the human visual system can effortlessly make sense of a novel scene even if the salient patterns are heavily altered (e.g. recognizing humans by their reflections in a strongly distorted mirror). This is possible as the human visual system is capable to generalize across different levels of

C. Palm et al. (Hrsg.), *Bildverarbeitung für die Medizin 2021*,
Informatik aktuell, https://doi.org/10.1007/978-3-658-33198-6_51

image manipulations such as contrast reduction, additive noise, or novel eidolon-distortions. However, ANN algorithms are typically very sensitive to these kind of image characteristics. Consider following example: A properly configured ResNet-152 [2] trained on standard color images and tested on a similar test distribution performs close to or even surpasses human observer performance [3]. Introducing the same type of noise in both training and testing datasets does not interfere with the performance of the network. However, if the network is trained on images with e.g. salt-and-pepper noise and tested on images with e.g. uniform noise, the performance is at chance level, even though both noise types do not seem much different to human observers [3]. Since such changes deep in the human brain are poorly understood, drawing inspirations from artificial neural networks has become a way to "unlock" the world of organisms [4].

Dasgupta et al. have presented a neural algorithm derived from the biological structure of fruit flies' olfactory system [5]. The fruit fly's brain has an elegant and efficient way of performing similarity searches. Unlike the common locality-sensitive hashing methods, which reduce the dimension of the input item and assign short "hashes" to each item such that similar items are more likely to be assigned to same or similar hash tag, the fruit fly brain expands the dimension. The brain then stores only 5 % of the expanded neurons with top activity as the hash tag for that odor [5]. Only a limited number of hash length – the percentage of the neurons with top activity that stored by the system – was investigated and the relationship between the length of the hash and the size of the projections is still unclear.

The main goal of this work is to apply this concept in the form of fixed BRPs [5] and localized connectivity [6] to neural networks. With this we hope to reduce training time while preserving the same performance and having a more generalized model. To investigate whether this approach can mimic the process of biological visual systems, experiments are performed by training the models on clear images and testing on noisy images.

2   Material and methods

2.1   Model

An illustration of the basic concept of this work is depicted in Fig. 1. The first step is to normalize the input image by converting the pixel intensities from range $[0, 255]$ to range $[0, 1]$. Z-score normalization is not necessary because all the pixels are in the same intensity range i. e. the values have equal contribution. The rescaling of the input is not necessary but encouraged to improve time efficiency.

The second step is to project the inputs to the hidden layer using sparse, binary random weights (either one or zero) with localized receptive fields (Fig. 1). Theoretically, if the number of hidden neurons is infinite, we can have an infinite large amount of different filter kernels (localized receptive fields) to project the patches from the input to the hidden layers. Thus, we can have activations for all possible patterns. A fruit fly projects 50 projection neurons (PNs) to 2000 Kenyon cells (KCs), which is a 40-fold expansion of neurons [5]. Likewise, the number of hidden neurons is a multiple-fold expansion of the input neurons which contains 784 neurons, due to the image size of 28 × 28.

The third step is the Winner-Takes-All procedure (Fig. 1, 3rd step). A fraction i. e. $a\%$ of the highest-activating neurons remain activated and the rest of the neurons are inhibited i. e. set to zero. a here is the hash length which indicates the number of the activated neurons. With the increase in neurons in the hidden layer, not all neurons contain meaningful information. Since the filters are generated in a random manner, those "nonsense" filters, which are not correlated to the actual pattern of the input, would generate low values in the hidden layer. Based on the choice of hash-length a, the Winner-Takes-All procedure can assign different input into different "Tags", which are better separable in higher-dimensional space.

The final step is to train a classifier i. e. a fully connected layer as a read-out layer for the generated "Tags" to actually classify (Fig. 1, 4th step). Weights for this layer are initialized using He et al. initialization [7] and are trained using back-propagation.

2.2 Dataset

To further investigate the capability of BRPs, MNIST images with additive Gaussian noise are generated for test purpose. Additive Gaussian noise is generated by randomly drawing numbers from a Gaussian distribution as follow to avoid negative values

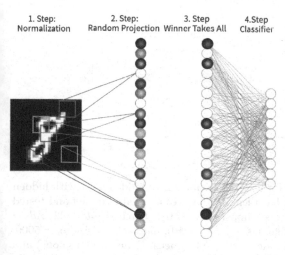

1. Step: Normalization   2. Step: Random Projection   3. Step Winner Takes All   4.Step Classifier

Fig. 1. An illustration of the basic neural network. Left column: an input image from the MNIST data set with five localized receptive fields selected by randomly chosen pixel center, respectively. Middle left column: the hidden layer of the basic network. It consists of hidden neurons with different intensities. Middle right column: the same hidden layer but only 20% of the neurons with higher activations are still activating and the remaining 80% are inhibited. Right column: the output layer with 10 output neurons, indicating 10 target classes. Darker circles indicate higher activations while white circles indicate inhibition.

$$\mathcal{N}'_{i,j} = I \cdot \frac{\mathcal{N}^*_{i,j}}{2} \tag{1}$$

$$\mathcal{N}^*_{i,j} \sim \mathcal{N}(2,1) \tag{2}$$

where $\mathcal{N}'_{i,j}$ denotes the noise added to the original image at position (i,j), I denotes the noise intensity, $\mathcal{N}^*_{i,j}$ is the basic noise value generated by a Gaussian distribution. Test results are shown in Fig.3 where all models are trained on 12000 original MNIST images and tested on images with different noise intensities. Each noise intensity contains 2000 images with the same level of additive Gaussian noise.

3   Results

Models with proper parameter settings using fixed BRPs yield almost the same level of performance as a fully-connected and fully trained network with the same hidden layer size (Fig. 2). The curve has shown that a hash length in the range of $(5\%, 30\%)$ leads to similar high-performance (at around 95%). As the hash length increases, the performance first slowly decreases (from 35% to 60%), then

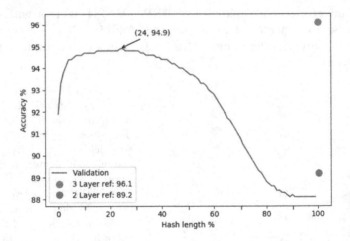

Fig. 2. Average validation accuracy for a model with a single hidden layer with hidden layer size $n_h = 5000$, dependent on hash length (%) over 50 trials, trained and tested on MNIST without noise. Parameters: drop rate $d = 0.9$, batch size $b = 32$, *Adam* optimizer, learning rate $lr = 0.001$, patch size $p = (10, 10)$, hidden layer size $n_h = 5000$. Each model is taken from the best model during 200 epochs. Orange dot(top one) and green dot(bottom one) on the right side of the figure indicate 3 layer reference i. e fully connected and fully trained single hidden layer network with the same hidden layer size $n_h = 5000$, and 2 layer reference i. e a fully trained network directly propagate from input layer to output layer with no hidden layer, respectively.

dramatically decreases(from 60% to 85%), and then remains relatively constant (around 88%).

As can be seen in Fig. 3, models using fixed BRPs start at almost the same accuracy compared to the reference model where each layer is fully connected with the next layer and fully trained. As the noise intensity increases, the difference between the performance in terms of accuracy of both BRPs and Ref models becomes more apparent. All results suggest that using BRPs leads to more robust performance in terms of classifying noisy images.

For the cost of the computations, 90% of the weights between the localized input layer and hidden layer are zero. The number of multiplication operations here with localized receptive fields are reduced by 98%. The remaining 2% of the weights are all ones, therefore a floating point matrix multiplication is "converted" to accumulations, which further reduce the computational cost. Furthermore, the parameters needed to be trained are greatly reduced by fixation of the weights between input layer and hidden layer, leading to a reduction of the training time.

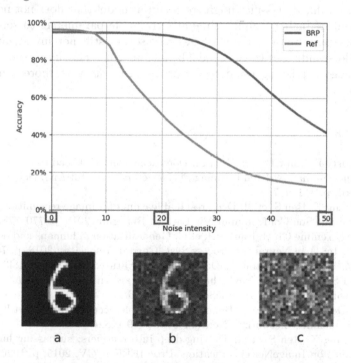

Fig. 3. Test accuracy on noisy images. BRP: model with a single hidden layer with BRPs where only the weights from the readout layer are trained. Ref: a fully-connected and fully trained reference model with the same architecture. Hidden layer size $n_h = 5000$. Image a, b and c: image with zero noise intensity, a noise intensity of 20 and a noisy intensity of 50, respectively. Training parameters are described as in the caption of Fig 2

4 Discussion

In this work we analyze the impact of the use of binary random projections on either the noise robustness and efficiency of neural networks. This analysis leads to the following conclusions: an artificial neural network does not need to be fully trained. Networks using localized receptive fields and fixed BRPs perform equally well compared to networks with all-to-all trained connectivity. This method helps to reduce a large amount of trainable parameters and training time while preserving the performance on the task and improving the ability of being noise-invariant, allowing memory and computational benefits.

As certain steps have not be covered in the frame for this work, the following denotes suggestions for further work on this topic. It is suggested to further test the performance of BRPs for convolutional neural networks. With enough differently initialized kernels, it is possible to achieve the same performance as a fully trained model. Furthermore, as investigated by Hoffer et al. a classifier can be fixed with little to none loss of accuracy for most tasks [8]. The combination of BRPs and a fixed classifier might result in a model that does not need to be trained at all, reducing training time and trainable parameters to zero. Other type of noise e. g Impulse noise, Poisson noise are still not investigated. For further understanding of the method's behaviour when classifying different type of noisy images, it is suggested to perform more tests with more complicated architectures.

References

1. Chakraborty B, Shaw B, Aich J, et al. Does deeper network lead to better accuracy: a case study on handwritten Devanagari characters. Proc Int Anal Doc Syst (DAS). 2018 April; p. 411–417.
2. He K, Zhang X, Ren S, et al. Deep residual learning for image recognition. In: Proc IEEE Comput Soc Conf Comput Vis Pattern Recognit; 2016. p. 770–778.
3. Geirhos R, Temme CRM, Rauber J, et al. Generalisation in humans and deep neural networks. In: Adv Neural Inf Process Syst. Curran Associates; 2018. p. 7538–7550.
4. LeCun Y, Bengio Y, Hinton G. Deep learning. Nature. 2015 May;521:436–444.
5. Dasgupta S, Stevens CF, Navlakha S. A neural algorithm for a fundamental computing problem. Science. 2017;358(6364):793–796.
6. Illing B, Gerstner W, Brea J. Biologically plausible deep learning - But how far can we go with shallow networks? Neural Netw. 2019;118:90–101.
7. He K, Zhang X, Ren S, et al. Delving deep into rectifiers: surpassing human-level performance on ImageNet classification. Proc IEEE ICCV. 2015; p. 1026–1034.
8. Hoffer E, Hubara I, Soudry D. Fix your classifier: the marginal value of training the last weight layer. Proc Conf Learn Represent. 2018; p. 5145–5153.

M3d-CAM

A PyTorch Library to Generate 3D Attention Maps for Medical Deep Learning

Karol Gotkowski[1], Camila Gonzalez[1], Andreas Bucher[2],
Anirban Mukhopadhyay[1]

[1]Graphisch-Interaktive Systeme, Technical university of Darmstadt
[2]Institut für Diagnostische und Interventionelle Radiologie, Universitätsklinikum
Frankfurt
karolgotkowski@gmx.de

Abstract. Deep learning models achieve state-of-the-art results in a wide array of medical imaging problems. Yet the lack of interpretability of deep neural networks is a primary concern for medical practitioners and poses a considerable barrier before the deployment of such models in clinical practice. Several techniques have been developed for visualizing the decision process of DNNs. However, few implementations are openly available for the popular PyTorch library, and existing implementations are often limited to two-dimensional data and classification models. We present M3d-CAM, an easy easy to use library for generating attention maps of CNN-based PyTorch models for both 2D and 3D data, and applicable to both classification and segmentation models. The attention maps can be generated with multiple methods: Guided Backpropagation, Grad-CAM, Guided Grad-CAM and Grad-CAM++. The maps visualize the regions in the input data that most heavily influence the model prediction at a certain layer. Only a single line of code is sufficient for generating attention maps for a model, making M3d-CAM a plug-and-play solution that requires minimal previous knowledge.

1 Introduction

Deep learning has become a central focus of medical image computing. Yet the lack of interpretability and black-box internal workings of deep neural networks, believed by many to be a primary drawback of deep learning methods [1, 2], is of particular concern in the medical field. Within the clinical routine, deep learning models would most likely act as decision support systems for practitioners. Such a system would only be used insofar it is trusted by the practitioner and he or she can follow the decision process. Fortunately, significant progress has been made in the development of interpretability techniques [3]. For image data, the generation of attention maps, that show which input regions network layers consider when making a prediction, are highly popular.

© Der/die Autor(en), exklusiv lizenziert durch
Springer Fachmedien Wiesbaden GmbH, ein Teil von Springer Nature 2021
C. Palm et al. (Hrsg.), *Bildverarbeitung für die Medizin 2021*,
Informatik aktuell, https://doi.org/10.1007/978-3-658-33198-6_52

Despite this, few implementations are available that are suited for the particularities of medical data. In this work we aim to close this gap by presenting *M3d-CAM*, an easy-to-use library for generating attention maps that can be seamlessly integrated into any medical imaging project. The library is suited for any CNN-based PyTorch [4] classification or segmentation model and is compatible with both two- and three-dimensional data.

With this work we aim to simplify the generation of attention maps, thus increasing the interpretability of classification and segmentation models. We hope that this in turn raises the trust of medical practitioners in deep learning.

2   Materials and methods

M3d-CAM works through injection into a given model, appending certain functions to it. The model itself will work as usual and its predictions remain untouched. M3d-CAM itself works behind the scenes and generates attention maps every time `model.forward` is called. The most important functions of M3d-CAM are explained in the following sections.

2.1   Injection

To inject a model with M3d-CAM one simply needs to insert the single line `model = medcam.inject(model)` after model initialization, as shown in code example 1. This will add all the necessary functionality to the model. Additionally, `inject` offers multiple parameters that can be adjusted. As an example one can define an `output_dir` and set `save_maps=True` to save every generated attention map. One can also set a desired `backend` which is used for generating the attention maps such as Grad-CAM. These backends are explained in more detail in section 2.4. Furthermore, it is possible to choose the layer of interest with `layer`. Hereby one can specifically define a single layer, a set of layers, every layer with *full* or the highest CNN-layer with *auto* for the most comfort.

2.2   Layer retrieval

As the layer names of a model are often unknown to the user, M3d-CAM offers the method `medcam.get_layers(model)` for quickly acquiring every layer name of a model.

It should be noted that attention maps cannot be generated for every type of layer. This is the case for fully-connected, bounding box and other special kinds of layers. While the attention for theses layers can be computed, it is not possible to project them back to the original input data.

2.3   Evaluation

M3d-CAM supports the evaluation of attention maps with respect to ground truth masks. This can be done by calling `model.forward(input,mask)`, including the mask in the forward call. The attention map is then internally evaluated by the `medcam.Evaluator` class with a predefined metric by the user. Alternatively, one can call the `medcam.Evaluator` class directly. By calling `model.dump()` or respectively `medcam.Evaluator.dump()` the evaluation results are saved as an excel table.

2.4 Backends

M3d-CAM supports multiple methods for generating attention maps. For simplicity we will refer to them as *backends*. We show examples of how the different backends perform (Sec. 3).

2.4.1 Grad-CAM. [5] works by first propagating the input through the entire model. In a second step a desired class in the output is isolated by setting every other class to zero. The output of this isolated class is then backpropagated through the model up to the desired layer. Here, the layer gradients are extracted and together with the feature maps of the same layer the attention map is computed. The approach of generating an attention map from a specific preferably high layer gives a good compromise between high-level semantics and detailed spatial information. Furthermore, by isolating a specific class Grad-CAM becomes class-discriminant.

```
# Import M3d-CAM
from medcam import medcam

# Init your model and dataloader
model = MyCNN()
data_loader = DataLoader(dataset, batch_size=1, shuffle=False)

# Inject model with M3d-CAM
model = medcam.inject(model, output_dir="attention_maps", save_maps=True)

# Continue to do what you're doing...
# In this case inference on some new data
model.eval()
for i, batch in enumerate(data_loader):
    # Every time forward is called, attention maps are generated and
    # saved
    output = model(batch)
    # more of your code...
```

Fig. 1. Example of injecting a model with M3d-CAM.

2.4.2   Guided backpropagation. [6] works by first propagating the input through the entire model similar to Grad-CAM. In a second step the output is backpropagated through the entire model. However, only the non-negative gradients are passed to the next layer as negative gradients correspond to suppressed pixels deemed not relevant by the authors. The advantage of Guided Backpropagation is that the attention is pixel-precise. The downsides are that it is neither class- nor layer-discriminant.

2.4.3   Guided Grad-CAM. is another backend presented by Selvaraju et al. [5], which is a combination of Guided Backpropagation and Grad-CAM in an effort to combine the best of both approaches. When generating attention maps with both backends the resulting attention maps can be combined through simply multiplying them element-wise. The only downside of Guided Grad-CAM is the need of performing backpropagation two times.

2.4.4   Grad-CAM++. is an extension of Grad-CAM introduced by Chattopadhay at al. [7]. It differs from the naive Grad-CAM in that it weights the gradients before combining them with the feature maps. This results in more precise attention maps, especially when dealing with multiple instances of the same class in an image.

3   Results

In this section, we qualitatively illustrate the attention maps extracted by M3d-CAM for three examples (Fig. 2). The first row shows the original images. The first displays a chest X-Ray used on the task of classification by employing a CovidNet [8], the second a lung CT slice on the task of 2D segmentation with an Inf-Net [9] and the third a 3D prostate CT image on the task of 3D segmentation by employing a nnUNet [10].

The result of applying the Grad-CAM backend is a heatmap-like image of the attention at the desired layer (Fig. 3). For Guided Backpropagation, the result is a noise-like image depicting the model attention (Fig. 4). The result

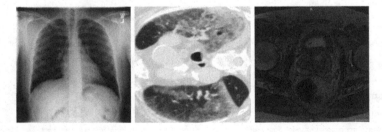

Fig. 2. From left to right: A chest X-Ray from the COVID-19 image data collection [11], a lung CT slice also from [11] and 3D prostate CT image from the Medical Decathlon dataset [12].

of combining both approaches in the Guided Grad-CAM approach is a noise-like class and layer discriminant pixel-precise attention map (Fig. 5). Finally, Grad-CAM++ produces heatmaps similar the original Grad-CAM but that more precisely depict the gradient weighting. Examples of these attention maps are shown in Figure 6.

4   Discussion

In this work we present M3d-CAM, a plug-and-play interpretability suite suited for PyTorch classification and segmentation models. The library implements a number of backend methods to extract attention maps, and supports both two- and three-dimensional data. With this contribution we hope to simplify the application of interpretability techniques to accelerate trust in medical deep learning models.

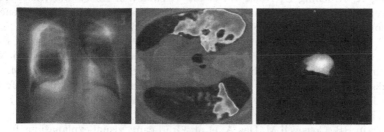

Fig. 3. The resulting Grad-CAM attention maps.

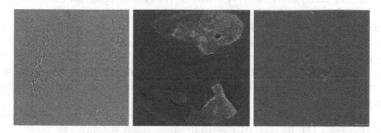

Fig. 4. The resulting Guided Backpropagation attention maps.

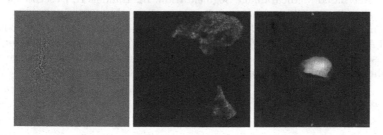

Fig. 5. The resulting Guided Grad-CAM attention maps.

Fig. 6. The resulting Grad-CAM++ attention maps.

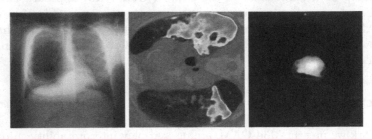

References

1. Hooker S, Erhan D, Kindermans PJ, et al. A benchmark for interpretability methods in deep neural networks. In: Advances in Neural Information Processing Systems; 2019. p. 9737–9748.
2. Huang X, Kroening D, Ruan W, et al. A survey of safety and trustworthiness of deep neural networks: verification, testing, adversarial attack and defence, and interpretability. Computer Science Review. 2020;37:100270.
3. Xu F, Uszkoreit H, Du Y, et al. Explainable AI: a brief survey on history, research areas, approaches and challenges. In: CCF International Conference on Natural Language Processing and Chinese Computing. Springer; 2019. p. 563–574.
4. Paszke A, Gross S, Massa F, et al. PyTorch: an imperative style, high-performance deep learning library. In: Advances in Neural Information Processing Systems; 2019. p. 8024–8035.
5. Selvaraju RR, Cogswell M, Das A, et al. Grad-cam: visual explanations from deep networks via gradient-based localization. Proc IEEE ICCV. 2017; p. 618–626.
6. Springenberg JT, Dosovitskiy A, Brox T, et al. Striving for simplicity: the all convolutional net. arXiv preprint arXiv:14126806. 2014;.
7. Chattopadhay A, Sarkar A, Howlader P, et al. Grad-cam++: generalized gradient-based visual explanations for deep convolutional networks. In: 2018 IEEE Winter Conference on Applications of Computer Vision (WACV). IEEE; 2018. p. 839–847.
8. Linda Wang ZQL, Wong A. COVID-Net: a tailored deep convolutional neural network design for detection of COVID-19 cases from chest radiography images; 2020.
9. Fan DP, Zhou T, Ji GP, et al. Inf-Net: automatic COVID-19 lung infection segmentation from CT images. IEEE TMI. 2020; p. 2626–2637.
10. Isensee F, Petersen J, Klein A, et al. Abstract: nnU-Net: Self-adapting Framework for U-Net-Based Medical Image Segmentation. In: Handels H, Deserno TM, Maier A, et al., editors. Bildverarbeitung für die Medizin 2019; 2019. p. 22–22.
11. Cohen JP, Morrison P, Dao L. COVID-19 image data collection. arXiv 200311597. 2020;Available from: https://github.com/ieee8023/covid-chestxray-dataset.
12. Simpson AL, Antonelli M, Bakas S, et al. A large annotated medical image dataset for the development and evaluation of segmentation algorithms; 2019.

Coronary Plaque Analysis for CT Angiography Clinical Research

Felix Denzinger[1,2,5], Michael Wels[2,5], Christian Hopfgartner[3], Jing Lu[2],
Max Schöbinger[2], Andreas Maier[1,4], Michael Sühling[2]

[1]Pattern Recognition Lab, Friedrich-Alexander-Universität Erlangen-
Nürnberg, Erlangen
[2]Computed Tomography, Siemens Healthineers, Forchheim, Germany
[3]ISO-Gruppe, Nuremberg, Germany
[4]Machine Intelligence, Friedrich-Alexander-Universität Erlangen-Nürnberg, Erlangen
[5]Contributed equally to this work.
felix.denzinger@fau.de

Abstract. The analysis of plaque deposits in the coronary vasculature is
an important topic in current clinical research. From a technical side
mostly new algorithms for different sub tasks – e.g. centerline extraction or vessel/plaque segmentation – are proposed. However, to enable
clinical research with the help of these algorithms, a software solution,
which enables manual correction, comprehensive visual feedback and tissue analysis capabilities, is needed. Therefore, we want to present such
an integrated software solution. A MeVisLab-based implementation of
our solution is available as part of the Siemens Healthineers syngo.via
Frontier and OpenApps research extension. It is able to perform robust
automatic centerline extraction and inner and outer vessel wall segmentation, while providing easy to use manual correction tools. Also, it allows for annotation of lesions along the centerlines, which can be further
analyzed regarding their tissue composition. Furthermore, it enables research in upcoming technologies and research directions: it does support
dual energy CT scans with dedicated plaque analysis and the quantification of the fatty tissue surrounding the vasculature, also in automated
set-ups.

1 Introduction

Cardiovascular diseases (CVDs) are the leading cause of natural death [1]. Therefore, the interest in clinical research in this area is high. Most CVDs are related
to atherosclerotic plaque deposits and the composition of these plaques plays an
important role in the patient outcome and risk stratification [2]. Modern cardiac computed-tomography angiography (CCTA) provides means to assess the
morphology of plaque deposits in the coronary arteries.

However, exact quantitative analysis of these deposits is tedious without
appropriate tools. If these tools are not available, clinical researchers are not

able to efficiently evaluate plaque deposits on larger patient cohorts, hindering them from contributing to progress in evidence-based medicine. Also, clinical studies need to be reproducible, which is easier to achieve – especially for studies with the focus on plaque analysis, with a high amount of processing steps – when most of the pipeline is automated. This also leads to a reduction of the amount of inter- and intra-observer variance.

To overcome these hurdles, we want to present a software solution and an associated semi-automatic general workflow for quantitative and semantic coronary artery plaque analysis from CCTA data with a focus on the underlying algorithms. As a semi-automatic approach it allows more efficient, accurate and reproducible plaque analysis. By allowing appropriate user-interaction at each processing step, the system is prevented from generating flawed final results.

Furthermore, two major topics in upcoming and current research in the area of CCTA are supported: dual energy (DE) CT scans are automatically detected as such, registered onto each other and the composition of the plaque deposits can be analyzed using information from two energy spectra. Also, the composition of the fatty tissue surrounding the vasculature was shown to be correlated with inflammation and consequently plaque aggregation and cardiac death [3]. In our software solution we additionally enable automated segmentation of the regions of interest for this analysis.

Since we present a tool-chain for clinical research this paper explains the individual elements of this software solution and highlights some related already published applications in clinical research.

2   Material and methods

2.1   General workflow

Starting from a CCTA volume as input, our tool-chain consists of the following steps: fully automatic heart isolation and coronary artery centerline detection, including centerline correction, then – if needed – tools for a manual correction of these pre-processing results, next, selection of the vessel branch and section of interest with a consecutive fully automatic vessel wall segmentation, and finally an analysis of the plaque composition and quantification using manually

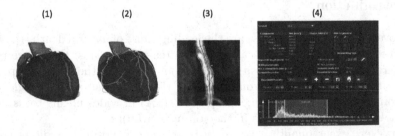

Fig. 1. Processing steps of our solution: (1) heart isolation, (2) centerline extraction, (3) ROI definition and segmentation, (4) plaque deposition analysis and annotation.

set Hounsfield unit (HU) thresholds. The workflow of our prototype software solution is depicted in Fig. 1. As soon as the volume is loaded the heart and its anatomies are fully-automatically detected with the method described by Zheng et al. [4], which utilizes marginal space learning and steerable features and is described to be robust and fast ($\approx$ 4 seconds per volume). The heart isolation is needed for further fully-automatic coronary artery centerline extraction. The method used for this step is described by Zheng et al. [5] as a both model- and data-driven approach, which takes the prior information about vessel specific regions of interest (ROIs) in order to allow robust centerline extraction also for occluded vessels. This method is as of today still the best performing fully-automatic approach on the Rotterdam Coronary Centerline Extraction Challenge leaderboard [6]. If the result of the centerline extraction step is not satisfactory it can be corrected by a simple interactive tool and additional centerlines can be manually drawn or created considering image evidence with a single seed point.

The vessel section to be analyzed can be selected by clicking on the start and end point on the centerline. The created markers can be shifted along the centerline if one is not satisfied with the initial selection. Next, the segmentation of both the inner and outer vessel wall within the area of interest can be triggered. For the inner wall segmentation the approach described in [7] is utilized. It is based on ray-casting and the analysis of a subsequent Markov random field graph with convex priors. The described approach is known to be robust and accurate on a subvoxel level as its the current leader on the Rotterdam Coronary Lumen Segmentation Challenge leaderboard [8].

For the outer vessel wall an adaptive self-learning edge-model using a combination of 3D and 2D active contour models is used [9]. By adaptation of the threshold for this approach the outer vessel wall segmentation can be widened or narrowed in real-time on cross-sectional views and then applied for the whole region of interest. Especially the outer wall segmentation is reader-dependent, and often not clearly defined, since there is a lack of contrast enhancement due to soft plaques within the arterial walls. Therefore, this is a good compromise between robustness and flexibility allowing a fast adaptation.

In order to correct or adapt the resulting inner and outer wall segmentation a quasi-real-time interactive method is used [10]. By describing the inner and outer vessel wall as implicit surfaces with radial basis functions, manual corrections in the curved or axial 2D views of the vessel can be directly propagated to the 3D surface and corrected accordingly.

2.2 Plaque analysis

The resulting plaque region then can be analyzed, e.g. with respect to its composition. Since the exact thresholds for different tissue types vary for different tube voltages, the thresholds between the mostly used tissue classes – lipid-rich, fibrotic and calcified – can be adapted directly in the histogram of the HU values. Additionally, this HU histogram of the ROI can be directly exported to enable further analysis of the value distribution. Moreover, an important factor in assessing coronary plaques are high risk plaque features. These include the degree of stenosis, positive remodeling, low HU attenuation and the so-called napkin ring sign. The degree of stenosis and remodeling can be determined for each individual section of the annotated lesion by taking the proximal and distal markers as weighted reference for each position. While low HU attenuation plaques can be derived from the plaque composition histogram the napkin ring sign can be annotated manually.

In the last decade DE scanners were introduced, which can provide a better tissue contrast in some areas due to two different energy spectra. According to literature [11], calcified plaques get well detected by single energy CT scans but lipid-rich and fibrotic tissue are harder to differentiate. Since this differentiation is especially important for the classification of high-risk plaques, the interest in plaque analysis with DE scans is high. Therefore, our presented software solution does support DE scans. Solely a prior registration of the two DE scans is needed to enable the same processing pipeline as described above. The plaque deposits can then be first examined regarding whether they are calcified or not with a single energy volume and then their composition can be further analyzed combining information from the two scans and thresholding the DE index. This follows the ideas proposed by [12].

Another rising topic in CCTA clinical research is the analysis of perivascular fat [3]. The HU distribution of the fat surrounding the coronary vasculature was shown to be correlated with inflammation leading to plaque aggregation. To enable research in this direction, we support the creation of ROIs which expand radially to the vessel dependent on either the inner or outer vessel wall. The radius of these ROIs can be freely set. Since in literature standardized ROIs exist, we provide an automated mode which creates one ROI for each main branch according to the definition in the literature.

3 Results

Since multiple sources provide such a software solution, we want to briefly differentiate our solution to other available tools. An overview of this can be seen in Table 1. While many other approaches do support standard pre-processing, segmentation and correction capabilities, our solution provides DE support, which no other solution to the best of our knowledge does. Also only the solution of Cedars Sinai does include perivascular tissue analysis but not in the automated setting we do.

Due to the nature of this paper, we will not provide quantitative results. In total 16 publications utilized our software solution up until today. Due to space restrictions, we are only able to highlight some of these here. First, we want to present work of Tesche et al. [13]. They used our solution to correlate different CCTA derived plaque characteristics with the questions whether lesions are intra-operatively determined to be haemodynamically significant. In their study they examined 37 lesions of 37 patients but they have increased the number of patients in later studies. Furthermore, the research of Ratiu et al. [14] aims

Table 1. Comparison to other available approaches. The features of alternate solutions are collected from public sources and are to the best of our knowledge. All available approaches contain tools for semi-automated vessel segmentation, centerline correction, plaque composition analysis and segmentation correction.

	Ours	Cedars Sinai AutoPlaq[1]	Medis QAngio CT[2]	Canon CT SUREPlaque[3]	GE VesselIQ Xpress[4]	Philips CT CCA[5]
Automated Pre-processing	Yes	No	Yes	Semi	Yes	Yes
Dual Energy Support	Yes	No	No	No	No	No
Perivascular Tissue Analysis	Yes	Yes	No	No	No	No
Automated Segment Labeling	No	Unknown	Yes	No	Yes	Yes

towards analyzing the lesion geometry as an additional indicator for high risk plaque segments. Morariu et al. [15] are currently conducting a trial examining also the characteristics of plaque deposits after initial myocardiac infarction. They plan to collect up to 100 patients with major adverse cardiac events as potential endpoint.

4 Discussion

In this paper we described a software solution which enables plaque and tissue analysis-related clinical research in the field of coronary artery diseases. In the workflow of this prototype all necessary processing steps for coronary plaque analysis exist and easy manual correction is able for all steps. The majority of fields of research which are currently in the focus are covered by our solution. These include the support of DE scans and the analysis of perivascular tissue, which are hardly supported by most other available solutions. The fully automatic labelling of the branch segments will be part of further improvement to the software. We presented already conducted clinical studies with our software solution, which proofs the applicability of described workflows and components in this important clinical research field.

---

[2] https://www.cedars-sinai.org/research/labs/dey.html
[3] https://medisimaging.com/apps/plaque-burden/
[4] https://www.vitalimages.com/product-information/ct-sureplaque/
[5] https://www.gehealthcare.co.uk/products/advanced-visualization/all-applications/autobone-vesseliq-xpress
[6] https://www.philips.co.uk/healthcare/product/HCAPP006/-ct-comprehensive-cardiac-analysis-cca-

References

1. Mendis S, Davis S, Norrving B. Organizational update: the World health organization global status report on noncommunicable diseases 2014. Stroke. 2015;46(5):e121–e122.
2. Naghavi M. From vulnerable plaque to vulnerable patient: a call for new definitions and risk assessment strategies. Part II. Circulation. 2003;108:1772–1778.
3. Antonopoulos AS, et al. Detecting human coronary inflammation by imaging perivascular fat. Sci Transl Med. 2017;9(398).
4. Zheng Y, Barbu A, Georgescu B, et al. Four-chamber heart modeling and automatic segmentation for 3-D cardiac CT volumes using marginal space learning and steerable features. IEEE Trans Med Imaging. 2008;27(11):1668–1681.
5. Zheng Y, Tek H, Funka-Lea G. Robust and accurate coronary artery centerline extraction in CTA by combining model-driven and data-driven approaches. Proc MICCAI. 2013; p. 74–81.
6. Schaap M, Metz CT, van Walsum T, et al. Standardized evaluation methodology and reference database for evaluating coronary artery centerline extraction algorithms. Med Image Anal. 2009;13(5):701–714.
7. Lugauer F, Zheng Y, Hornegger J, et al. Precise lumen segmentation in coronary computed tomography angiography. Proc MICCAI. 2014; p. 137–147.
8. Kirişli H, et al. Standardized evaluation framework for evaluating coronary artery stenosis detection, stenosis quantification and lumen segmentation algorithms in computed tomography angiography. Med Image Anal. 2013;17(8):859–876.
9. Grosskopf S, Biermann C, Deng K, et al. Accurate, fast, and robust vessel contour segmentation of CTA using an adaptive self-learning edge model. In: Medical Imaging 2009: Image Processing. vol. 7259. International Society for Optics and Photonics; 2009. p. 72594D.
10. Wels M, Lades F, Hopfgartner C, et al. Intuitive and accurate patient-specific coronary tree modeling from cardiac computed-tomography angiography. In: The 3rd interactive MIC Workshop; 2016. p. 86–93.
11. Danad I, Ó Hartaigh B, Min JK. Dual-energy computed tomography for detection of coronary artery disease. Expert Rev Cardiovasc Ther. 2015;13(12):1345–1356.
12. Barreto M, Schoenhagen P, Nair A, et al. Potential of dual-energy computed tomography to characterize atherosclerotic plaque: ex vivo assessment of human coronary arteries in comparison to histology. J Cardiovasc Comput Tomogr. 2008;2(4):234–242.
13. Tesche C, et al. Coronary CT angiography derived morphological and functional quantitative plaque markers correlated with invasive fractional flow reserve for detecting hemodynamically significant stenosis. J Cardiovasc Comput Tomogr. 2016;10(3):199–206.
14. Ratiu M, et al. Impact of coronary plaque geometry on plaque vulnerability and its association with the risk of future cardiovascular events in patients with chest pain undergoing coronary computed tomographic angiography: the GEOMETRY study: Protocol for a prospective clinical trial. Medicine. 2018;97(49).
15. Morariu M, et al. Impact of inflammation-mediated response on pan-coronary plaque vulnerability, myocardial viability and ventricular remodeling in the postinfarction period-the VIABILITY study: Protocol for a non-randomized prospective clinical study. Medicine. 2019;98(17).

Robust Slide Cartography in Colon Cancer Histology
Evaluation on a Multi-scanner Database

Petr Kuritcyn[1], Carol I. Geppert[2], Markus Eckstein[2], Arndt Hartmann[2],
Thomas Wittenberg[1], Jakob Dexl[1], Serop Baghdadlian[1], David Hartmann[1],
Dominik Perrin[1], Volker Bruns[1], Michaela Benz[1]

[1]Fraunhofer Institute for Integrated Circuits IIS
[2]Institute of Pathology, University Hospital Erlangen,
Friedrich-Alexander-Universität Erlangen-Nürnberg (FAU)
`petr.kuritcyn@iis.fraunhofer.de`

Abstract. Robustness against variations in color and resolution of digitized whole-slide images (WSIs) is an essential requirement for any computer-aided analysis in digital pathology. One common approach to encounter a lack of heterogeneity in the training data is data augmentation. We investigate the impact of different augmentation techniques for whole-slide cartography in colon cancer histology using a newly created multi-scanner database of 39 slides each digitized with six different scanners. A state of the art convolutional neural network (CNN) is trained to differentiate seven tissue classes. Applying a model trained on one scanner to WSIs acquired with a different scanner results in a significant decrease in classification accuracy. Our results show that the impact of resolution variations is less than of color variations: the accuracy of the baseline model trained without any augmentation at all is 73% for WSIs with similar color but different resolution against 35% for WSIs with similar resolution but color deviations. The grayscale model shows comparatively robust results and evades the problem of color variation. A combination of multiple color augmentations methods lead to a significant overall improvement (between 33 and 54 percentage points). Moreover, fine-tuning a pre-trained network using a small amount of annotated data from new scanners benefits the performance for these particular scanners, but this effect does not generalize to other unseen scanners.

1 Introduction

Histopathology involves the microscopic examination of tissue sections. The sections undergo various preparation steps before analysis: fixation, embedding, sectioning, staining and digitization [1]. Each step introduces some form of variation into the resulting whole-slide image. A trained pathologist can cope with these variances; however, a human analysis is prone to subjectivity and inter-observer variance. Computational pathology aims to support pathologists in their decision-making process by automating in a very objective and validated fashion the calculation of scores or extraction of parameters hidden to the human eye. Deep learning approaches achieve very good results in many applications [2]. However, training robust models for the analysis of histopathological slides is still a challenge. The algorithm's accuracy suffers from the high variability encountered in slides in the field [2]. Sources of heterogeneity are different assays, unstandardized preparation protocols, different characteristics of the scanner components - most relevantly it's camera and microscope objective - and finally color post-processing steps. There are two main approaches to counter the problem of variances in WSIs: (i) normalization of images during runtime and (ii) representing the variance already in the training database.

The first approach aims to provide a standardized input to the classifier by adjusting the slide's color and scale to match the properties of the reference slides the network was trained on. Earlier solutions rely on a normalization based on color deconvolution of the underlying staining components [3]. The disadvantage of these solutions is that they frequently produce unrealistic color alterations and are not robust against severe stain variations. More recent techniques use machine learning algorithms to improve the normalization quality by taking into account morphological properties in addition to the color [1, 4]. Two prominently employed network architectures for transferring the reference slides' style are sparse auto-encoders or generative adversarial networks (GANs) [5]. These methods produce more reliable results, however, they are computationally expensive and prone to false color estimations in unseen regions.

The second approach requires a sufficiently heterogeneous multi-centric dataset. When this is not available, a viable workaround is to introduce variance synthetically using domain-specific data augmentation. Native image patches can be duplicated and altered in terms of their geometry and color with the goal of increasing the network's capability to generalize to unseen data. Geometric transformations leave the color information intact and modify only morphological information. Patches can be rotated, flipped, scaled or images can be artificially blurred to simulate out-of-focus scans. Color augmentations, on the other hand, include variations of the color's hue, saturation, gamma, etc. This can help to mimic different stain protocols or color alterations of WSI scanners. A color augmentation tool specific to the domain of histopathology is a stain variation [6], where the hematoxylin and eosin components are separated using a color deconvolution in order to vary their color properties independently. Training and evaluating classifiers on slides that stem from one and the same laboratory and scanner can result in overly optimistic accuracy estimations. On the contrary, evaluating on a multi-centric dataset frequently shows poor performance [7]. Telez et al. compared for different applications the performance gain from stain normalization and stain augmentation and conclude that the latter is more beneficial [2].

Previous research has largely focused on the variance introduced by variations in the staining protocol. In this work, we investigate the effects of variations that stem from the use of different slide-scanners.

Table 1. WSI resolution, size of test database and number of patches.

Scanner	Resolution in μm per pixel	number of test patches	number of patches for fine-tuning
3DHISTECH MIDI	0.22	1,381,316	40,230
Fraunhofer iSTIX	0.17	2,123,364	49,005
Fraunhofer SCube	0.27	857,511	38,528
PreciPoint M8	0.35	514,397	35,524
Hamamatsu Nanozoomer S210	0.22	1,424,716	-
Hamamatsu Nanozoomer S360	0.23	1,298,056	-

2 Materials and methods

2.1 Materials

The dataset used for the baseline cartography network comprises 161 hematoxylin and eosin (HE) stained colon sections from the Institute of Pathology at the University Hospital Erlangen. First, all samples were digitized with a 3DHISTECH MIDI scanner (20x magnification, 0.22 μm per pixel) and annotated manually by accurately outlining the contours of seven different tissue classes: tumor, necrosis, inflammation, connective combined with adipose tissue, muscle tissue, mucosa and mucus. Based on the annotated WSIs, labelled non-overlapping patches of pixel size 224x224 are generated. Patches that do not intersect with a manual annotation or contain no or only little foreground are discarded. The number of patches per class and slide is limited to 10,000 (using random sampling) in order to limit the overall dataset size while ensuring that information from all available slides is used. The training database comprises 2,173,515 patches from 92 slides. The validation set contains 719,010 patches from a disjoint set of 30 slides. These two datasets were used to train the CNN, while the remaining 39 glass slides were additionally digitized with four other automated scanners and with a manual microscope using the real-time stitching software iSTIX. The resolution as well as the color varies significantly between the different scanners (Tab. 1, Fig. 1).

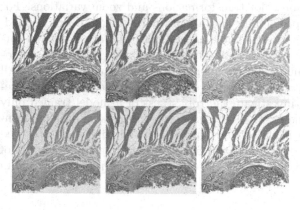

Fig. 1. Digitized slide scanned with MIDI, M8, iSTIX (upper row, from left to right), S210, S360, SCube (lower row, from left to right).

For each slide, the annotations are transferred from the original scan to the new scans by co-aligning the WSIs. The main steps for the registration are the adjustment of resolution, calculation of features, brute-force-matching of the slides' feature points and finally the estimation of a global transformation (translation and rotation). Afterwards, for each scanner a test database with labelled patches (224x224) from 30 slides is generated without limiting the number of patches per class/slide. Due to the different resolution and background detection, the amount of image patches varies among the scanner datasets. A set of nine slides is excluded from these datasets and reserved for additional fine-tuning experiments for three scanners (M8, SCube, iSTIX). Moreover, tiles from the original scanner are included in a mixed database for fine-tuning comprising 163,287 patches.

2.2 Methods

CNNs are a common choice to solve image classification tasks. One popular CNN architecture is Xception, which was introduced by Chollet [8]. Its main characteristics are a depthwise separable convolution with residual connections. We slightly adapted the architecture by introducing two dropout layers between the fully connected layers at the top and replacing the logistic regression with softmax. Moreover, our input image size is 224x224 (instead of 299x299) in order to obtain more image patches that lie entirely within the bounds of the manual annotations. All experiments were carried out using the TensorFlow framework (version 2.2). For training, cross entropy loss and Adam optimizer with a learning rate of 0.001 and an exponential decay was applied. Image patches are zero-centered and the batches are generated with respect to class labels ensuring that each class is equally represented on average in a batch. Class imbalances are compensated by oversampling of underrepresented classes. A dropout rate of 0.5 was chosen.

First, a baseline experiment is carried out, where no data augmentation is employed. Afterwards several data augmentation techniques are applied during training and the robustness of the resulting model is evaluated on our six per-scanner test databases. Based on the observation that the slides vary mainly in color and in scale, we focus on color transformations and zoom variations. For each augmentation type, a probability and a valid parameter range is defined. We investigate variations of saturation, hue and contrast and apply gamma correction to the image patches. Additionally, the hematoxylin and eosin components are separated [6] and manipulated independently (HE augmentation). All experiments that employ data augmentation start with the weights of the baseline training. Moreover, we investigate the robustness of a model trained only on grayscale image tiles. Finally, we combine the most promising data augmentation types in a single run in order to evaluate if their individually observed benefits add up. In addition, the impact of fine-tuning with a small number of scanner-specific images is evaluated for three of the scanners individually and in combination (Tab. 1).

Table 2. Classification accuracies (number of true positive classifications divided by the total number of classified patches) for different models on each scanner test set.

Model	Classification accuracy on					
	3DHISTECH MIDI	PreciPoint M8	Fraunhofer iSTIX	SCube	Hamamatsu S210	S360
Baseline	0.939	0.394	0.290	0.731	0.354	0.361
Grayscale	0.908	0.849	0.680	0.885	0.864	0.882
HE + Gamma	0.925	0.696	0.432	0.884	0.663	0.727
Hue + Sat + HE	0.918	0.891	0.621	0.896	0.880	0.901
Hue + Sat + Bright + Cont	0.933	0.894	0.493	0.858	0.863	0.917
M8 fine-tuning	0.610	0.939	0.519	0.759	0.668	0.780
iSTIX fine-tuning	0.566	0.642	0.821	0.614	0.576	0.533
SCube fine-tuning	0.894	0.592	0.386	0.936	0.489	0.536
Mixed fine-tuning	0.902	0.917	0.852	0.904	0.778	0.799
Zoom	0.931	0.418	0.310	0.750	0.343	0.344
Gamma	0.921	0.398	0.370	0.848	0.305	0.331
HE	0.932	0.679	0.401	0.831	0.637	0.680
Hue	0.927	0.861	0.410	0.852	0.821	0.896
Saturation	0.934	0.452	0.365	0.856	0.422	0.459
Brightness	0.918	0.494	0.371	0.815	0.372	0.397
Contrast	0.927	0.455	0.336	0.796	0.368	0.380

3   Results

Results obtained on the scanner-specific test sets are listed in Tab. 2. The baseline and grayscale models are trained without any data augmentation. Starting point for the fine-tuning is the model trained on the MIDI scanner with HE and gamma augmentation.

4   Discussion

A baseline experiment confirms earlier observations that a trained CNN shows poor performance on unseen data from another scanner. In our experiments, the influence of changes in resolution is less critical than the deviation in color: the accuracy of the baseline model on SCube scans (73%), which are similar in color but have a different resolution, is significantly higher than that on Hamamatsu scans (35%), which share the same resolution with the original MIDI scans. The highest impact on the results is gained by employing the HE and hue augmentations. On the contrary, zoom augmentation yields only little benefit. Surprisingly, the grayscale model shows comparatively robust results and evades the problem of color variation - the highest burden for robust models. A combination of multiple methods (hue, saturation and HE augmentations) lead to a significant overall improvement. By fine-tuning the model using a small set of patches from the newly targeted scanner, the overall accuracy could be raised to a level close to that obtained on the native dataset for all new scanners except iSTIX. A likely explanation is that the manual scanning concept inherently suffers from stronger variances and the overall quality is inferior to that of high-end automated scanners (more out-of-focus areas, stitching artefacts).

Fine-tuning the network with additional patches from four scanner datasets ("mixed") yields a solid performance on all scanners. However, this model does not generalize as well as the model trained on a data augmented (hue, saturation and HE color augmentation together) database and shows worse results on the unseen Hamamatsu datasets: 78-80% against of 88-90%. In future work we will focus on extending the augmentation range and developing an automated approach for increasing the robustness of a pre-trained CNN.

Acknowledgement. This work was supported by the Bavarian Ministry of Economic Affairs, Regional Development and Energy through the Center for Analytics – Data – Applications (ADA-Center) within the framework of „BAYERN DIGITAL II" (20-3410-2-9-8). A part of the employed scanners and the deep learning cluster were funded by the Federal Ministry of Education and Research under the project reference numbers 16FMD01K, 16FMD02 and 16FMD03. Hamamatsu scans courtesy of Hamamatsu Photonics Deutschland GmbH.

References

1. Bejnordi BE, Litjens G, et al.   Stain specific standardization of whole-slide histopathological images. IEEE Trans Med Imaging. 2016;35(2):404–415.
2. Tellez D, Litjens G, Bándi P, et al. Quantifying the effects of data augmentation and stain color normalization in convolutional neural networks for computational pathology. Med Image Anal. 2019;58:516–24.
3. Reinhard E, Adhikhmin M, Gooch B, et al. Color transfer between images. IEEE Comput Graph Appl. 2001;21(5):34–41.
4. Khan AM, Rajpoot N, Treanor D, et al. A nonlinear mapping approach to stain normalization in digital histopathology images using image-specific color deconvolution. IEEE Trans Biomed Eng. 2014;61(6):1729–1738.
5. Zanjani FG, et al. Stain normalization of histopathology images using generative adversarial networks. Proc IEEE Int Symp Biomed Imaging. 2018; p. 573–577.
6. Tellez D, Balkenhol M, Otte-Höller I, et al. Whole-slide mitosis detection in H E breast histology using PHH3 as a reference to train distilled stain-invariant convolutional networks. IEEE Trans Med Imaging. 2018;37(9):2126–2136.
7. Leo P, Lee G, Shih NNC, et al. Evaluating stability of histomorphometric features across scanner and staining variations: prostate cancer diagnosis from whole slide images. J Med Imaging (Bellingham). 2016;3(4):1–11.
8. Chollet F. Xception: deep learning with depthwise separable convolutions. Conf Comput Vis Pattern Recognit. 2017; p. 1800–1807.

Digital Staining of Mitochondria in Label-free Live-cell Microscopy

Ayush Somani[1], Arif Ahmed Sekh[2], Ida S. Opstad[2], Åsa Birna Birgisdottir[3], Truls Myrmel[3], Balpreet Singh Ahluwalia[2], Krishna Agarwal[2], Dilip K. Prasad[4], Alexander Horsch[4]

[1]Department of Mathematics and Computing, IIT (ISM) Dhanbad, India
[2]Department of Physics and Technology, UiT The Arctic University of Norway
[3]Department of Clinical Medicine, UiT The Arctic University of Norway
[4]Department of Computer Science, UiT The Arctic University of Norway
alexander.horsch@uit.no

Abstract. Examining specific sub-cellular structures while minimizing cell perturbation is important in the life sciences. Fluorescence labeling and imaging is widely used. With the advancement of deep learning, digital staining routines for label-free analysis have emerged to replace fluorescence imaging. Nonetheless, digital staining of sub-cellular structures such as mitochondria is sub-optimal. This is because the models designed for computer vision are directly applied instead of optimizing them for microscopy data. We propose a new loss function with multiple thresholding steps to promote more effective learning for microscopy data. We demonstrate a deep learning approach to translate the label-free brightfield images of living cells into equivalent fluorescence images of mitochondria with an average structural similarity of 0.77, thus surpassing the state-of-the-art of 0.7 with L1. We provide insightful examples of unique opportunities by data-driven deep learning-enabled image translations.

1 Introduction

The study of function and structure of nanoscale sub-cellular organelles such as mitochondria is considered vital for understanding sub-cellular mechanisms [1]. Its small size can fall below the diffraction limit [2] and poses a considerable challenge. Mitochondria specific live-cell friendly fluorescent dyes [3] and high resolution microscopes yield high contrast imaes [4]. Nonetheless, there are trade-offs involved with the use of fluorescent dyes. Such dyes are chemical additions to the living cell system. They perturb the natural function and sometimes even damages the cells [5]. Furthermore, the phenomenon of photobleaching limits the photon-budget and long-term imaging [6]. Therefore, it is of high interest to explore label-free microscopy solutions such as brightfield differential interference and phase-contrast microscopy which use the inherent optical contrast of the sub-cellular structures in the image formation [7]. Unfortunately, the images obtained by these modalities encode the entire cell content, which makes the data difficult to interpret for studies concentrating on only a small portion of the sub-cellular content [8].

This study introduces a deep learning-based approach for digital staining of mitochondria in label-free brightfield microscopy images of living cells. We implement a conditional generative adversarial network (cGAN) [9] to transfer the unstained embryonic heart-derived cell-line to their corresponding mitochondria stained images (Fig. 1). The highlight of our work is a novel loss function.

2   Materials and methods

2.1   Data acquisition

The rat cardiomyoblast cell-line H9c2 (cells derived from embryonic heart tissue; Sigma Aldrich) was cultured in DMEM with 10% FBS on MatTek glass-bottom dishes. The cells were transiently transfected $24 - 48$ hours to express the mitochondrial fluorescence marker eGFP-OMP25-TM. During acquisition, the cells were kept at $37°C$, 5% $CO2$, atmospheric oxygen, and a cell-culture medium (DMEM with 10% FBS). Time-lapse microscopy data were acquired using a DeltaVision OMX V4 Blaze imaging system (GE Healthcare Life Sciences, Marlborough, MA, USA) equipped with a 60X 1.42NA oil-immersion objective (Olympus) and sCMOS cameras. A total of five cells were imaged. Images were acquired by shifting the focal plane along the z-axis and repeating the acquisition of aligned pairs of brightfield and fluorescence images as separate channels using 2s as the temporal rate of revisiting the same plane. Each image is of size 1024×1024 pixels, where each pixel is of size 80 nm. For ensuring a good correlative imaging set-up, the images of the two modes were recorded using two different cameras with inbuilt pre-calibration for registration. Images of five cells were used for the approach. Each aligned image pair was randomly cropped into 25 smaller patches (256×256 pixels). The patches with mitochondrial region less than 20% were discarded, obtaining a total of 8480 correlated pairs of images, which were then proportionally split into 70-20-10% training, validation, and test sets. We had $5,936$ correlated image pairs for training and 848 correlated pairs of images for testing through this exercise.

Fig. 1.   Proposed method for label-free to digitally labeled image translation.

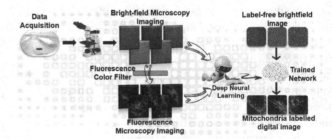

2.2   cGAN architecture

The learning of non-linear mapping from label-free microscopy images to standard fluorescent stained image pair is accomplished using cGAN [9], which is an extension of the generative adversarial network (GAN). The model comprises of subsequent learning of a Generator network (G) and a Discriminator network (D), as shown in Fig. 2 using U-Net [10] as the backbone. G is an encoder-decoder network assigned to generate labeled images from the passed real brightfield image, inferring the probability distribution generating the data. The generator loss function computes the loss by comparing the generated image with the corresponding ground truth real fluorescence image. This generated image is then passed to the discriminator network with a comparatively more straightforward task of learning the rules to distinguish between the images generated by the generator network and the ground truth real of fluorescence images. The discriminator loss function seeks to maximize the probability of how realistic the generated image looks against the input target pair. This follows a zero-sum game of adversarial learning of the G-D network. When both function's losses attain a Nash equilibrium, we expect that the generator can generate close-to-reality digitally labeled images. Pix2pix [11] is used in this work, a variant of aligned image-to-image translation using cGAN. The primary motivation for choosing this model is the flexibility and adaptability to a wide variety of tasks without explicitly defining the relationship. The model learns the explicit density function describing the probability distribution.

2.3   Training details

The networks for all the combinations were trained from scratch for 200 epochs, and results were compared using Adam optimizer. Image rescaling was avoided to preserve the image spatial context. ReLu activation was employed and no dropouts were included.

3   Proposed loss function

The design or adoption of an optimal generator loss function is critical for the model's performance and often a challenging endeavor. MinMax and L1 norm

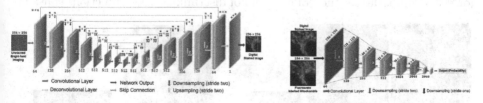

Fig. 2. Pipeline to train a deep neural network; left: generator; right: discriminator network.

based loss function are some conventional loss functions successfully used for low-noise medical images [12]. Sub-cellular fluorescence microscopy has a dominance of noisy and empty background due to the nature of fluorescence. This results in the conventional loss functions prioritizing learning on the noisy background and sub-optimally learning the foreground pixels which are few in relative numbers. For example, Fig. 3(A) shows an actual fluorescence image, (B) is a digital candidate image generated by the generator, (C) the 3D rendering of pixel-by-pixel L1 loss shows that the sum of loss in background pixels can be higher compared to the foreground object due to large fraction of noisy background. If the generator minimizes the L1 loss, learning of the noisy background is prioritized. We propose to use a weighted loss function, in which the weight matrix shown in (D) when multiplied with the L1 loss (C) allows to make the net loss more sensitive to the foreground, as shown in (E). The details of the proposed weighted L1 loss appear in the following paragraph.

We propose using a custom multiple thresholding-normalized (TN) loss function [13] that effectively mitigates the problem mentioned above. The proposed loss aims to reduce the contribution (and not completely neglect it) of the noisy background to the loss estimation as compared to the foreground. Since the TN-based loss is not strictly zero in the background, learning of the low-intensity features such as out-of-focus light is still incorporated, only with lesser priority. We compute the weight matrix based on the three-sigma rule to a normal curve that can be derived from Chebyshev's inequality for a wide class of probability distributions. For a normal distribution with mean μ and standard deviation σ, the rule states that $\mu \pm \sigma$ contains $\sim 66.7\%$ of the image measurements, $\mu \pm 2\sigma$ covers 95% measurements and $\mu \pm 3\sigma$ covers 99.7% of the image measurements. The image is subsequently divided into three parts based on μ and σ and shifts the normalization to 0-20%, 20-70% and 70-100%, respectively. The eq. 1 below describes the computation of the weight matrix using the target image F

$$I_{\text{weight}} = \sum_{n=1}^{3} \sum_{i=m_{n-1}}^{m_n} \left(a_n \frac{F(x_i, y_i) - M_{n-1}}{M_n - M_{n-1}} + b_n \right) \tag{1}$$

where $m_0 = 0$, $M_0 = \min(F)$, $m_1 = M_1 = \mu + \sigma$, $m_2 = M_3 = \mu + 3\sigma$, $m_3 = 255$, $M_3 = \max(F)$. Further, heuristically chosen coefficients $a_1 = 0.2, b_1 = 0, a_2 = 0.5, b_2 = 0.2$, and $a_3 = 0.3, b_3 = 0.7$.

In order to choose the loss function for the discriminator network, we performed a comparative study of a variety of discriminator loss functions consider-

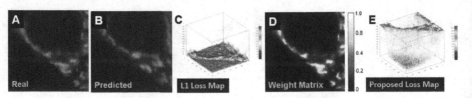

Fig. 3. Illustration of the proposed T-N based loss function.

Table 1. Study of loss functions for the discriminator network in terms of SSIM.

Generator	Dice + BCE	Jaccard	Focal loss	Mean square error
L1	0.3292	0.3921	0.4058	0.4292
TN-weighted L1	0.5212	0.5877	0.6521	0.6874

ing two options for the generator loss function: the conventional L1 loss and the TN weighted L1 loss (Table 1). We found that mean square error loss and focal loss provided a better convergence for both options of the generator loss. MSE loss providing the best result compared to other experimented losses was considered for the discriminator. This pixel-wise loss function emphasis the difference between the foreground and background statistical pixel data for learning.

4 Results

Structural similarity index (SSIM) and peak signal-to-noise ratio (PSNR) were used for performance evaluation. We performed a comparative study for three set-ups, namely T-N(1), T-N(16), and L1, where T-N(x) represents the proposed loss function with batch size x. L1 represents the L1 based vanilla loss function used in state-of-the-art mitochondria labeling [14]. Quantitative results and representative examples are shown in Fig. 4. We consistently observed that the proposed method provides better SSIM than the state-of-the-art, with median SSIM of 0.77 (TN) being significantly better than the state-of-the-art (0.7 of L1). PSNR shows a similar trend, although not as prominently as SSIM. In terms of computation time, the digital staining takes 34 milliseconds per image of size 256×256 on average, using a standard desktop computer equipped with a single GPU. Even with a relatively moderate computer, the fast inference time suggests that the proposed digital staining can be easily integrated with an automated microscope.

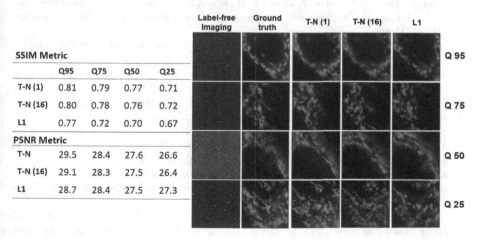

SSIM Metric

	Q95	Q75	Q50	Q25
T-N (1)	0.81	0.79	0.77	0.71
T-N (16)	0.80	0.78	0.76	0.72
L1	0.77	0.72	0.70	0.67

PSNR Metric

	Q95	Q75	Q50	Q25
T-N	29.5	28.4	27.6	26.6
T-N (16)	29.1	28.3	27.5	26.4
L1	28.7	28.4	27.5	27.3

Fig. 4. Quartile comparision of different learning methods.

5 Discussion and conclusion

We presented a method for artificially labelling mitochondria from a label-free brightfield microscopy image. The proposed TN loss function integrated with the adversarial network approach performs significantly better than the state-of-the-art. We envision this method to save researchers time, labor and costs, and enable better studies of cells without photo-toxicity, photo-bleaching, and perturbation of the natural cell composition. Since the method is data-driven, it does not need prior information regarding the experimental settings such as the camera, precise microscopy modality or the dyes used during experimentation. The model's precision can likely be further enhanced by training the network on a larger dataset with a higher number and variety of cells. We note that the presented digital staining approach can, in a straight forward manner, also be combined with other microscopy modalities by following a similar approach.

References

1. Samanta S, He Y, Sharma A, et al. Fluorescent probes for nanoscopic imaging of mitochondria. Chem. 2019;5(7):1697–1726.
2. Swayne TC, Gay AC, Pon LA. Methods cell biol.. vol. 80. Academic Press; 2007.
3. Chazotte B. Labeling mitochondria with fluorescent dyes for imaging. Cold Spring Harb Protoc. 2009;2009(6).
4. Kandel ME, Hu C, Kouzehgarani GN, et al. Epi-illumination gradient light interference microscopy for imaging opaque structures. Nat Commun. 2019;10(1):1–9.
5. Hoebe R, Van Oven C, Gadella TW, et al. Controlled light-exposure microscopy reduces photobleaching and phototoxicity in fluorescence live-cell imaging. Nat Biotechnol. 2007;25(2):249–253.
6. Christiansen EM, Yang SJ, Ando DM, et al. In silico labeling: predicting fluorescent labels in unlabeled images. Cell. 2018;173(3):792–803.
7. Zahedi A, On V, Phandthong R, et al. Deep analysis of mitochondria and cell health using machine learning. Sci Rep. 2018;8(1):1–15.
8. Vicar T, Balvan J, Jaros J, et al. Cell segmentation methods for label-free contrast microscopy: review and comprehensive comparison. BMC Bioinformatics. 2019;20(1):360.
9. Mirza M, Osindero S. Conditional generative adversarial nets. arXiv preprint arXiv:14111784. 2014;.
10. Ronneberger O, Fischer P, Brox T; Springer. U-net: convolutional networks for biomedical image segmentation. CoRR. 2015; p. 234–241.
11. Isola P, Zhu JY, Zhou T, et al. Image-to-image translation with conditional adversarial networks. Proc IEEE Comput Soc Conf Comput Vis Pattern Recognit. 2017; p. 5967–5976.
12. Armanious K, Jiang C, Fischer M, et al. MedGAN: medical image translation using GANs. Comput Med Imaging Graph. 2020;79:101684.
13. Kotte S, Kumar PR, Injeti SK. An efficient approach for optimal multilevel thresholding selection for gray scale images based on improved differential search algorithm. Ain Shams Med J. 2018;9(4):1043–1067.
14. Ounkomol C, Seshamani S, Maleckar MM, et al. Label-free prediction of three-dimensional fluorescence images from transmitted-light microscopy. Nat Methods. 2018;15(11):917–920.

Influence of Inter-Annotator Variability on Automatic Mitotic Figure Assessment

Frauke Wilm[0,1], Christof A. Bertram[0,2], Christian Marzahl[1],
Alexander Bartel[3], Taryn A. Donovan[4], Charles-Antoine Assenmacher[5],
Kathrin Becker[6], Mark Bennett[7], Sarah Corner[8], Brieuc Cossic[9],
Daniela Denk[10], Martina Dettwiler[11], Beatriz Garcia Gonzalez[7],
Corinne Gurtner[11], Annabelle Heier[12], Annika Lehmbecker[12], Sophie Merz[2,12],
Stephanie Plog[7], Anja Schmidt[12], Franziska Sebastian[12], Rebecca C. Smedley[8],
Marco Tecilla[13], Tuddow Thaiwong[8], Katharina Breininger[1], Matti Kiupel[8],
Andreas Maier[1], Robert Klopfleisch[2], Marc Aubreville[1,14]

[0]Both authors contributed equally
[1]Pattern Recognition Lab, Computer Sciences, Friedrich-Alexander-Universität Erlangen-Nürnberg, Erlangen, Germany
[2]Institute of Veterinary Pathology, Freie Universität Berlin, Germany
[3]Institute for Veterinary Epidemiology and Biostatistics, Freie Universität Berlin
[4]Department of Anatomic Pathology, Animal Medical Center, New York, USA
[5]Department of Pathobiology, University of Pennsylvania, Philadelphia, USA
[6]Department of Pathology, University of Veterinary Medicine Hannover, Germany
[7]Synlab's VPG Histology, Bristol, UK
[8]Veterinary Diagnostic Laboratory, Michigan State University, Lansing, USA
[9]Pharmacology & Preclinical Development, Idorsia Pharmaceuticals Ltd, Switzerland
[10]International Zoo Veterinary Group, Keighley, UK
[11]Institute of Animal Pathology, Vetsuisse Faculty, University of Bern, Switzerland
[12]IDEXX Vet Med Labor GmbH, Kornwestheim, Germany
[13]F. Hoffmann-La Roche Ltd, Basel, Switzerland
[14]Technische Hochschule Ingolstadt, Ingoldstadt, Germany
frauke.wilm@fau.de

Abstract. Density of mitotic figures in histologic sections is a prognostically relevant characteristic for many tumours. Due to high inter-pathologist variability, deep learning-based algorithms are a promising solution to improve tumour prognostication. Pathologists are the gold standard for database development, however, labelling errors may hamper development of accurate algorithms. In the present work we evaluated the benefit of multi-expert consensus (n = 3, 5, 7, 9, 11) on algorithmic performance. While training with individual databases resulted in highly variable F_1 scores, performance was notably increased and more consistent when using the consensus of three annotators. Adding more annotators only resulted in minor improvements. We conclude that databases by few pathologists and high label precision may be the best compromise between high algorithmic performance and time investment.

© Der/die Autor(en), exklusiv lizenziert durch
Springer Fachmedien Wiesbaden GmbH, ein Teil von Springer Nature 2021
C. Palm et al. (Hrsg.), *Bildverarbeitung für die Medizin 2021*,
Informatik aktuell, https://doi.org/10.1007/978-3-658-33198-6_56

1 Introduction

Histologic examination of tumour specimens is used to derive important information with regards to patient prognosis and selection of appropriate treatment. For numerous tumour types, including canine mast cell tumours, cellular proliferation is one of the most meaningful prognostic parameters. As part of the recommended grading schemes, cells undergoing division (mitotic figures) must be counted in histologic sections. However, identification of mitotic figures has a high degree of inter-observer variability due to inconsistent classification of mitotic figures (as opposed to mitotic-like impostors) or overlooking/omitting mitotic figure candidates [1, 2]. In order to improve reproducibility and accuracy of enumerating mitotic figures, promising deep learning-based algorithms for the automated analysis of digitised histologic sections have been developed [1, 3, 4, 5]. However, as pathologists are the gold standard for dataset development, visual and cognitive limitations of human experts may hamper the consistency of datasets and subsequently algorithmic performance [2].

All available datasets on mitotic figures from human and canine tumours have used not more than two pathologists as annotators for initial labelling in histologic images [2, 3, 4, 5, 6]. Disagreement between the labels of these two pathologists was reported in up to 68.2 % [3]. Divergent labels between these two pathologists were reviewed for final consensus by one [5] or two [3, 4] additional pathologists or by reassessment of the same experts [2, 6]. Although consensus by multiple pathologists is expected to counterbalance the high inter-rater variability, influence on algorithmic performance has not been examined.

This study aims to evaluate the ideal number of expert opinions required for the development of deep learning-based mitotic figure detection algorithms with high accuracy. For this purpose, a well established object detection algorithm was trained with labels derived from a consensus of a range of pathologists ($n = 1$-11) and evaluated against reference annotations derived from the total consensus of twelve pathologists.

2 Material and methods

For this investigation, datasets were created from 50 histologic images of canine mast cell tumours from 50 patients. Use of these samples was approved by the local governmental authorities (State Office of Health and Social Affairs of Berlin, approval ID: StN 011/20). Histologic sections were created with routine methods (haematoxylin and eosin stain) and digitised at a resolution of 0.25 μm per pixel (400 x magnification) using an Aperio ScanScope CS2 (Leica, Germany) scanner.

2.1 Creation of databases

Independent databases were created by twelve veterinary pathologists (each at least three years of experience in histopathology) using the SlideRunner annotation software (https://github.com/DeepPathology/SlideRunner). For each of the

50 slides, a field of interest in the tumour area with a standard size of 2.37 mm^2 was selected and annotators marked centroid coordinates of all mitotic figures recognised in these tumour regions. Each pathologist identified between 1,324 and 4,412 mitotic figures (total number of annotations: 32,917). The dataset was split into 35 training, 5 validation and 10 test images with similar variability in mitotic figure density in the selected regions.

2.2   Deep learning-based mitotic figure detection

For mitotic figure detection we customised a publicly available RetinaNet implementation [1] with a ResNet18 stem. For network training, 2,500 patches (1,024 x 1,024 pixels at highest resolution) each containing at least one mitotic figure were randomly drawn from the 35 training images. The network was trained with a variable number of databases created by the pathologists. The training and validation reference was individually defined as the majority vote of this subgroup. The training was split into two phases. First, only the randomly initialised network heads were trained (batch size: 12) for five epochs using a maximal learning rate of 10^{-3}. Afterwards, the complete model was trained for an additional ten epochs and a maximal learning rate of 10^{-4}. During this second phase, 1,500 patches from the validation set were used for model selection.

Four different training set-ups were evaluated: (1) The network was trained with each individual pathologist's database and the model performance was compared to the annotator's performance on the test set. To ensure stability, the F_1 score was computed as median of three independent training runs. (2) The network was trained on the consensus of an increasingly larger, randomly chosen subset of pathologists. In order to obtain unambiguous agreement, these increases consisted only of odd increments. For each addition, ten training runs were averaged to determine the influence of the random selection of annotators. For the last two experiments (3) and (4) the annotators were sorted in descending order by their label agreement compared to the majority vote measured by the F_1 score. The model was then trained on (3) the first n pathologists ($\hat{=}$ highest agreement) and (4) on the last n pathologists ($\hat{=}$ lowest agreement).

By using the consensus, we only trained with mitotic figures with at least 50 % agreement. We modified the loss computation by weighting the sample with the percentage of pathologists that agreed upon the respective sample (> 50-100 %).

2.3   Model evaluation

The test set was generated from ten test slides and comprised all mitotic figure labels upon which the majority of all twelve pathologists (i.e. at least seven pathologists) agreed. For model performance evaluation, the F_1 score was computed. As previously defined by Bertram et al. [6], a mitotic figure detection was counted as true positive if the Euclidean distance of the reference and predicted bounding box centroids was at most 25 pixels ($\hat{=}$ 6.25 μm, i.e. approximately the average cell radius of neoplastic mast cells). The detector confidence threshold was chosen based on the highest performance on the validation set.

3 Results

Label accuracy of the twelve pathologists compared to the majority vote was highly variable with F_1 scores ranging from 0.64 to 0.85 (median: 0.77) for the whole dataset and from 0.68 to 0.86 (median: 0.77) for the test cases. In Fig. 1 the labelling performance of each annotator is compared to the F_1 scores of the RetinaNet, which was trained on mitotic figure labels of the same pathologists. For the five pathologists with the lowest label agreement on the reference annotations, the algorithmic approach showed similar performance on the test dataset. Regardless of the label performance of the annotators, the algorithmic F_1 score was capped at around 0.74 for the network architecture used. A more detailed analysis showed that higher algorithmic performance was associated with high annotation precision, while labelling sensitivity seemed to have a negligible influence.

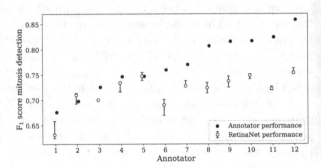

Fig. 1. Labelling performance (F_1 score) of individual annotator compared to the performance of networks trained with annotations from each respective pathologist (median and range of three training runs) evaluated on the majority vote test set.

Tab. 1 summarises the network performance when training the algorithm with databases of an increasingly larger subset of annotators. Compared to a single annotator, models trained with multi-expert labels resulted in an overall higher performance and a lower variability as measured by the interquartile range. Fig. 2 shows that training with databases that have the highest agreement with the majority vote yielded the best results. However, this arrangement benefited the least from higher numbers of annotators (as opposed to using the databases with the lowest agreement).

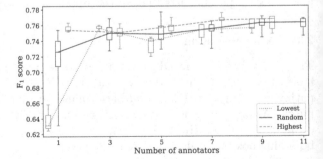

Fig. 2. Performance (F_1 score) of models trained with different combinations of annotators. Whiskers represent the minimum and maximum F_1 score from the training runs.

Table 1. Comparison of F_1 scores of models trained with different reference annotations based upon the majority vote from different combinations of annotators.

Database	Number of annotators	Training Runs	Median	Minimum	Maximum	Interquartile Range
Each once	1	18 x 3	0.726	0.625	0.763	0.038
Random	3	10	0.75	0.728	0.769	0.016
Random	5	10	0.749	0.729	0.777	0.017
Random	7	10	0.756	0.730	0.765	0.008
Random	9	10	0.763	0.745	0.771	0.008
Random	11	10	0.763	0.746	0.769	0.010
Highest agreement	3	5	0.751	0.73	0.762	0.010
Highest agreement	5	5	0.759	0.748	0.770	0.007
Highest agreement	7	5	0.767	0.75	0.776	0.003
Highest agreement	9	5	0.768	0.749	0.771	0.016
Lowest agreement	3	5	0.756	0.753	0.76	0.003
Lowest agreement	5	5	0.74	0.720	0.745	0.018
Lowest agreement	7	5	0.754	0.736	0.761	0.017
Lowest agreement	9	5	0.756	0.749	0.768	0.012

4 Discussion

The high variability between annotators in the present study is consistent with previous studies [2, 3, 7] and warrants a detailed evaluation of label consistency and the impact on algorithmic performance, as was the goal of the present study. Generally, our results show that the use of a consensus of a higher number of pathologists for training the algorithm yields better and more consistent results. In particular, F_1 scores were noticeably variable when training the algorithm with single annotators (interquartile range: 0.038). A consensus by three pathologists was highly beneficial for more consistent training results (interquartile range: 0.016). Increasing the number of randomly selected annotators further only improved the median F_1 score by a small amount (+0.013). Nevertheless, we have also shown that even training with a single annotator can result in high performance. Of note, a high annotation precision of individual pathologists, i.e. few false positive labels, seemed to be more important than high labelling sensitivity, i.e. few false negatives labels, for training of high-performing models. This analysis, however, might have been biased by the ground truth definition as consensus of the majority of pathologists. Our results emphasise that high annotation accuracy and consensus by a small number of pathologists may result in the best trade-off between algorithmic performance and labour intensity of dataset development. Further enhancement of label consistency may be achieved with repeated screening of images or algorithmically augmented labelling [6]. An interesting approach to reduce subjectivity for future mitotic figures datasets was recently introduced by Tellez et al. [8]. In this study, a specific immunohistochemical marker of mitotic figures was used to derive object labels and labels were assigned to images with standard histologic stain via image registration.

The major limitation of the conducted experiments was the pathologist-defined ground truth. Although pathologists are the current gold standard for labelling histologic images, they have high inter-rater variability which hampers not only training of data-driven algorithms (as proven in the present study) but also biases performance evaluation. The finding that algorithms trained with multi-expert databases outperformed many pathologists on the test set was attributed to the fact that algorithms yielded high sensitivity. Furthermore, the experiments in the present work were limited to a standard object detection architecture with relatively low complexity. Compensation for noisy labels and higher F_1 scores may be achieved with a more complex model, such as by adding a second classification stage [1, 6], and larger training datasets. Further improvement of data-derived algorithms may be accomplished with advanced deep learning methods that incorporate label accuracy during training.

Acknowledgement. FW gratefully acknowledges financial support received by Merck KGaA. CAB gratefully acknowledges financial support received from the Dres. Jutta & Georg Bruns-Stiftung für innovative Veterinärmedizin.

References

1. Aubreville M, Bertram CA, Marzahl C, et al. Deep learning algorithms out-perform veterinary pathologists in detecting the mitotically most active tumor region. Sci Rep. 2020;10(16447):1–11.
2. Bertram CA, Veta M, Marzahl C, et al. Are pathologist-defined labels reproducible? Comparison of the TUPAC16 mitotic figure dataset with an alternative set of labels. In: Interpretable and Annotation-Efficient Learning for Medical Image Computing. IMIMIC 2020, MIL3ID 2020, LABELS 2020. Lecture Notes in Computer Science. Springer; 2020. p. 204–213.
3. Veta M, Van Diest PJ, Willems SM, et al. Assessment of algorithms for mitosis detection in breast cancer histopathology images. Med Image Anal. 2015;20(1):237–248.
4. Veta M, Heng YJ, Stathonikos N, et al. Predicting breast tumor proliferation from whole-slide images: the TUPAC16 challenge. Med Image Anal. 2019;54:111–121.
5. Roux L, Racoceanu D, Capron F, et al. MITOS & ATYPIA-detection of mitosis and evaluation of nuclear atypia score in breast cancer histological images. IPAL, Agency Sci. Technol Res Inst Infocom Res, Singapore, Tech Rep. 2014;.
6. Bertram CA, Aubreville M, Marzahl C, et al. A large-scale dataset for mitotic figure assessment on whole slide images of canine cutaneous mast cell tumor. Scientific Data. 2019;6(1):1–9.
7. Veta M, Diest PJV, Jiwa M, et al. Mitosis counting in breast cancer: object-level interobserver agreement and comparison to an automatic method. PloS one. 2016;11(8).
8. Tellez D, Balkenhol M, Otte-Höller I, et al. Whole-slide mitosis detection in H&E breast histology using PHH3 as a reference to train distilled stain-invariant convolutional networks. IEEE Trans Med Imaging. 2018;37(9):2126–2136.

Automatic Vessel Segmentation and Aneurysm Detection Pipeline for Numerical Fluid Analysis

Johannes Felde[1], Thomas Wagner[2], Hans Lamecker[1], Christian Doenitz[3], Lina Gundelwein[1]

[1]1000shapes GmbH, Wiesenweg 10, 12247 Berlin, Germany
[2]Regensburg Center of Biomedical Engineering, OTH and University Regensburg, Galgenbergstr. 30, 93053 Regensburg, Germany
[3]Universitätsklinikum Regensburg, Franz-Josef-Strauß-Allee 11, 93053 Regensburg, Germany
johannes.felde@1000shapes.com

Abstract. Computational Fluid Dynamic calculations are a great assistance for rupture prediction of cerebral aneurysms. This procedure requires a consistent surface, as well as a separation of the blood vessel and aneurysm on this surface to calculate rupture-relevant scores. For this purpose we present an automatic pipeline, which generates a surface model of the vascular tree from angiographies determined by a marker-based watershed segmentation and label post-processing. Aneurysms on the surface model are then detected and segmented using shape-based graph cuts along with anisotropic diffusion and an iterative Support Vector Machine based classification. Aneurysms are correctly detected and segmented in 33 out of 35 test cases. Simulation relevant vessels are successfully segmented without vessel merging in 131 out of 144 test cases, achieving an average dice coefficient of 0.901.

1 Introduction

Intracranial aneurysms are a common cerebrovascular disease, in which a weakness of the vessel wall causes widening or ballooning of cerebral arteries. A small percentage of intracranial aneurysms rupture and consequently cause subarachnoid hemorrhage with high mortality and disability rates. Due to the catastrophic nature of aneurysm rupture on the one hand side, but low rupture risk and significant risk of complication during treatment on the other side, rupture risk assessment is an important step during clinical decision making. Different scores based on clinical, morphological and hemodynamic parameters like Normalized Wall Shear Stress (WSS) and Oscillatory Shear Index (OSI) [1] to evaluate the rupture risk, can be computed on a patient individual geometry of the vascular tract with the help of Computational Fluid Dynamics (CFD) simulations. Sufficient smoothness and resolution of the reconstructed geometry have to be ensured, to prevent introduction of non-physiological flow structures. The definition of the rupture risk scores require a differentiation between aneurysm wall and parent vessel wall. Therefore, an aneurysm detection mechanism is required. These requirements, in combination with problems like resolution-related merging of blood vessels, pose a great challenge to the development of a fully automated segmentation pipeline for CFD analyses. Solutions that cover both problems are either semi-automatic [2] with a manual selection of seeds for a region growing, or they are only designed to detect the aneurysm and not to generate a CFD usable surface [3].

2   Methods

In this section, we describe our automatic seed extraction combined with a marker-based watershed segmentation and discuss our extension of the approach by Lawonn et al. [4] to segment and detect more complex aneurysms.

2.1   Dataset

The training data for aneurysm detection consist of 50 surface meshes provided by Pozo et al. [5] as well as 109 surface meshes from MICCAI 2020 Cerebral Aneurysm Detection challenge (CADA) [6]. The aneurysm detection and segmentation is evaluated on 35 labeled 3D Rotational Angiography (3DRA) images provided by Universitätsklinikum Regensburg (UKR). For the evaluation of the vessel segmentation, this test set is extended by 109 labeled 3DRA images from CADA challenge.

2.2   Marker-based watershed vessel tree segmentation

The vessel tree is segmented using a watershed segmentation initialized with markers defining the foreground (vessels) and background (exterior).

2.2.1   Skeletonization. After normalizing the image data and applying an anisotropic diffusion filter to reduce image noise while preserving strong edges, the image is thresholded using an automatically calculated Otsu threshold. This results in a segmentation containing artifacts and fused vessels. A coarse vascular tree skeleton is extracted following [7] and used to mask the image data to the region of interest, accelerating the following computations.

2.2.2   Marker-based watershed segmentation. The markers for the marker-based watershed segmentation are positioned on the large, relevant vessels of the coarse vessel tree. Therefor, the vascular tree is traversed starting from the internal carotid artery which is the vessel with the largest volume. At each node inflow direction vector v_{in} and the outflow direction vectors v_{out_n} of the incident edges are computed. Edges are grouped to vessel tracts by similar direction and radius, if they fulfill the properties: $1 - \frac{\mathbf{v_{in}} \cdot \mathbf{v_{out_n}}}{\|\mathbf{v_{in}}\| \|\mathbf{v_{out_n}}\|} > t_{\cos}$ and $\frac{\bar{r}_{in}}{\bar{r}_{out_n}} < r_{\mathrm{ratio}}$, where $t_{\cos} = 0.6$ and $r_{\text{ratio}} = 0.7$ have been heuristically determined. On each vessel tract, exceeding the empirically determined values for length of 15 mm and average radius of 2.5 mm, a marker is placed. Thin vessels that are not relevant for the CFD simulation are thus not marked and will not be segmented. The exterior marker for labeling the non exterior area is placed on a voxel with intensity 0. The marker-based watershed segmentation is computed on the gradient of the masked image resulting in a voxelwise classification with different labels for each grouped vessel.

2.2.3 Post-processing. In order to differentiate between voxel contact areas representing touching vessel walls from those representing vessel bifurcations, we consider the local diffusion of the contact area voxels, defined by the linear diffusion C_l and planar diffusion C_p introduced by Westin et al. [8]. Assuming a more elliptical expansion for removable voxels, their C_l tends to be larger and C_p smaller than for the mostly circular cross sectioned vessel bifurcations. To determine C_l and C_p, the positions of the contact voxels are used to construct a covariance matrix with computation of singular values $\lambda_1 \geq \lambda_2 \geq \lambda_3$: $C_l = \frac{\lambda_1 - \lambda_2}{\lambda_1 + \lambda_2 + \lambda_3}$ and $C_p = \frac{2(\lambda_2 - \lambda_3)}{\lambda_1 + \lambda_2 + \lambda_3}$. The contact voxels are removed, if C_l exceeds and C_p goes below the predefined thresholds $t_{C_l} = 0.66$ and $t_{C_p} = 0.37$.

2.3 Aneurysm detection and segmentation

A modified version of Lawonn et al. [4] algorithm pipeline for detection of aneurysms based on the vascular surface geometry is used. We changed the order of the processing steps and introduced new features to the classifier to reduce false positives and ensure a stable classification of abnormal aneurysms.

2.3.1 Surface pre-processing. The surface mesh is generated from the watershed segmentation using generalized marching cubes. To prevent possible numeric mis-calculations, it is ensured that only manifold surface parts are present.

2.3.2 Aneurysm candidate generation. Initial binary labeling of the surface triangles $\{T_j\}$ is performed by solving the combinatorial optimization problem described in [4] using the Boykov et al. graph cut algorithm [9] based on the surface shape index [10] values S_i. A subsequent connected component analysis to group coherent triangle fields with the same label is performed. Grouped fields with aneurysm label and an average shape index $\bar{S}_i < t_S$ are discarded and labeled as vessel, where $t_S = 0.78$ is determined heuristically.

2.3.3 Growing of aneurysm candidates. As aneurysms are not perfectly spherical, but contain concave regions (Fig. 1), parts of it might be labeled as vessel. Hence, we perform an anisotropic diffusion on the aneurysm field borders, smoothing and expanding them towards the concave regions and merging close separated fields following [4]. Based on the resulting diffusion field, represented by the continuous function $\mathbf{u}$, threshold T_{opt} assigning triangles to the aneurysm label is optimized by minimizing the length of the derived border curve. A second analysis of connected labels is performed in order to classify each grown or merged connected field in the next stage.

2.3.4 Candidate classification. A Support Vector Machine (SVM) is used to reclassify the candidates in order to reduce the error rate. In total, six features are extracted from the mesh data including average shape index $\overline{S_i}$ and spherical diffusion on all field points as well as planar diffusion and linear diffusion on the field contour points, as proposed in [4]. Additionally, the variance of the shape index is used to distinguish aneurysms with both, concave and convex regions and thus similar $\overline{S_i}$ as tubular structures from vessels. Furthermore, to prevent misclassification of spherical vessel tips as aneurysms, linear diffusion of all points per field is used, exploiting the tubular characteristics of the vessels. Using mesh data of [5] and [6], 326 aneurysm candidate fields were calculated, comprising 141 aneurysm and 185 vessel fields. For each field the six features were extracted and used for a SVM training with a nonlinear RBF kernel. Optimal regularization parameter $C = 10$ and influence parameter $\gamma = 2.88$ were determined by a grid search with a 5-cross validation, achieving an accuracy of 94%. The grown candidate fields are classified with the trained SVM. Merged aneurysm fields now classified as label, probably consist of a true positive aneurysm candidate merged with a false positive and are thus separated again in a re-optimiziation process. It includes a threshold T_{limit} determination, by reducing threshold T_{opt} on $\mathbf{u}$, until the merged fields are separated. These separated fields, created by T_{limit}, are re-classified with the SVM, resulting in the final classification.

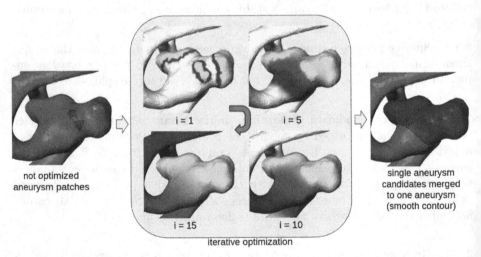

Fig. 1. Optimization of the graph cut segmented aneurysm candidate fields yields a single aneurysm with a smooth contour.

3   Results

The pipeline was qualitatively evaluated with respect to correct vessel and aneurysm segmentation on the 35 UKR cases. For quantitative evaluation of the vessel segmentation the dice value was calculated for the 35 UKR and 109 CADA cases.

3.1   Segmentation

The proposed segmentation yields dice coefficients of 0.9292 ± 0.02 for UKR and 0.8728 ± 0.043 for the more heterogeneous CADA challenge image data. 33 of 35 UKR and 98 of 109 CADA image data segmentations showed no merged vessels in simulation relevant vessels, i.e. all vessels upstream of the aneurysm as well as at least 5 times the carrier vessel diameter downstream of the aneurysm. Touching aneurysms and vessels are correctly segmented as separate structures by our algorithm, opposed to the merged structure retrieved by Otsu segementation (Fig. 2). Generally over-segmentation rather than under-segmentation is observed.

3.2   Aneurysm detection

From the 35 aneurysms, 33 were correctly detected and segmented. The aneurysms with spherical shape are easily recognized and segmented, as seen in Fig. 4(a) and 4(b), but also aneurysms with deep concave regions, are correctly segmented as a result of the improvement as seen in Fig. 4(c) and 4(d). Only two small aneurysms (Fig. 4(e)) were not detected.

4   Discussion

We have presented a fully automated segmentation of the middle cerebral arteries and an automatic aneurysm detection resulting in surface models for CFD analysis. We segment the arterial tree with a high reliability using a marker-based watershed segmentation with subsequent separation of merged vessels. In future

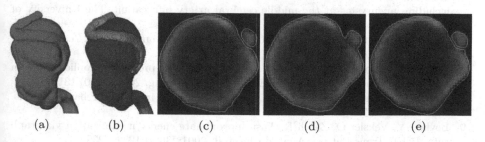

(a)   (b)   (c)   (d)   (e)

Fig. 2. Difficult CADA case A095 [6]: (a) Ground truth (GT) surface. (b) Proposed segmentation. (c) GT segmentation slice. (d) Otsu segmentation slice. (e) Proposed segmentation slice.

Fig. 3. Segmentation results for aneurysms with: (a) Normal sphere like structure. (b) Large sphere like structure. (c) Deep concave region. (d) Deep concave region with two sphere like blobs. (e) Missing segmentation.

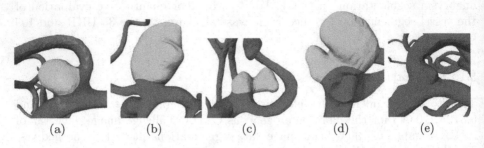

|(a)|(b)|(c)|(d)|(e)|

work we want to extend this method to fusiform aneurysms and further improve the separation of merged vessels. For the former, new features have to be added to the aneurysm detection algorithm. For the latter we plan to improve the skeletonization method which currently traces the centerline between two thin neighboring vessels, resulting in the segmentation to label them as one merged vessel tract. A recalculation of the skeleton on the watershed segmentation with a subsequent computation of a minimal spanning tree will help splitting merged vessels.

References

1. Xiang J, Natarajan SK, Tremmel M, et al. Hemodynamic–morphologic discriminants for intracranial aneurysm rupture. Stroke. 2011;42(1):144–152.
2. Seo JH, Eslami P, Caplan J, et al. A highly automated computational method for modeling of intracranial aneurysm hemodynamics. Front Physiol. 2018;9:681.
3. Rahmany I, Laajili S, Khlifa N. Automated computerized method for the detection of unruptured cerebral aneurysms in DSA images. Curr Med Imaging. 2018;14(5):771–777.
4. Lawonn K, Meuschke M, Wickenhöfer R, et al. A geometric optimization approach for the detection and segmentation of multiple aneurysms. In: Computer Graphics Forum. vol. 38. Wiley Online Library; 2019. p. 413–425.
5. Pozo Soler J, Frangi AF, Consortium Tn. Database of cerebral artery geometries including aneurysms at the middle cerebral artery bifurcation. The University of Sheffield; 2017.
6. CADA challenge dataset; 2020. Available from: https://cada.grand-challenge.org/Dataset/.
7. Fouard C, Malandain G, Prohaska S, et al. Blockwise processing applied to brain microvascular network study. IEEE Trans Med Imaging. 2006;25(10):1319–1328.
8. Westin CF. Geometrical diffusion measures for MRI from tensor basis analysis. Proc ISMRM'97. 1997;.
9. Boykov Y, Veksler O, Zabih R. Fast approximate energy minimization via graph cuts. IEEE Trans Pattern Anal Mach Intell. 2001;23(11):1222–1239.
10. Koenderink JJ, Van Doorn AJ. Surface shape and curvature scales. Image Vis Comput. 1992;10(8):557–564.

Abstract: Widening the Focus

Biomedical Image Segmentation Challenges and the Underestimated Role of Patch Sampling and Inference Strategies

Frederic Madesta[0,1,3], Rüdiger Schmitz[0,1,2,3], Thomas Rösch[2], René Werner[1,3]

[0]Both authors contributed equally
[1]Department of Computational Neuroscience, UKE, Hamburg, Germany
[2]Department for Interdisciplinary Endoscopy, UKE, Hamburg, Germany
[3]Center for Biomedical Artificial Intelligence (bAIome), Hamburg, Germany
f.madesta@uke.de

The field of biomedical computer vision has considerably been influenced by image analysis challenges, which are mainly dominated by deep learning-based approaches. Much effort is put into challenge-specific optimization of model design, training schemes and data augmentation techniques. The paper [1] aims to widen the focus beyond model architecture and training pipeline design by shedding a light on inference efficiency and the role of patch sampling strategies for large images that cannot be processed at once. First, examining MICCAI challenge datasets of previous years, we demonstrate that inference patch overlap can considerably influence segmentation performance. This is contrasted with the status quo in challenge reporting, with inference strategies being rarely detailed at all. Second, dataset-specific patch overlap effects are shown to be aetiologically related to varying intra-patch segmentation accuracy. Third, we introduce novel strategies for inference-time patch sampling that outperform the de facto standard, namely ordered, sliding window-like cropping, in terms of convergence speed and stability (Fig. 1). The proposed Monte Carlo-based strategies are built on uncertainty mechanisms and local image entropy. Finally, we provide practical guidance on inference strategy optimization.

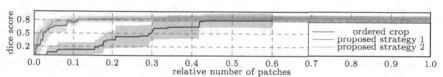

Fig. 1. Dice convergence curves for different patch sampling strategies (mean ± SD).

References

1. Madesta F, Schmitz R, Rösch T, et al. Widening the Focus: biomedical image segmentation challenges and the underestimated role of patch sampling and inference strategies. Proc MICCAI 2020. 2020; p. 289–298.

© Der/die Autor(en), exklusiv lizenziert durch
Springer Fachmedien Wiesbaden GmbH, ein Teil von Springer Nature 2021
C. Palm et al. (Hrsg.), *Bildverarbeitung für die Medizin 2021*,
Informatik aktuell, https://doi.org/10.1007/978-3-658-33198-6_58

End-to-end Learning of Body Weight Prediction from Point Clouds with Basis Point Sets

Alexander Bigalke[1], Lasse Hansen[1], Mattias P. Heinrich[1]

[1]Institut für Medizinische Informatik, Universität zu Lübeck

alexander.bigalke@uni-luebeck.de

Abstract. The body weight of a patient is an important parameter in many clinical settings, e.g. when it comes to drug dosing or anesthesia. However, assessing the weight through direct interaction with the patient (anamnesis, weighing) is often infeasible. Therefore, there is a need for the weight to be estimated in a contactless way from visual inputs. This work addresses weight prediction of patients lying in bed from 3D point cloud data by means of deep learning techniques. Contrary to prior work in this field, we propose to learn the task in an end-to-end fashion without relying on hand-crafted features. For this purpose, we adopt the concept of basis point sets to encode the input point cloud into a low-dimensional feature vector. This vector is passed to a neural network, which is trained for weight regression. As the originally proposed construction of the basis point set is not ideal for our problem, we develop a novel sampling scheme, which exploits prior knowledge about the distribution of input points. We evaluate our approach on a lying pose dataset (SLP) and achieve weight estimates with a mean absolute error of 4.2 kg and a mean relative error of 6.4 % compared to 4.8 kg and 7.0 % obtained with a basic PointNet.

1 Introduction

The precise knowledge of a patient's body weight is a crucial requirement in several clinical scenarios, including anesthesia or drug dosage. In emergency situations, however, patients are often unable to communicate their weight due to unconsciousness, dementia or neurological disorder. Weighing the patient on-site with an ordinary scale is infeasible in case of severe injuries, and bed scales are expensive and not always available. For these reasons, weight is often estimated by clinical staff although this procedure has been shown to be error-prone in clinical studies [1].

To obtain more accurate weight estimates, several works use a multiple linear regression model to infer body weight from biometric measurements such as height, and waist and hip circumference [2]. Since manual measurements of these quantities are time-intensive and infeasible in case of certain injuries, it is difficult to integrate this approach into clinical routine. Instead, a fully automatic and contactless weight estimate is desirable.

Springer Fachmedien Wiesbaden GmbH, ein Teil von Springer Nature 2021
C. Palm et al. (Hrsg.), *Bildverarbeitung für die Medizin 2021*,
Informatik aktuell, https://doi.org/10.1007/978-3-658-33198-6_59

This can be achieved by deriving the weight estimate from visual sensor data using methods from computer vision. For this purpose, the use of depth sensors is particularly suitable. Firstly, depth maps and corresponding point clouds carry rich geometric information which is of eminent importance for accurate weight estimates. Secondly, patients are unidentifiable on depth maps which prevents any privacy concerns.

This work addresses the task of weight estimation of patients lying in bed from 3D point cloud data by means of deep learning techniques. Contrary to prior work in this field, we aim to learn weight prediction in an end-to-end fashion.

1.1 Related work

More generic work in the field of weight estimation from visual data predicts the weight of free-standing subjects from RGB-D data [3]. The proposed method segments the subject from the background and extrapolates biometric measures from the silhouette. The deduced measures are fed into a neural network to regress the subject's weight.

Several works address weight estimation from point clouds of lying patients in a clinical environment [4, 5]. Libra3D [4] fits a mesh to the point cloud whereby the patient's back is modeled with help of the bed plane. Based on the mesh, the volume of the patient is calculated and multiplied with a fixed empirically determined density to obtain a weight estimate. The authors of [5] extend this work by additionally extracting more abstract features from the point cloud, which are forwarded by a neural network for weight regression. All of these works rely on hand-crafted features and are not trained end-to-end.

In recent years, end-to-end learning from point clouds has become viable owing to deep learning architectures that directly operate on raw point sets. The pioneering PointNet [6] applies a shared multi-layer perceptron to each point individually and achieves permutation invariance through a symmetric max pooling operation.

1.2 Contribution

To our knowledge, this is the first work to learn weight prediction from 3D point clouds in an end-to-end fashion. Since learning weight regression directly from raw point clouds using a PointNet architecture [6] is a complex task, we suggest to simplify the problem by considering input point clouds relative to a fixed reference. To achieve this, we adopt the idea of basis point sets (BPS) [7] to encode the input point cloud. The resulting feature vector is subsequently fed into a fully connected neural network to regress the weight. Based on the observation that the construction of the BPS in [7] is not ideal for our specific problem, we propose an adapted sampling scheme to incorporate prior knowledge about the distribution of input points. We experimentally validate our approach on the SLP dataset [8] and significantly outperform several baselines, including a PointNet architecture [6].

2   Materials and methods

Our method receives a point cloud cropped around the bed as input and outputs the patient's weight in kg. The point cloud is initially pre-processed, subsequently encoded by means of a BPS and finally processed by a neural network for weight prediction (Fig. 1). We assume the patient to be uncovered and in a supine position, which can easily be realized in clinical workflow.

2.1   Pre-processing

In the pre-processing step, the patient needs to be segmented from the bed. First, we use the RANSAC algorithm [9] to fit a plane to the mattress and keep only the points above the plane as it was done in [4]. Most of the kept points belong to the patient, but there may remain point clusters belonging to other objects on the bed. To remove those points, we cluster the cloud using DBSCAN [10] and only keep the largest cluster.

2.2   Basis point set and neural network

After pre-processing, we are left with a set of patient point clouds $X_i \in \mathbb{R}^{N_i \times 3}$, $(i = 1, ..., p)$, each comprising N_i points $x_{ij} \in \mathbb{R}^3$. We encode the clouds with help of a BPS as elaborated in [7]. In [7], each cloud is initially normalized to fit a unit sphere which entails a loss of scale information. Since scale is indispensable for weight estimation, we only mean-center each cloud. Subsequently, a BPS

$$B = [b_1, ..., b_k], b_j \in \mathbb{R}^3, \|b_j\| \leq r \tag{1}$$

is constructed by uniform sampling of k points from a sphere of radius r. This set is fixed for all point clouds in training and test set. We select $k = 2048$ and set the radius to the maximal radius of all point clouds in the training set, i.e. $r = \max_i(\max_j \|x_{ij} - (\sum_k x_{ik})/N_i\|)$.

Given the BPS B, an input point cloud X_i is encoded by computing the distance from each basis point to the nearest point in the input cloud, yielding a k-dimensional feature vector

$$f_i^B = [\min_{x_{ij} \in X_i} d(b_1, x_{ij}), ..., \min_{x_{ij} \in X_i} d(b_k, x_{ij})] \in \mathbb{R}^k \tag{2}$$

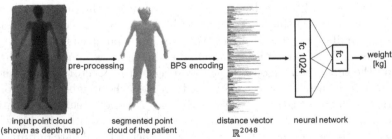

Fig. 1. Overview of our proposed pipeline for weight estimation from point clouds.

This feature vector is subsequently fed into a neural network, consisting of the following sequence of layers: BN, FC(1024), ReLU, BN, Dropout(p=0.8), FC(1). The network parameters are optimized by minimizing a mean squared error loss between predicted weight and ground truth.

2.3   Adapted sampling of basis points

In Fig. 2(a), a BPS obtained by uniform sampling in the sphere is shown relative to an input point cloud. We observe that many basis points are far away from the patient and thus encode less detailed information. As all patients have a similar orientation and occupy similar regions of the sphere, we conclude that the uniform distribution of basis points is not ideal for our specific problem. We believe that a more expressive basis can be constructed by incorporating prior knowledge about the distribution of input points. To achieve this, we propose to sample the basis points from a unified point cloud which comprises all clouds from the training set. As this basis is prone to overfitting, we subsequently add Gaussian noise with a standard deviation of $\sigma = 0.3$ to the sampled basis points. The resulting BPS is depicted in Fig. 2(b).

3   Results

3.0.1   Dataset. We evaluate our method on a subset of the SLP dataset [8]. The subset comprises depth maps of 109 subjects which are lying in bed in a supine position without a cover. Each subject takes 15 different poses while staying in supine position, yielding an overall of 1635 frames. For each frame, a bounding box around the bed is obtained with the help of depth thresholding, and the corresponding image crop is transformed to a point cloud using the internal

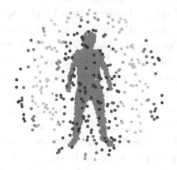

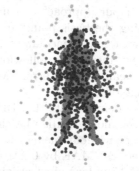

(a) Uniform sampling in the sphere.

(b) Sampling from training points.

Fig. 2. Comparison of two basis point sets constructed with different sampling schemes. We visualize a slice of the sphere around the input point cloud of a patient, which is shown in gray for reference. Basis points are shown in colour to represent the distance to the closest input point. The basis points constructed by our sampling scheme (b) are substantially more concentrated around the patient.

Table 1. Results for weight estimation on the SLP dataset.

Method	MAE [kg]	MRE [%]	in 10 % range [%]
Mean	9.46	14.6	40.8
Median	9.54	14.3	44.9
PointNet [6]	5.42 ± 0.4	8.0 ± 0.5	70.7 ± 3.2
PointNet [6] & median	4.84 ± 0.48	7.1 ± 0.6	74.7 ± 5.3
BPS random sampling	4.91 ± 0.09	7.5 ± 0.1	74.0 ± 0.8
BPS adapted sampling	4.69 ± 0.08	7.1 ± 0.1	76.1 ± 1.0
BPS adapted sampling & median	$\mathbf{4.19 \pm 0.12}$	$\mathbf{6.4 \pm 0.2}$	$\mathbf{78.6 \pm 2.9}$

camera parameters. The weight of the subjects ranges from 43.7 to 105.1 kg with a mean of 68.0 kg and a standard deviation of 12.7 kg. We use the first 60 subjects for training and results are reported for the remaining 49 subjects.

3.0.2 Implementation Details. For pre-processing, we run RANSAC with a threshold of 1 cm for 1000 iterations. DBSCAN is used with $\epsilon = 2.5$ cm and minpts = 5. Network parameters are optimized with the ADAM optimizer. The initial learning rate is set to 0.001 and halved every 40 epochs. We use a batch size of 16 and train for 200 epochs. Each experiment is repeated ten times and we report mean and standard deviation.

3.0.3 Baselines. As baseline, we train a basic PointNet [6] to directly regress the weight from the point cloud of the patient. Additionally, we estimate the weight of each test subject with a constant value which corresponds to the mean/median weight of all subjects from the training set of the same sex as the test subject.

Results are presented in Tab. 1. We compare the baseline methods to three variants of our approach: 1) uniform sampling of basis points in the sphere, 2) sampling the basis points from training points, 3) same as 2), but for each subject, we take the median of the predicted weights for all 15 frames. For each method, we report the following metrics on the test set: mean absolute error (MAE), mean relative error (MRE), percentage of subjects within a relative error range of ± 10 %.

Results demonstrate that BPS with random sampling halves both MAE and MRE of the mean/median baselines and considerably improves on the PointNet architecture without median filtering as well. Applying our adapted sampling further reduces MAE by 0.22 kg and MRE by 0.4 % points. Finally taking the median of 15 independent weight estimates for the same subject yields another improvement of 0.5 kg in MAE and 0.7 % points in MRE. That way, we achieve an overall MAE of 4.19 kg, MRE of 6.4 % and the weight of 78.6 % of the subjects is estimated within a 10 % error range. This constitutes a relative performance gain in MAE of 56 % compared to the mean/median baseline and of 13.4 % in relation to the corresponding PointNet model.

4   Discussion

This work successfully applied the concept of BPS [7] to learn body weight prediction from point clouds of lying patients in an end-to-end fashion. We optimized the method for the specific problem at hand by introducing a customized sampling scheme for basis construction which takes the prior distribution of input points into account and thus contributed a meaningful performance gain. Finally, the experiments showed that a further increase of accuracy can be achieved by statistical averaging over several independent weight estimates for the same subject. Altogether, our method achieves a higher accuracy (MAE=4.2 kg, MRE=6.4 %) than weight estimates by clinical staff, which exhibit MAEs between 5.7 and 8.7 kg in [2] and MREs of 7.7 to 11.0 % in [1]. That way, our work demonstrates the potential of end-to-end deep learning in the context of weight estimation and thus encourages further research in this direction. Future work could, for instance, incorporate semantic labels or point descriptors into the encoding or address the construction of an even more tailored basis set.

Acknowledgement. This work was supported by the Federal Ministry for Economic Affairs and Energy of Germany (FKZ: 01MK20012B).

References

1. Menon S, Kelly AM. How accurate is weight estimation in the emergency department? Emerg Med Australas. 2005;17(2):113–116.
2. Lorenz MW, Graf M, Henke C, et al. Anthropometric approximation of body weight in unresponsive stroke patients. J Neurol Neurosurg Psychiatry. 2007;78(12):1331–1336.
3. Velardo C, Dugelay JL. What can computer vision tell you about your weight? Procs IEEE EUSIPCO. 2012; p. 1980–1984.
4. Pfitzner C, May S, Merkl C, et al. Libra3D: Body weight estimation for emergency patients in clinical environments with a 3D structured light sensor. IEEE Int Conf Robot Autom. 2015; p. 2888–2893.
5. Pfitzner C, May S, Nüchter A. Neural network-based visual body weight estimation for drug dosage finding. Med Imaging 2016 Image Process. 2016;9784:97841Z.
6. Qi CR, Su H, Mo K, et al. Pointnet: Deep learning on point sets for 3D classification and segmentation. Proc IEEE Comput Soc Conf Comput Vis Pattern Recognit. 2017; p. 652–660.
7. Prokudin S, Lassner C, Romero J. Efficient learning on point clouds with basis point sets. Proc IEEE Int Conf Comput Vis Workshop. 2019; p. 0–0.
8. Liu S, Ostadabbas S. Seeing under the cover: A physics guided learning approach for in-bed pose estimation. Proc Springer Int Conf Med Image Comput Comput Assist Interv. 2019; p. 236–245.
9. Fischler MA, Bolles RC. Random sample consensus: a paradigm for model fitting with applications to image analysis and automated cartography. Commun ACM. 1981;24(6):381–395.
10. Ester M, Kriegel HP, Sander J, et al. A density-based algorithm for discovering clusters in large spatial databases with noise. Kdd. 1996;96(34):226–231.

Abstract: Deep Learning Algorithms Out-perform Veterinary Pathologists in Detecting the Mitotically Most Active Tumor Region

Marc Aubreville[1,2], Christof A. Bertram[3], Christian Marzahl[2],
Corinne Gurtner[4], Martina Dettwiler[4], Anja Schmidt[5],
Florian Bartenschlager[3], Sophie Merz[3], Marco Fragoso[3], Olivia Kershaw[3],
Robert Klopfleisch[3], Andreas Maier[2]

[1]Technische Hochschule Ingolstadt, Germany
[2]Pattern Recognition Lab, Friedrich-Alexander-Universität Erlangen-Nürnberg,
Germany
[3]Institute of Veterinary Pathology, Freie Universität Berlin, Germany
[4]Department of Infectious Diseases and Pathobiology, Vetsuisse Faculty, University of
Bern, Bern, Switzerland
[5]Vet Med Labor GmbH - Division of IDEXX Laboratories, Ludwigsburg, Germany
marc.aubreville@thi.de

Manual count of mitotic figures, which is determined in the tumor region with the highest mitotic activity, is a key parameter of most tumor grading schemes. The mitotic count has a known high inter-rater disagreement and is strongly dependent on the area selection due to uneven mitotic figure distribution. In our work[1], we assessed the question, how significantly the area selection could impact the mitotic count. On a data set of 32 cases of H&E-stained canine cutaneous mast cell tumor, fully annotated for mitotic figures, we asked eight veterinary pathologists to select a field of interest for the mitotic count, and retrieved the mitotic count for that area from the data set. Additionally, we evaluated three deep learning-based methods for the assessment of highest mitotic density. We found that the predictions by all models were, on average, better than those of the experts. Further, we found considerable differences in position selection between pathologists, which could partially explain the high variance that has been reported for the manual mitotic count. To achieve better inter-rater agreement, we propose to use a computer-based area selection for support of the pathologist in the manual mitotic count.

References

1. Aubreville M, Bertram CA, Marzahl C, et al. Deep learning algorithms out-perform veterinary pathologists in detecting the mitotically most active tumor region. Sci Rep. 2020;10(1):16447.

© Der/die Autor(en), exklusiv lizenziert durch
Springer Fachmedien Wiesbaden GmbH, ein Teil von Springer Nature 2021
C. Palm et al. (Hrsg.), *Bildverarbeitung für die Medizin 2021*,
Informatik aktuell, https://doi.org/10.1007/978-3-658-33198-6_60

Abstract: Maximum A-posteriori Signal Recovery for OCT Angiography Image Generation

Lennart Husvogt[1,2], Stefan B. Ploner[1], Siyu Chen[2], Daniel Stromer[2],
Julia Schottenhamml[1], Yasin Alibhai[3], Eric Moult[2], Nadia K. Waheed[3],
James G. Fujimoto[2], Andreas Maier[1]

[1]Pattern Recognition Lab, Friedrich-Alexander-Universität Erlangen-Nürnberg
[2]Research Laboratory of Electronics, Massachusetts Institute of Technology, USA
[3]New England Eye Center, Tufts School of Medicine, Boston, USA
`lennart.husvogt@fau.de`

Optical coherence tomography angiography (OCTA) is a clinically promising modality to image retinal vasculature. For this end, optical coherence tomography (OCT) volumes are repeatedly scanned and intensity changes over time are used to compute OCTA images. Because of patient movement and variations in blood flow, OCTA data are prone to noise. To address this issue, we propose a novel iterative maximum a posteriori (MAP) signal recovery algorithm which generates OCTA volumes with reduced noise and improved image quality [1]. The proposed algorithm is based on the OCTA signal model and maximum likelihood estimate (MLE) by Ploner et al. [2]. The MLE was extended into a MAP estimate by using wavelet shrinkage and total variation minimization as regularizers. Reconstruction results are compared against ground truth OCTA data which were merged from six co-registered OCTA scans [3]. Significant improvements in signal-to-noise ratio and structural similarity were observed. The presented method is, to the best of our knowledge, the first use of Bayesian statistics for OCTA image generation.

References

1. Husvogt L, Ploner SB, Chen S, et al. Maximum a-posteriori signal recovery for optical coherence tomography angiography image generation and denoising. Biomed Opt Express. 2021;12(1):55–68.
2. Ploner SB, Riess C, Schottenhamml J, et al. A joint probabilistic model for speckle variance, amplitude decorrelation and interframe variance (IFV) optical coherence tomography angiography. Proc BVM. 2018; p. 98–102.
3. Ploner SB, Kraus MF, Moult EM, et al. Efficient and high accuracy 3-D OCT angiography motion correction in pathology. Biomed Opt Express. 2021 Jan;12(1):125–146.

Abstract: Simultaneous Estimation of X-ray Back-scatter and Forward-scatter using Multi-task Learning

Philipp Roser[1,4], Xia Zhong[2], Annette Birkhold[3], Alexander Preuhs[1],
Christopher Syben[1], Elisabeth Hoppe[1], Norbert Strobel[5],
Markus Kowarschik[3], Rebecca Fahrig[3], Andreas Maier[1,4]

[1]Pattern Recognition Lab, Friedrich-Alexander-Universität Erlangen-Nürnberg
(FAU), Germany
[2]Diagnostic Imaging, Siemens Healthcare GmbH, Erlangen, Germany
[3]Advanced Therapies, Siemens Healthcare GmbH, Forchheim, Germany
[4]Erlangen Graduate School in Advanced Optical Technologies (SAOT), Germany
[5]Institute of Medical Engineering, University of Applied Sciences
Würzburg-Schweinfurt, Germany
philipp.roser@fau.de

Scattered radiation is a major concern that affects X-ray image-guided pro-cedures in two ways. First, in complicated procedures, backscatter significantly contributes to the patient's (skin) dose. Second, forward scatter reduces con-trast in projection images and introduces artifacts in 3-D reconstructions. While conventionally used anti-scatter grids improve image quality by blocking X-rays, its attenuation must be compensated by a higher input dose. When quantify-ing the skin dose, backscatter is usually considered by applying predetermined scalar backscatter factors or linear point spread functions to the patient's skin entrance dose. However, since patients have different shapes, the generalization of conventional methods is limited. Here, we propose a novel approach that combines traditional techniques with multi-task learning to estimate the for-ward and backscatter simultaneously. In a simulation study including head and thorax data, we jointly estimated forward and backscatter with 94 % accuracy on average and outperformed the associated single-task approaches. In the fu-ture, the inclusion of a first-order scatter estimate based on the patient model is a promising approach to increase the overall performance and the physical plausibility [1].

References

1. Roser P, Zhong X, Birkhold A, et al. Simultaneous estimation of X-ray back-scatter and forward-scatter using multi-task learning. Proc MICCAI. 2020 October; p. 199–208.

© Der/die Autor(en), exklusiv lizenziert durch
Springer Fachmedien Wiesbaden GmbH, ein Teil von Springer Nature 2021
C. Palm et al. (Hrsg.), *Bildverarbeitung für die Medizin 2021*,
Informatik aktuell, https://doi.org/10.1007/978-3-658-33198-6_62

Deep Learning-based Spine Centerline Extraction in Fetal Ultrasound

Astrid Franz, Alexander Schmidt-Richberg, Eliza Orasanu, Cristian Lorenz

Philips GmbH Innovative Technologies, Röntgenstr. 24-26, D-22335 Hamburg
astrid.franz@philips.com

Abstract. Ultrasound is widely used for fetal screening. It allows for detecting abnormalities at an early gestational age, while being time and cost effective with no known adverse effects. Searching for optimal ultrasound planes for these investigations is a demanding and time-consuming task. Here we describe a method for automatically detecting the spine centerline in 3D fetal ultrasound images. We propose a two-stage approach combining deep learning and classic image processing techniques. First, we segment the spine using a deep learning approach. The resulting probability map is used as input for a tracing algorithm. The result is a sequence of points describing the spine centerline. This line can be used for measuring the spinal length and for generating view planes for the investigation of anomalies.

1 Introduction

Ultrasound is the modality of choice for fetal screening as it is able to show fetal anatomy in sufficient detail, while at the same being time and cost effective with no known adverse effects. Fetal screening allows for detecting abnormalities at an early gestational age, such that therapeutically suitable interventions can be planned and performed as required. Currently, the trend goes towards using 3D ultrasound, since a 3D image contains much more spatial information about the location of several organs with respect to each other and it allows for a variety of workflow optimizations.

One of the main fetal scans takes place in the second trimester between 18 and 22 weeks gestational age, when specific recommended standard measurements are determined, see for instance [1]. The localization of the abdominal cross-sectional plane with the corresponding measurement of the abdominal circumference is described in [2]. Another structure that is investigated is the fetal spine. First, the length of the spine provides an insight into the fetal growth. Second, a variety of spinal anomalies as spina bifida, meningocele, diastematomyelia, vertebral segmentation anomalies, sacral agenesis, spinal dysgenesis, spondylothoracic or spondylocostal dysplasia can be detected in 3D fetal ultrasound scans [3]. 3D ultrasound of the fetal spine has great diagnostic benefit, as it allows the operator to manipulate data in any plane after the completion of the exam. State-of-the-art fetal ultrasound examination is based on a manual search for optimal view planes, which is a demanding and time-consuming task. Hence an automatic detection of the spine centerline would be of huge benefit, since it allows for an automatic generation of view planes which are well-suited for the investigation of spinal anomalies.

2   Materials and methods

Here we describe a method for automatically detecting the spine centerline in 3D fetal ultrasound images. We propose a two-stage approach combining deep learning and classic image processing techniques. First, we segment the spine using an F-NET approach, as described in [4]. The resulting probability map is used as input for a tracing algorithm, similar to the one described in [5], where this was used for rib centerline tracing in CT. The result is a sequence of points describing the spine centerline.

2.1   Data

Our data consists of 400 3D fetal ultrasound scans with a gestational age ranging from 15 weeks to 41 weeks (mean gestational age 26 weeks). The in-plane voxel size ranges from 0.12 mm to 0.51 mm (mean 0.25 mm) and the slice thickness from 0.30 mm to 0.93 mm (mean 0.51 mm). The data includes a wide range of typical ultrasound artifacts, such as shadows. These artifacts make it impossible to segment the spine directly, since some parts of the spine are extinguished. In all these datasets, the spinal canal is manually annotated by setting 5 to 10 landmarks, which can be done with reasonable effort. These landmarks are automatically connected by straight lines. Based on these centerline annotations, we generated label masks by dilating with a certain radius, given in number of voxels. Since this dilation radius is a crucial parameter in the whole spine segmentation pipeline, we varied this parameter between 0 and 50. To get a feeling of the thickness of the spine label map with respect to the dilation radius, Fig. 1(b) shows in blue as example a dilation radius 15. As can be seen, this radius nicely covers the spinal canal and parts of the surrounding bone. A dilation radius of 50 would cover the whole spine.

2.2   Preprocessing

As a preprocessing step, the images are isotropically resampled. Since the size of the fetus greatly varies with respect to the gestational age, we do not use a fixed voxel size, but choose a voxel size which is linearly growing with respect to the gestational age, starting with 0.4 mm at a gestational age of 14 weeks and ending at 1.6 mm at a gestational age of 42 weeks. These values were chosen with respect to fetal growth curves [6]. The spinal length in such resampled images averages at about 140 voxels, independent of the gestational age.

Table 1. Voxel size (vs), padding (p) and size of the receptive field (rf) of the F-NET at different resolution levels.

Gestational age	Resolution 1			Resolution 2			Resolution 3		
	vs	p	rf	vs	p	rf	vs	p	rf
14 weeks	0.4 mm	4	3.2 mm	0.8 mm	9	15.2 mm	1.6 mm	19	62.4 mm
42 weeks	1.6 mm	4	14.4 mm	3.2 mm	9	60.8 mm	6.4 mm	19	249.6 mm

2.3 Spine probability map generation

For spine detection, we first apply an F-NET as described in [4]. This is a fully convolutional network architecture that processes images at multiple scales and different fields of view in order to combine detailed voxel-level features with features that take large context into consideration, while requiring significantly less memory to store hidden layers than previously proposed U-NET architectures using shortcut connections [4]. The segmentation results were nearly independent of the F-NET parameters such as kernel size and number of feature extraction blocks, hence we used the standard settings of [4], namely kernel size 3 and number of feature extraction blocks 3. However, we reduced the number of resolution levels from the standard settings of 4 to 3, since the receptive field at resolution level 3 has a size of 25 cm at a gestational age of 42 weeks (Tab. 1) and hence contains nearly the complete fetal torso. Thus the resolution level 4 would not add any more information. In this way, we could enlarge the patch size, i.e. the number of voxels the network can process in parallel, and hence speed up the computation.

2.4 Centerline tracing

The result of the previous step is a probability map describing the probability of the class spine. This probability map is used as input for an iterative tracing algorithm, as described in [5]. During the tracing, a probability weighted covariance matrix $\Sigma_i \in \mathbb{R}^{3\times3}$ of the voxel coordinates in a spherical region around the point of interest c_i is evaluated to estimate the tracing direction. Furthermore, the same sphere is used to calculate a probability-weighted center of mass. The tracing starts off with the point $c_0 \in \mathbb{R}^3$ having largest probability. If other points share this probability, the first one found is taken. First at c_0 the radius of the averaging sphere is chosen such that the fraction of voxels $F_{p>0.5}$ with probability $p > 0.5$ is between predefined limits $F_{\min} < F_{p>0.5} < F_{\max}$, where limits have been chosen empirically to be $F_{\min} = 0.02$ and $F_{\max} = 0.06$. Then, keeping the chosen radius of the averaging sphere, points are iteratively added to the centerline by repeating the following steps for $i = 0, 1, 2, \ldots$:

1. Calculate the probability weighted covariance matrix at c_i. The eigenvector $t_i \in \mathbb{R}^3$ corresponding to the largest eigenvalue of Σ_i is used as estimation of the tangent direction.
2. Starting from c_i, move in tangential direction t_i until a probability value < 0.5 or a maximal moving distance $d_{\max} = 15$ voxels is reached. If before

reaching d_{max}, the probability drops below < 0.5, a look-ahead mechanism tries to bridge the gap in walking direction up to a maximal distance $d_{\mathrm{gap}} = 10$ voxels.

3. Calculate the weighted mean vector $c_{i+1} \in \mathbb{R}^3$ in a spherical region around the current position and add this point to the list of spine centerline points.

This pipeline is iterated until the moving distance falls below a predefined threshold. Tracing from the initial point c_0 is performed in both possible directions, and the results are concatenated.

2.5   Evaluation metrics

For evaluating the results, we used three different evaluation metrics. We used the Dice coefficient for evaluating the F-NET segmentation, described in Sec. 2.3. The Dice coefficient measures the overlapping region of the thickened ground truth annotation and the probability map generated by the F-NET. It is a number between 0 and 1, where 0 means no overlap at all and 1 means full overlap.

The false negative rate (FNR) describes the fraction of the ground truth line which is not contained in the resulting traced spine centerline. We used a predefined outlier distance of 10 mm to define which points are found, i.e. a point of the ground truth annotation is considered to be found if there is a point in the traced spine centerline with a distance of at most 10 mm. The FNR is given in % throughout this paper. For computing the FNR, both the ground truth line and the detected centerline are approximated by 100 tightly-spaced points, and for each of these 100 ground truth points it is checked if a detected centerline point is in the range of the outlier distance.

For each of the 100 tightly-spaced points of the detected spine centerline, which is not a false negative as defined before, the distance to the ground truth line is computed. This distance is averaged yielding a mean distance of the detected spine centerline to the ground truth annotation.

2.6   Experiment set-up

For evaluation, we split our dataset in five folds of 80 images each to perform a five-fold cross validation: we used four folds, i.e. 320 datasets, for network training, applied the resulting segmentation network to the remaining fold of 80 test datasets, and subsequently traced the centerline of the resulting probability maps for the test datasets. One example case is shown in Fig. 1.

3   Results

The evaluation measures (Sec. 2.5) for a variety of dilation radii used for constructing ground truth label masks out of the annotated spine centerlines are shown in Fig. 2.

Fig. 3 shows the distribution of the Dice coefficient, the mean distance and the FNR for all our 400 cases for a dilation radius of 15 as a box-whisker-plot, both for training and test.

4   Discussion

As can be seen in Fig. 2(a), the Dice coefficient is increasing with growing dilation radius. This is to be expected since the more voxels a structure has, the less a voxel mismatch will count towards the overlap. For elongated structures with fewer voxels, this measure is not well-suited for describing the segmentation accuracy: As soon as the detected centerline is off by a few millimeters, the Dice coefficient drops drastically. In the example of Fig. 1, the Dice coefficient is 0.539, although the spine centerline is correctly detected: The FNR is 0 meaning that all spine centerline points are detected within the outlier distance of 10 mm, and the mean distance of the detected centerline to the ground truth line in this case is 1.014 mm. Hence for the application of detecting the spine centerline, the FNR and the mean distance are better suited for evaluating the result. These two measures show a drastic decrease when the dilation radius goes from 0 to 5, and then stay nearly constant, where the FNR shows a minimum at a dilation

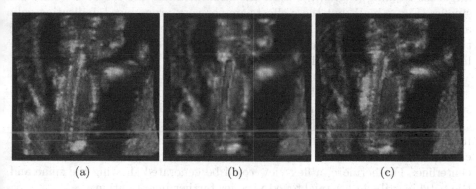

(a)   (b)   (c)

Fig. 1. Example of a test case: (a) ground truth annotation of the spine centerline, (b) thickened ground truth centerline (blue) and FNET segmentation result (red), (c) traced centerline resulting from the FNET probability map. The images (a) and (c) are a flattened view following the annotated line and are therefore not a slice of the original dataset, whereas (b) is an image slice containing most of the thickened ground truth centerline.

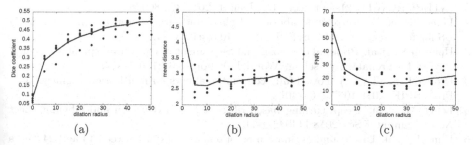

(a)   (b)   (c)

Fig. 2. (a) Dice coefficient, (b) mean distance and (c) FNR as a function of the dilation radius. The points indicate the values for the five folds, the line is the mean over all folds.

268   Franz et al.

Fig. 3. Box-whisker-plots for the (a) Dice coefficient, (b) mean distance and (c) FNR for a dilation radius of 15.

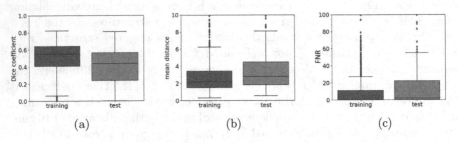

(a)   (b)   (c)

radius of approx. 15 (Fig. 2(c)). Hence a dilation radius of 15 seems to be reasonable for this application.

Fig. 3 concentrates on a dilation radius of 15. Clearly the Dice coefficient is larger for training (Fig. 3(a)), while the mean distance and the FNR values are smaller (Fig. 3(b,c)), but these effects are not very pronounced, indicating only a slight over-fitting effect. Half of the test cases have a FNR below 3, meaning that in half of the test cases at least 97% of the annotated ground truth spine line is found by our algorithm.

Hence our presented fully automatic two-stage approach for detecting the spine centerline in 3D fetal ultrasound scans yields promising results. The resulting spine centerline can be used for selecting dedicated view planes. They can be presented to the physician for investigating the spine, for instance for measuring the length or detecting anomalies. An estimation of the spinal length can even automatically be proposed by calculating the length of the detected centerline. Furthermore, a flex view could be generated showing the spine and the outgoing ribs in a straightened view for further investigation.

References

1. Papageorghiou AT, et al. International standards for fetal growth based on serial ultrasound measurements: The fetal growth longitudinal study of the INTERGROWTH-21st project. The Lancet. 2014;384:869–879.
2. Lorenz C, et al. Automated abdominal plane and circumference estimation in 3D US for fetal screening. Procs SPIE. 2018;10574:105740I.
3. Upasani V, et al. Prenatal diagnosis and assessment of congenital spinal anomalies: Review for prenatal counseling. World J Orthop. 2016;7:406–417.
4. Brosch T, Saalbach A. Foveal fully convolutional nets for multi-organ segmentation. Procs SPIE. 2018;10574:105740U.
5. Lenga M, et al. Deep learning based rib centerline extraction and labeling. Lect Notes Computer Sci. 2018;11404:99–113.
6. Ulm M, et al. Ultrasound evaluation of fetal spine length between 14 and 24 weeks of gestation. PND. 1999;19:637–641.

Abstract: Studying Robustness of Semantic Segmentation under Domain Shift in Cardiac MRI

Peter M. Full[1,2], Fabian Isensee[1], Paul F. Jäger[1], Klaus Maier-Hein[1]

[1]Division of Medical Image Computing, German Cancer Research Center (DKFZ), Heidelberg, Germany
[2]Medical Faculty Heidelberg, Heidelberg University, Heidelberg, Germany
`p.full@dkfz-heidelberg.de`

Cardiac magnetic resonance imaging (cMRI) is an integral part of diagnosis in many heart related diseases. Recently, deep neural networks (DNN) have demonstrated successful automatic segmentation, thus alleviating the burden of time-consuming manual contouring of cardiac structures. Moreover, frameworks such as nnU-Net provide entirely automatic model configuration to unseen datasets enabling out-of-the-box application even by non-experts. However, current studies commonly neglect the clinically realistic scenario, in which a trained network is applied to data from a different domain such as deviating scanners or imaging protocols. This potentially leads to unexpected performance drops of deep learning models in real life applications. In this work, we systematically study challenges and opportunities of domain transfer across images from multiple clinical centres and scanner vendors. In order to maintain out-of-the-box usability, we build upon a fixed U-Net architecture configured by the nnU-net framework to investigate various data augmentation techniques and batch normalization layers as an easy-to-customize pipeline component and provide general guidelines on how to improve domain generalizability abilities in existing deep learning methods. Our proposed method ranked first at the *Multi-Centre, Multi-Vendor & Multi-Disease Cardiac Image Segmentation Challenge (M&Ms)*. We expect our experimental insights to be helpful for clinical scenarios in which externally trained DNNs are deployed on in-house data with potentially differing scanner vendors or imaging protocols. In such scenarios, our approach is able to improve segmentation quality by bridging domain gaps between data sets and as a consequence reduces time-efforts and costs associated with generating manually annotated in-domain datasets at clinical sites. [1]

References

1. Full PM, Isensee F, Jäger PF, et al. Studying robustness of semantic segmentation under domain shift in cardiac MRI. STACOM. 2020;.

© Der/die Autor(en), exklusiv lizenziert durch
Springer Fachmedien Wiesbaden GmbH, ein Teil von Springer Nature 2021
C. Palm et al. (Hrsg.), *Bildverarbeitung für die Medizin 2021*,
Informatik aktuell, https://doi.org/10.1007/978-3-658-33198-6_64

On Efficient Extraction of Pelvis Region from CT Data

Tatyana Ivanovska[1], Andrian O. Paulus[1], Robert Martin[2], Babak Panahi[3], Arndt Schilling[2]

[1]Department for Computational Neuroscience, Georg-August Universität Göttingen
[2]Clinic for Trauma Surgery, Orthopaedics and Plastic Surgery, University Medicine Göttingen
[3]Institute for Diagnostic and Interventional Radiology, University Medicine Göttingen
tiva@phys.uni-goettingen.de

Abstract. The first step in automated analysis of medical volumetric data is to detect slices, where specific body parts are located. In our project, we aimed to extract the pelvis regionfrom whole-body CT scans. Two deep learning approaches, namely, an unsupervised slice score regressor, and a supervised slice classification method, were evaluated on a relatively small-sized dataset. The result comparison showed that both methods could detect the region of interest with accuracy above 93%. Although the straightforward classification method delivered more accurate results (accuracy of 99%), sometimes it tended to output discontinuous regions, which can be solved by combination of both approaches.

1 Introduction

For efficient analysis of medical images, it is beneficial to pre-extract the region of interest for further processing steps. This allows for the reduction of the amount of data, so that subsequent computations are boosted and possible errors are reduced. This is especially important if the number of slices comprising the region of interest is relatively small, when compared to the complete sequence size.

In the literature, the approach of labeling the anatomical regions is referred as bodypart recognition. It serves as an initialization module for anatomy detection or segmentation algorithms [1]. Classical approaches utilized extensions to Generalized Hough Transform (GHT) [2] for such a task. For instance, Seim et al. [3] followed the approach of Khoshelham [2] to localize the pelvic bone for further segmentation. However, Seim et al. stated that the performance of the GHT strongly depends on the quality of the template shape and the speed is rather low, since it is a brute force method. Since the ultimate goal of our project is to analyze data with multiple fractures and mislocated bones, such a method might fail in localization of the pelvis region.

Deep learning methods that do not require any prior knowledge of the data can be roughly separated into two categories: supervised classifiers, which are trained on labeled images, and unsupervised regressors, where the anatomical

Springer Fachmedien Wiesbaden GmbH, ein Teil von Springer Nature 2021
C. Palm et al. (Hrsg.), *Bildverarbeitung für die Medizin 2021*,
Informatik aktuell, https://doi.org/10.1007/978-3-658-33198-6_65

landmarks are learned from the slice ordering. Roth et al. [4] used labeled CT scans from 1675 patients to train a convolutional neural network (CNN) to differentiate between 5 classes (neck, lung, liver, pelvis, legs). Yan et al. [1] proposed a multi-stage deep learning framework to discover local discriminative patches and build local classifiers to differentiate between 12 anatomical classes using data from 675 patients. Yan, Lu, and Summers [5] proposed an unsupervised body part regressor that constructs a coordinate system for the human body and outputs a continuous score for each axial slice, representing the normalized position of the body part in the slice. These so-called slice scores are learned from intrinsic structural slice ordering information in CT volumes. The main advantage of this approach is that it does not require labeled data for training.

For our application, the pelvis region detection is required in the first step, and other anatomical classes can be disregarded at the moment. We utilized whole-body computed tomography (CT) data [6] of $\approx$ 100 patients. As this was a relatively small dataset, the goal of our study was to explore the priority approach for extraction of pelvis with limited data. We analyzed two deep learning approaches. The first method is an unsupervised body-part regressor proposed by Yan, Lu and Summers [5]. The second method uses a classical VGG-based convolutional neural network [7] for slice classification task, which can be considered a simplified version of the approach by Roth et al. [4]. We applied both methods to our dataset, present the results, and analyze the findings.

2 Materials and methods

The study was approved by the local ethics committee of University Medicine Göttingen (RefNo: 1-5-19). Anonymized whole-body CT data of 93 patients were included into the project.

Several example slices from different patients are presented in Fig. 1. The data were converted to a standardized slice thickness of 5 mm. The spatial resolution was 512×512 and the number of slices varied for each patient. The average slice number was 236 ± 56, and the median slice value was 234. It can be observed that pelvis region occupies 43 ± 2.2 slices, i. e. $\approx \frac{5}{6}$ of the slices can be potentially disregarded in subsequent processing steps.

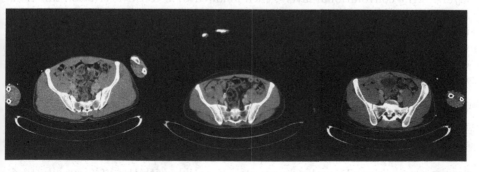

Fig. 1. Three example slices depicting pelvis region.

The data were split into training, validation, and test sets patient-wise. 10 and 9 patients were put to the test and validation sets, respectively, the 74 scans were used for training. Pelvis region in each dataset was identified by an experienced observer.

2.1 Methods

The unsupervised Body Part Regressor is a novel learning method that learns the body part knowledge from inter-slice relationships in a self-organization process [5]. It has six convolutional layers from a standard network (VGG16), a global average pooling layer and a fully connected layer, which outputs the score. A novel loss function that consists of two terms serves for efficient learning. Yan, Lu and Summers collected around 800 CT data from 420 subjects. They also provided an open source implementation of their method [8]. We re-implemented the method in pytorch using the original source code and the implementation by G. Chartrand [9], which was trained and evaluated on the IRCAD dataset [10]. It was suggested in the original publication to reduce the width and height of slices. We have also observed in our experiments that usage of smaller input image sizes produces more accurate results. Therefore, the original data were resized to 64×64. The image intensities in Hounsfield units [11] were clipped to a range of $[-300, 300]$ to provide more contrast to soft tissues. Thereafter, intensities were scaled to a range of $[0, 1]$ and tripled in order to create a multichannel image. One third of the training volumes were augmented by shifting the individual slices to the left and right, as well as up- and downwards. The amount of shifting are randomly chosen for each individual volume and ranged from $[10, 70]$ pixels. Training runs were initialized using the same parameters found in [9], with the exception of the batch composition. Here, batches consisted of 12 different volumes each represented by 14 equidistantly spaced slices. After obtaining the scores, a histogram-based method was applied to compute the slice values for each region in a volume. For more details, we refer to the original work [5].

The VGG-based Slice Classifier was built using VGG11 [7], the lightest model from the VGG family. The model consisted from 11 weight layers and 5 pooling layers: eight convolutional layers, each followed by a ReLU activation function, five max pooling operations, each reducing feature map by 2, and three fully connected layers. All convolutional layers had 3×3 kernels. The first convolutional layer produced 64 channels and then, as the network deepened, the number of channels doubled after each max pooling operation until it reached 512. On the following layers, the number of channels did not change.

We replaced the last classification layer to a layer for 2 class classification, and used the Imagenet weights. The standard augmentation tools, such as scaling, rotation, horizontal and vertical flips were applied to the data. The input image size was $224 \times 224 \times 3$. CT data preprocessing steps were the following: the intensities in Hounsfield units were clipped to a range of $[0, 3000]$; each volume was z-score normalized. To make the inputs compatible with the VGG architecture,

Table 1. $\mu \pm \sigma$ metrics for validation and test sets for both approaches.

TP	FP	TN	FN	A	P	R	F1
Unsupervised Body Part Regressor							
Validation Set							
36 ± 6.4	7.2 ± 5.8	174 ± 57	7.6 ± 6	0.93 ± 0.05	0.84 ± 0.1	0.83 ± 0.1	0.83 ± 0.1
Test Set							
34 ± 4.9	4.8 ± 7.1	174 ± 44.5	9.8 ± 4.8	0.93 ± 0.05	0.9 ± 0.1	0.78 ± 0.1	0.82 ± 0.08
VGG Classifier							
Validation Set							
42.6 ± 3.1	0.7 ± 0.9	187 ± 57.4	0.2 ± 0.4	0.99 ± 0.02	0.98 ± 0.02	0.99 ± 0.01	0.99 ± 0.01
Test Set							
43.4 ± 1.8	0.3 ± 0.5	179 ± 41	0.3 ± 0.5	0.99 ± 0.01	0.99 ± 0.01	0.99 ± 0.01	0.99 ± 0.08

the original images dimensions (512×512) were resized to 224×224, and intensities were scaled to a range of $[0, 1]$, the images were copied 3 times to be used as a multichannel image, and then normalized using $mean = [0.485, 0.456, 0.406]$ and $std = [0.229, 0.224, 0.225]$.

2.2 Evaluation measures

The following values were used for evaluation: true positives (TP), false positives (FP), true negatives (TN), false negatives (FN), which refer to correctly and incorrectly classified slices, where pelvis region is located. From these values the following metrics were computed: accuracy $A = \frac{TP+TN}{TP+TN+FP+FN}$, precision $P = \frac{TP}{TP+FP}$, recall $R = \frac{TP}{TP+FN}$, and F1 score $F1 = \frac{2TP}{2TP+FP+FN}$.

3 Results and discussion

The unsupervised regressor was trained for 50 epochs with the following parameters: batch dimensions $g = 12$, $m = 14$, Adam optimizer with $lr = 0.0001$. The VGG classifier was trained starting from ImageNet weights for 20 epochs using Adam optimizer with $lr = 0.0001$ and batches of 64 images. The results are summarized in Table 1.

As it can be observed in Table 1, the VGG classifier produced highly accurate results with maximally two false positive and one negative slices per patient. In most cases misclassifications appear at the beginning or the end of pelvis region. An illustrative example is presented in Fig. 2. Actually, the errors of the predictions (left and right slices in Fig. 2) contain some minor parts of the pelvic bones, and thus, the expert had possibly not always marked them for all datasets consistently. We leave the investigation of inter- and intra-observer variability for future work. The standard deviation in TP and TN is explained by the fact that the number of slices occupied by pelvis region differed for each patient.

Although the unsupervised regressor was able to find the correct regions as presented in Fig. 3, the results had significantly lower rates than by the supervised classification method (Tab. 1). This is probably explained by the fact that we used about 10 times less data for training, when compared to the original publication, namely, 73 vs. 800 volumes.

However, the classification-based approach suffered from one drawback: since the method considers only 2D slices and no 3D information is taken into account, it can potentially produce disjoint regions, e. g., miss some slices within or detect something outside the region of interest. For instance, the classifier in some rare cases detected several slices in the shoulder region and marked them as pelvis, since it visually reminded the lateral parts of pelvic bones. The probability values of the classification were similar to the ones at the end of the pelvis region and no straightforward thresholding was possible. This problem could be solved by using a combined approach, where the results from both methods are

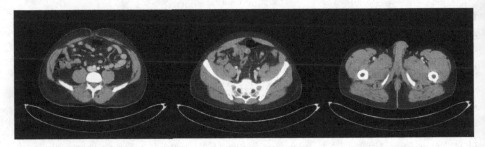

Fig. 2. Predictions of the VGG-based classifier. Left: false positive slice at the beginning of pelvis; middle: correct prediction; right: false negative slice at the end of pelvis.

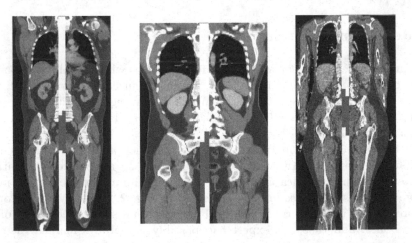

Fig. 3. Results of the unsupervised regressor detection overlaid with data from three patients are shown. The algorithm detection of pelvis region is marked in red, the expert readings are shown in green.

considered together, since the unsupervised method produces one continuous region by definition. We plan to add more training data to the unsupervised regressor and leave the extension for future work. Moreover, we also plan to investigate, how well such an approach would perform, when more regions in the body must be localized.

4 Conclusion

In this study we compared two deep learning approaches for the task of body part detection: an unsupervised regressor and a slice classification network, to label pelvic bones in whole-body CT data with a relatively small dataset. Even with this small amount of data, the accuracy was already high. This suggests, that given more training data and combining both methods, such an approach will presumably lead to efficient and reliable reduction of data for analysis of CTs of the pelvis.

References

1. Yan Z, Zhan Y, Peng Z, et al. Multi-instance deep learning: discover discriminative local anatomies for bodypart recognition. IEEE Trans Med Imaging. 2016;35(5):1332–1343.
2. Khoshelham K. Extending generalized hough transform to detect 3d objects in laser range data. In: ISPRS Workshop on Laser Scanning and SilviLaser 2007, 12-14 September 2007, Espoo, Finland. International Society for Photogrammetry and Remote Sensing; 2007. .
3. Seim H, Kainmueller D, Heller M, et al. Automatic segmentation of the pelvic bones from CT data based on a statistical shape model. VCBM. 2008;8:93–100.
4. Roth HR, Lee CT, Shin H, et al. Anatomy-specific classification of medical images using deep convolutional nets. In: 2015 IEEE 12th International Symposium on Biomedical Imaging (ISBI); 2015. p. 101–104.
5. Yan K, Lu L, Summers RM. Unsupervised body part regression via spatially self-ordering convolutional neural networks. In: 2018 IEEE 15th International Symposium on Biomedical Imaging (ISBI 2018). IEEE; 2018. p. 1022–1025.
6. Furlow B. Whole-body computed tomography trauma imaging. Radiol Technol. 2017;89(2):159CT–180CT.
7. Simonyan K, Zisserman A. Very deep convolutional networks for large-scale image recognition. arXiv preprint arXiv:14091556. 2014;.
8. Yan L, Lu L, Summers RM;. https://github.com/rsummers11/.
9. Implementation in Keras by Gabriel Chartrand;. https://github.com/Gabsha/ssbr.
10. IRCAD Dataset;. https://www.ircad.fr/research/3dircadb/.
11. DenOtter TD, Schubert J. Hounsfield unit. In: StatPearls [Internet]. StatPearls Publishing; 2019. .

CT Normalization by Paired Image-to-image Translation for Lung Emphysema Quantification

Insa Lange[1], Fabian Jacob[2], Alex Frydrychowicz[2], Heinz Handels[1], Jan Ehrhardt[1]

[1]Institute of Medical Informatics, University of Lübeck
[2]Department for Radiology and Nuclear Medicine, University Hospital of Schleswig-Holstein
insa.lange@student.uni-luebeck.de

Abstract. In this work a UNet-based normalization method by paired image-to-image translation of Chest CT images was developed. Due to different noise-levels, emphysema quantification shows sincere subordination to the choice of the filterkernel. Images for training and testing of 71 patients were available, reconstructed using the smooth Siemens B20f filterkernel and the sharp B80f filterkernel. Results were evaluated in regard to the image quality, including a visual assessment by two imaging experts, the L1 distance, the emphysema quantification (emphysema index and Dice overlap of emphysema segmentations). Emphysema quantification was compared to classical normalization methods. Our approach lead to very good image quality in which the mean B20f L1 distance to the B80f could be reduced by about 88.5 % and the mean Dice was raised by 189 % after normalization. Classical methods were outperformed. Even though small differences between B20f and normalized B80f images were noticed, the normalized images were found to be overall of diagnostic quality.

1 Introduction

Chronic-obstructive pulmonary disease (COPD) is a very common widespread illness that is responsible for many deaths worldwide. Patients suffering from COPD are experiencing a limitation of airflow to the lungs often caused by an alveolar obstruction called lung emphysema. Thus, diagnosing COPD and evaluating progress of the disease is of great significance. Standard diagnostic methods are pulmonary function tests using spirometry, however, computed tomography (CT) is increasingly used to exactly locate affected areas in the lung.

Quantification of lung emphysema in Chest-CTs can be achieved by a simple threshold segmentation of emphysema areas inside the lung, meaning lung segmentations are needed. A widely accepted threshold is $< -950\,HU$ and a global emphysema index (EI) can be computed from the segmented emphysema volume (EV) and the total lung volume (TLV) by $EI = \frac{100\% \times EV}{TLV}$. Inconveniently, the calculated emphysema index strongly depends on the selected CT

Springer Fachmedien Wiesbaden GmbH, ein Teil von Springer Nature 2021
C. Palm et al. (Hrsg.), *Bildverarbeitung für die Medizin 2021*,
Informatik aktuell, https://doi.org/10.1007/978-3-658-33198-6_66

imaging parameters such as slice thickness or reconstruction kernel, which makes CT normalization methods necessary to achieve comparable results [1, 2].

This paper focuses on CT normalization with respect to the chosen reconstruction kernel. EI quantifications based on images reconstructed using smooth kernels (like Siemens B20f) seem to correspond well to pulmonary function tests [2]. In comparison, quantifications based on images reconstructed by sharp kernels (like Siemens B80f) will result in deviation of the EI, suggesting a much greater EV is present than it actually is. Previous work suggested filtering methods [3, 4] or frequency decomposition methods [2, 4], which didn't take the truncation artifact at $-1024\,HU$ into account, to normalize CT images reconstructed with different kernels to a consistent appearance. A more recent approach successfully applies image-to-image translation (Siemens: B50f → B30f) by Convolutional Neural Networks (CNNs) for this task [5].

The aim of this work is to investigate the possibilities and limitations of state-of-the-art image-to-image translation techniques for CT kernel normalization. For this purpose, we consider the challenging task of normalizing Siemens B80f images (very sharp kernel) and translating the images into B20f images (very smooth kernel). Our work should contribute to the question whether images generated in this way are suitable for clinical diagnostics. Therefore, we present a quantitative evaluation of the generated images and the calculated EI and Dice, as well as a visual assessment of image quality by an experienced radiologist and an in medical imaging specialized computer scientist.

2   Materials and methods

2.1   Materials

Imaging data of 71 patients were acquired on a 64-row MSCT (Somatom Definition AS+, Siemens) and reconstructed simultaneously with a soft (B20f) and a sharp kernel (B80f). Slice thickness varied between $0.7\,mm$ and $1\,mm$ and was resampled to $1\,mm$ for all reconstructions. The accustomed in-slice spacing and slice dimensions of 512×512 pixels were kept unchanged. Due to the simultaneous reconstruction, the images form a well suited basis for paired image-to-image translation techniques.

2.2   Image-to-image translation with UNet

In the past, both paired image-to-image translation, e.g. Pix2Pix [6], MedGAN [7] or MEGAN [8], and unpaired image-to-image translations, e.g. CycleGAN [9] produced remarkable results. Paired image translation methods apply pixel-wise error losses to corresponding images of each domain, whereas unpaired methods such as CycleGAN typically use distribution matching losses that often result in hallucinated features in the generated images [10]. This effect has been less observed in paired methods [10], and we believe that paired image-to-image translation with the same raw data for each image pair can be used for diagnostic purposes.

For the paired image-to-image translation of B80f images to B20f images a UNet architecture with three skip-connections, maxpooling for compression and 128 feature maps in maximal compression was build and multiple times trained in 100 epochs. In each training eleven to twelve patients were left out for testing and eleven to twelve patients for validation. Due to the great size of the CT data, images were cut into patches for training. For all of the chosen patients to be used in training the same number of randomly selected non-overlapping patches was added to the training dataset. L1 loss was used to compare to the original B20f.

2.3 Experiments

The quantitative analysis compares the original B20f images to the normalized B80f images. The differences in HU values (L1 distance), and computed EI, as well as the Dice overlap between the emphysema regions are computed. Our UNet-based approach is compared to a heuristic filter-based approach [4] and a frequency decomposition method [2]. Paired one-sided T-tests were performed.

For visual evaluation, either an original B20f image or a normalized B80f image was randomly selected. Two experts rated the selected images blinded: a clincal radiologist (>5 years experience) and a computer scientist specialized on medical image computing (>5 years experience). The radiologist used a radiological workstation with quality assured monitor for the evaluation. All images were assigned a score by both experts seperately, ranging from 0 (certain synthetic) to 5 (certain original), thus including three levels of certainty for each originals and synthetic images and leaving no rating score for undecided.

3 Results

Multiple CNN trainings were performed, so that each patient was part of the test set at some point. Fig. 1 shows an original B20f, original B80f and the normalized B80f image, as well as emphysema segmentations and resulting difference images of one patient. The normalized B80f image is barely distinguishable

Fig. 1. (left to right) original B20f, original B80f, normalized B80f; (top to bottom) image, image with emphysema segmentation, difference image to original B20f.

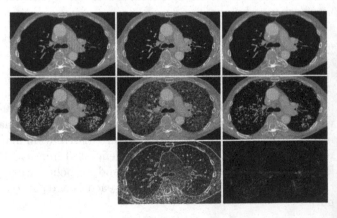

Table 1. Statistics of Dice and absolute differences in EI.

Images	Abs. difference in EI mean ± std	[min, max]	Dice mean ± std	[min, max]
B80f	17.32 ± 4.72	[5.78, 25.66]	0.19 ± 0.19	[0.01, 0.69]
UNet	0.93 ± 1.27	[0.01, 5.53]	0.55 ± 0.21	[0.03, 0.89]
Heuristic	1.90 ± 2.65	[0.04, 9.26]	0.43 ± 0.21	[0.00, 0.85]
Frequency-based	1.66 ± 2.26	[0.02, 9.36]	0.38 ± 0.25	[0.00, 0.85]
B80f, EI>5	17.17 ± 5.49	[5.78, 25.66]	0.41 ± 0.12	[0.25, 0.69]
UNet, EI>5	2.02 ± 1.45	[0.25, 5.53]	0.76 ± 0.07	[0.64, 0.89]
Heuristic, EI>5	4.31 ± 2.92	[0.39, 9.26]	0.63 ± 0.11	[0.47, 0.85]
Frequency-based, EI>5	3.44 ± 2.72	[0.35, 9.36]	0.61 ± 0.15	[0.19, 0.85]

from the original B20f and the typical over-segmentation of emphysema regions in B80f images is greatly reduced by the normalization. The computed EI for this patient is 17.45% (B20f), 34.76% (B80f) and 16.90% (normalized B80f), and computed Dice scores are 0.43 (B20f vs. B80f) and 0.73 (B20f vs. normalized B80f) showing an improved emphysema detection in the normalized images.

3.1 Quantitative results

The L1 distances averaged over all 71 patients and all voxels showed a remarkable reduction from (mean ± std) 84.5 HU ± 11.7 for B80f images to 9.7 HU ± 1.7 for normalized B80f images in comparison to the B20f images. Due to difficulties in the lung segmentation task, emphysema quantification was accomplished for only a subset of 50 patients. Emphysema quantification after UNet normalization was compared to the results of frequency decomposition and heuristic normalization.

While plotting the differences in EI calculations in Fig. 2 with and without normalization is barely showing any distinguishment between all three normalization methods, statistical calculations in Tab. 1 show an advantage of the UNet normalization method ($p<0.05$ compared to frequency-based normalization and $p<0.001$ for heuristic normalization and B80f).

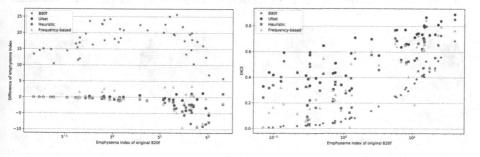

Fig. 2. Differences in EI compared to ground truth (left) and Dice values (right).

Looking at the Dice plot in this figure as well as the calculations in the same table, the UNet takes an obvious lead ($p<10^{-12}$ compared to both methods and B80f). Values suggest, that classical methods find a good EI compared to the baseline EI from B20f images. But as for exactly locating the airflow obstructions, those methods are not helpful and don't seem to gain any more information compared to performing a simple spirometry.

3.2   Visual assessment by experts

For 36 patients randomly either the original B20f or the normalized B80f image was selected, resulting in 16 original and 20 normalized images to be reviewed by the experts. Overall no image received a score of 0 or 5 to be certain original or synthetic. Mean scores and standard deviation for each group and both imaging experts as well as an overall score can be reviewed in Fig. 3.

4   Discussion

The aim of this work is to provide a CT normalization method for lung emphysema quantification and to evaluate its diagnostic usability. The quantitative evaluation of the L1 distances in Hounsfield units and of the differences in the computed EI show a remarkable agreement between the baseline B20f images and the normalized B80f images. Thus, average differences in the computed EI are reduced from 17.61 before normalization to 0.98 afterwards. However, the average Dice score shows only a moderate agreement of 0.58 between baseline and normalized images. It must be noted, though, that for patients with a low EI (≤ 5), the segmented emphysema regions consist of only a few isolated pixels. For patients with medium to high EI, moderate to very good agreements are observed (Dice: 0.64–0.89). The normalization approach by UNet clearly outperformed the heuristic and frequency-based normalization methods [2, 4] in regard to emphysema quantification, especially in Dice values.

The visual qualitative assessment of randomly selected original B20f and normalized B80f images has shown that neither the radiologist nor the computer scientist was able to distinguish between both image groups with absolute

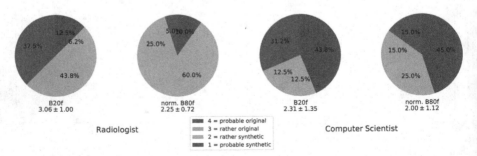

Fig. 3. Score distribution and mean ± std scores of visual assessment.

certainty. Although the computer scientist has many years of experience with medical image data, he could hardly distinguish between original and synthetic image data (58% of images correctly classified), whereas the radiologist tended to be able to differentiate between synthetic and original data (75% of images correctly classified). According to the radiologist, slight differences in the images can be detected at the emphysema borders.

In our opinion, a key lesson from this experiment is that a qualitative assessment of synthetically generated medical images should always be performed by experienced radiologists at clinical workstations. Nevertheless, according to an initial assessment by the radiologist, the normalized B80f images meet the diagnostic quality standards in radiology. A more in-depth analysis is necessary.

Even though difficult conditions for this research were chosen in translating very sharp and noisy images to very smooth images, high-quality images could be generated with a simple U-Net architecture with only three skip connections and a moderate size of the training set. A limitation of this study is that all image data for training and testing were acquired with the same type of CT scanner, so that for other settings new training data has to be acquired and the net has to be re-trained.

Building upon this research further CNN training with adjusted architecture can be expected in the attempt to minimize the differences in B20f and synthetic B20f images even more.

References

1. Bartel ST, Bierhals AJ, Pilgram TK, et al. Equating quantitative emphysema measurements on different CT reconstructions. Med Phys. 2011;38(8):4894–4902.
2. Gallardo-Estrella L, Lynch DA, Prokop M, et al. Normalizing computed tomography data reconstructed with different filter kernels: effect on emphysema quantification. Eur Radiol. 2016;26(2):478–486.
3. Ohkubo M, Wada S, Kayugawa A, et al. Image filtering as an alternative to the application of a different reconstruction kernel in CT imaging: feasibility study in lung cancer screening. Med Phys. 2011;38(7):3915–3923.
4. Ehrhardt J, Jacob F, Handels H, et al. Comparison of post-hoc normalization approaches for CT-based lung emphysema index quantification. Proc BVM. 2016; p. 44–49.
5. Jin H, Heo C, Kim JH. Deep learning-enabled accurate normalization of reconstruction kernel effects on emphysema quantification in low-dose CT. Phys Med Biol. 2019;64(13).
6. Isola P, Zhu JY, Zhou T, et al. Image-to-image translation with conditional adversarial networks. Proc CVPR. 2017; p. 1125–1134.
7. Armanious K, Jiang C, Fischer M, et al. MedGAN: medical image translation using GANs. Comput Med Imaging Graph. 2020;79.
8. Uzunova H, Ehrhardt J, Handels H. Memory-efficient GAN-based domain translation of high resolution 3D medical images. Comput Med Imaging Graph. 2020;89.
9. Zhu JY, Park T, Isola P, et al. Image-to-image translation with conditional adversarial networks. Proc ICCV. 2017; p. 2223–2232.
10. Cohen JP, Luck M, Honari S. Distribution matching losses can hallucinate features in medical image translation. Proc MICCAI. 2018;11070:529–536.

Ultrasound Breast Lesion Detection using Extracted Attention Maps from a Weakly Supervised Convolutional Neural Network

Dalia Rodríguez-Salas, Mathias Seuret, Sulaiman Vesal, Andreas Maier

Pattern Recognition Lab, FAU Erlangen-Nürnberg
dalia.rodriguez@fau.de

Abstract. In order to detect lesions on medical images, deep learning models commonly require information about the size of the lesion, either through a bounding box or through the pixel-/voxel-wise annotation of the lesion, which is in turn extremely expensive to produce in most cases. In this paper, we aim at demonstrating that by having a single central point per lesion as ground truth for 3D ultrasounds, accurate deep learning models for lesion detection can be trained, leading to precise visualizations using Grad-CAM. From a set of breast ultrasound volumes, healthy and diseased patches were used to train a deep convolutional neural network. On the one hand, each diseased patch contained in its central area a lesion's center annotated by experts. On the other hand, healthy patches were extracted from random regions of ultrasounds taken from healthy patients. An AUC of 0.92 and an accuracy of 0.87 was achieved on test patches.

1 Introduction

Early detection of high-risk breast lesions is crucial to prevent them from progressing to invasive diseases, and in turn breast cancer incidence and mortality can be likely reduced [1]. Although mammography imaging is the breast screening modality par excellence, breast ultrasound is often used as a supplementary screening modality and it provides a lower cost alternative for low- and middle-income countries. The increasing development of deep learning techniques for computer vision tasks in recent years has shown a clear raise on performance of automated breast lesion detection and classification systems [2].

In this work, we investigate the usage of a 3D convolutional neutral network (CNN) for detecting and localizing lesions in 3D ultrasound scans of breasts. The labels of our training data consists of lesion classes according to the American College of Radiology Breast Imaging Reporting and Data System system, as well as an estimation of the lesion central point for volumes containing a lesion. We consider our system as weakly-supervised because while the shape and dimensions of lesions are absent from our training data, we aim at visualizing these nevertheless. Weak supervision has the advantage of requiring less expensive ground truth, however this makes Machine Learning tasks more challenging.

For the detection of breast ultrasound lesions, more traditional machine learning techniques outnumber those using deep learning. Most of the works on lesion detection on breast imaging using deep learning techniques focus their efforts on 2D modalities such as mammogram and Magnetic Resonance Imaging.

Among the most recent works using traditional machine learning techniques, the one presented in [3] can be highlighted. They used a genetic algorithm to optimize a Random Forest classifier to generate candidate regions. A region is then classified as lesion depending on its probability built using pixel-level probabilities returned by the Random Forest. They achieved a sensitivity of 84.4% on a dataset of 56 samples breast ultrasounds.

In [2], the performance of different deep learning network architectures for localization was compared when trained on breast ultrasounds to detect lesions. YOLO [4], R-CNN [5], and SSD [6] were the base architectures used in their experiments, where SSD trained with patches of size 300×300 reached the best performance. Despite of working with ultrasound imaging and deep learning models, their work is not directly comparable to ours because 1) they work with 2D images sampled from the 3D volumes by the specialist, and 2) they counted with expert's annotations about the shape and size of the tumors.

Different works using deep learning techniques on breast ultrasound volumes target to classify whether the patient has a benign or malignant lesion. An overview of such works and a general overview of deep learning on ultrasound imaging can be found in [7].

The main contributions of this work are:

1. A system which detects and localizes lesions on breast ultrasound imaging.
2. A weakly supervised pipeline for lesion/abnormality detection and localization that can be extended to other medical imaging modalities.

2 Materials and methods

The dataset used in our experiments consists of 904 volumes obtained from 461 patients, as shown in Table 1. Note that patients with at least one lesion are counted in the lesion class, regardless of whether they might have no lesions in one of their breasts.

The core of our system is a 3D CNN, more specifically a Residual Neural Network [8]. While there are different standard versions of the Residual Neural Network, having from 18 to 152 layers, the dimensionality of our data allows us to use only the smallest ones for memory reasons. Indeed, convolving the data with filters requires significantly more memory in 3D than in 2D. Because the default Residual Neural Network architecture has 1000 units in its output layer, we replace them with a single unit, which has a sigmoid activation on top to facilitate binary classification.

To train the CNN, using whole volumes is impracticable for three main reasons. First, as mentioned before, memory requirements would be extremely high.

Table 1. Number of patients and samples in our dataset.

Dataset	Total	Train		Test		Per Class	
		Healthy	Lesion	Healthy	Lesion	Healthy	Lesion
Patients	461	141	189	61	70	202	255
Samples	904	393	253	163	95	556	348

Second, loading such an amount of data from the hard drive would be too slow to train a CNN in a reasonable amount of time. And, third, this can lead to over-fitting issues due to the small amount of training data that we have. Indeed, if the CNN is trained on large volumes, then it is more difficult for the network to learn what it is supposed to spot, and a greater number of training samples is then required. For these reasons, we train our CNN on 3D crops.

We get healthy crops by randomly sampling volumes labeled as healthy only, since there is no information about lesion size in the other volumes: crops containing only healthy tissues would have not guaranteed even if they had been extracted far from lesion centers. For positive samples, we extract crops centered on lesions. These crops are stored in new files, such that they can be obtained without loading the whole volumes in memory.

Two data augmentation methods are applied during the training. First, the crops that are stored in files, as described above, are created larger than what is given to the CNN, with a size of $28 \times 280 \times 280$. Random crops of the right size, i.e. $16 \times 160 \times 160$, are selected at run time, as illustrated in Fig. 1, which adds some variability to lesion locations during the training. Thus, the network learns to recognize lesions regardless of where in the input they are. The other augmentation which we use is flipping the data on horizontal and depth axes with a probability of 50%. This is justified by the fact that the shape of lesions is not constrained, and the CNN should have the same output regardless of their orientation.

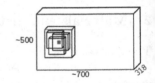

Fig. 1. Some variation is added in the training data by extracting random crops of size $16 \times 160 \times 160$ from a neighborhood around the lesion's patch sized $28 \times 280 \times 280$.

The CNN is trained for 250 epochs, and thanks to the crop size, we can give it batches of 14 samples. We use the binary cross-entropy as loss function, and update the weights of the network using Adam [9]. In practice, we found that an initial learning rate of 0.001 performs well.

It is then possible to use a trained CNN to produce heatmaps indicating how likely each part of a given volume are to belong to a given class. In this work, this is done with Gradient-weighted Class Activation Mapping [10]. Given an input processed by the CNN, the gradient of an output class, in our case the lesion class, is back-propagated to the output of the last convolutional layer. Averaging these gradients for each location in the convolution indicates how

Table 2. Accuracy and AUC.

Central point	Center		Center		Random	
Patch size	(28×280×280)		(16×160×160)		(16×160×160)	
Metric	AUC	Accuracy	AUC	Accuracy	AUC	Accuracy
5-fold CV	0.8536	0.7433	0.9307	0.8743	0.9253	0.8744
Variance	± 0.0876	± 0.0836	± 0.0267	± 0.0260	± 0.0371	± 0.0291
Test set	0.9139	0.8411	0.9357	0.8798	0.9253	0.8721

much this location contributes to the class output. Thus, we obtain a heatmap which has the same dimension as the output of the last convolutional layer of the CNN. This heatmap can then be resized, with interpolation, to match the size of the input. The heatmap and the input are then added with a weight of 0.3 for the heatmap and 0.7 for the input. Lastly a colormap is applied to the image to produce hot-spots on the regions which are more likely to be lesions.

3 Results

In Table 2, the AUC and accuracy for a threshold of 0.5 are reported for both the test-set evaluated on the network trained with the complete training set, and the validation sets under a 5-fold cross validation process for which the average and standard deviation are reported. For the evaluation, the complete patch of $28 \times 280 \times 280$, as well as smaller patches circumscribed by it of size $16 \times 160 \times 160$, either with the centered in the lesion patch or in random locations were given to the network.

In Fig. 2, the accuracy for the train- and test-set are plotted along the 250 epochs the network was trained for. On training patches, the two augmentation methods described in Section 2 were applied in each epoch. On testing patches, only random crops were extracted. The variation added to the testing patches was merely for experimental reasons, nevertheless, results without this variation are reported for the final model on Table 2.

Finally, in Fig. 3, the resulting heat-maps of using our network on patches of $9 \times H \times W$ as well as their overlapping (weighted addition) with their respective input is shown for four samples in the testing set. Where H and W are the height and width of the entire ultrasound volumes.

4 Discussion

Results in Table 2 show that the network performs better when using the smallest patches. This does not mean that the network is not capable of detecting lesions on bigger patches. As shown in Fig. 3, even in much bigger patches, the network focuses its attention on regions which are more likely to belong to a lesion. This behavior is not unexpected, despite of being trained on much smaller patches, the network's convolutional filters learn location variations of the input data

Fig. 2. Accuracy plot over 250 epochs for the training (blue) and test (orange) patches of size $28 \times 280 \times 280$. On training patches, random flip on the depth- and horizontal-axis as well as random crops of size $16 \times 160 \times 160$ were applied in each epoch. On test patches, only the random crop operation was used.

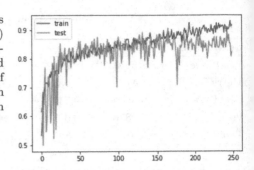

whenever those variations were shown on the training samples. A clear example of this, can be found in [11], where a CNN is trained on small patches of text and the generated heat-map on a entire page, it is capable to distinguish text areas from background or illustrations. We attribute the decrease on accuracy to the average pooling layer on the Residual Neural Network architecture: it is expected that the larger is the crop the more is the area without possible lesion. This implies that relatively low values will come out from the average pooling layer, even if a lesion is present in the patch.

In Fig. 3, the heat-maps indicate that our network does not only pay attention to the lesion but also on different locations -commonly other black areas-; nevertheless, the major attention corresponds to the lesion area.

An adequate metric to evaluate the localization pipeline has to be developed as metrics such as Intersection over Union (IoU), or similar, make little sense when having a single point of the lesion as ground truth. For instance, in Fig.3-d, the hot-spot of the heatmap clearly shows the localization of the lesion; however, it does not overlap with the center of the lesion annotated by experts.

4.1 Conclusion and future work

In this paper, it was shown that an accurate CNN for patch-level classification of lesions in ultrasound volumes can be trained with the information of a single cen-

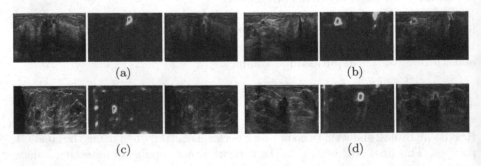

Fig. 3. Input, heat-map, and their overlapping for 4 ultrasounds in the test set. The displayed slice corresponds to the first coordinate of the estimated center of the lesion. In the input images, the center of the lesion which was annotated by experts is shown with a small red point.

tral point of the lesion. A key point of the pipeline resides on the augmentations used during the training phase: feeding the network with different random crops circumscribed in the extracted patches, gave the network enough information on the variability of the ultrasound volumes.

The generation of attention maps of our network using Grad-CAM provides information about the localization of the lesions. As future work, we plan to apply post-processing on the heat-maps to extract quantitative information of the size and localization of the lesions.

References

1. Morrow M, Schnitt SJ, Norton L. Current management of lesions associated with an increased risk of breast cancer. Nature rev Clin oncol. 2015;12(4):227.
2. Cao Z, Duan L, Yang G, et al. An experimental study on breast lesion detection and classification from ultrasound images using deep learning architectures. BMC Med Imaging. 2019 Jul;19(1):51.
3. Torres F, Escalante-Ramirez B, Olveres J, et al. Lesion detection in breast ultrasound images using a machine learning approach and genetic Optimization. In: Iberian Conference on Pattern Recognition and Image Analysis. Springer; 2019. p. 289–301.
4. Redmon J, Divvala S, Girshick R, et al. You only look once: unified, real-time object detection. Proc IEEE CCVPR. 2016; p. 779–788.
5. Girshick R, Donahue J, Darrell T, et al. Rich feature hierarchies for accurate object detection and semantic segmentation. Proc IEEE CVPR. 2014; p. 580–587.
6. Chen LC, Papandreou G, Kokkinos I, et al. Deeplab: semantic image segmentation with deep convolutional nets, atrous convolution, and fully connected crfs. IEEE Trans Pattern Anal Mach Intell. 2017;40(4):834–848.
7. Liu S, Wang Y, Yang X, et al. Deep learning in medical ultrasound analysis: a review. Engineering. 2019;5(2):261–275.
8. He K, Zhang X, Ren S, et al. Deep residual learning for image recognition. Proc IEEE CVPR. 2016; p. 770–778.
9. Kingma DP, Ba J. Adam: a method for stochastic optimization. arXiv preprint arXiv:14126980. 2014;.
10. Selvaraju RR, Cogswell M, Das A, et al. Grad-CAM: visual explanations from deep networks via gradient-based localization. Proc IEEE ICCV. 2017; p. 618–626.
11. Seuret M, Limbach S, Weichselbaumer N, et al. Dataset of pages from early printed books with multiple font groups. In: Proceedings of the 5th International Workshop on Historical Document Imaging and Processing; 2019. p. 1–6.

Abstract: Extracting and Leveraging Nodule Features with Lung Inpainting for Local Feature Augmentation

Sebastian Gündel[1,3], Arnaud A. A. Setio[1], Sasa Grbic[2], Andreas Maier[3], Dorin Comaniciu[2]

[1]Digital Technology and Innovation, Siemens Healthineers, Erlangen, Germany
[2]Digital Technology and Innovation, Siemens Healthineers, Princeton, NJ, USA
[3]Pattern Recognition Lab, Friedrich-Alexander-Universität Erlangen, Germany
sebastian.guendel@fau.de

Chest X-ray (CXR) is the most common examination for fast detection of pulmonary abnormalities. Recently, automated algorithms have been developed to classify multiple diseases and abnormalities in CXR scans. However, because of the limited availability of scans containing nodules and the subtle properties of nodules in CXRs, state-of-the-art methods do not perform well on nodule classification. To create additional data for the training process, standard augmentation techniques are applied. However, the variance introduced by these methods are limited as the images are typically modified globally. In this paper [1], we propose a method for local feature augmentation by extracting local nodule features using a generative inpainting network. The network is applied to generate realistic, healthy tissue and structures in patches containing nodules. The nodules are entirely removed in the inpainted representation. The extraction of the nodule features is processed by subtraction of the inpainted patch from the nodule patch. With arbitrary displacement of the extracted nodules in the lung area across different CXR scans and further local modifications during training, we significantly increase the nodule classification performance and outperform state-of-the-art augmentation methods.

References

1. Gündel S, Setio AAA, Grbic S, et al. Extracting and leveraging nodule features with lung inpainting for local feature augmentation. In: Liu M, Yan P, Lian C, et al., editors. Machine Learning in Medical Imaging. Cham: Springer International Publishing; 2020. p. 504–512.

© Der/die Autor(en), exklusiv lizenziert durch
Springer Fachmedien Wiesbaden GmbH, ein Teil von Springer Nature 2021
C. Palm et al. (Hrsg.), *Bildverarbeitung für die Medizin 2021*,
Informatik aktuell, https://doi.org/10.1007/978-3-658-33198-6_68

Abstract: Automatic Dementia Screening and Scoring by Applying Deep Learning on Clock-drawing Tests

Shuqing Chen[1], Daniel Stromer[1], Harb Alnasser Alabdalrahim[1],
Stefan Schwab[2], Markus Weih[2], Andreas Maier[3]

[1]Pattern Recognition Lab, Computer Science, FAU Erlangen-Nürnberg
[2]Department of Neurology, FAU Erlangen-Nürnberg
[3]Pattern Recognition Lab, FAU Erlangen-Nürnberg
shuqing.chen@fau.de

Dementia is one of the most common neurological syndromes in the world. Usually, diagnoses are made based on paper-and-pencil tests and scored by personal judgments of experts. This technique can introduce errors and has high inter-rater variability. In this study, the an automatic assessment of clock-drawing test (CDT) images was developed [1]. The CDTs were classified by the Shulmann system with scores varying from 1 to 6, increasing accordingly to the severity of dementia. To automatically classify the CDTs, our work is based on a comparison of three deep learning architectures including transfer learning of three pre-trained nets: VGG16, ResNet-152, and DenseNet-121. The dataset for our experiments consisted of 1315 individuals. To avoid the bias caused by the random data selection for the training with the limited amount of data, which also included several dementia types, we selected the training data and the validation data based on manifold learning methods. For training the network, we used optimization strategies such as adaptive moment estimation, stochastic gradient descent, root mean squared probability and a learning-rate scheduler. We discovered that using a varying learning rate yields in better results compared to a fixed learning rate during training. The outcome of our work is a standardized and digital estimation of the dementia screening result and severity level for an individual. We achieved off-diagonal accuracies of 96.65 % for screening and up to 98.54 % for scoring. Our proposed neural network achieved very high AUC and outperformed reported clinical screening results by up to 27 %, other machine-learning screening techniques by up to 24 %, and machine-learning scoring approaches up to 27 %. The algorithm can be easily integrated into hospitals' environments and care facilities to help monitoring the state of patients with dementia.

References

1. Chen S, Stromer D, Alabdalrahim HA, et al. Automatic dementia screening and scoring by applying deep learning on clock-drawing tests. Sci Rep. 2020;10(20854):1–11.

© Der/die Autor(en), exklusiv lizenziert durch
Springer Fachmedien Wiesbaden GmbH, ein Teil von Springer Nature 2021
C. Palm et al. (Hrsg.), *Bildverarbeitung für die Medizin 2021*,
Informatik aktuell, https://doi.org/10.1007/978-3-658-33198-6_69

Deep Learning Compatible Differentiable X-ray Projections for Inverse Rendering

Karthik Shetty[1], Annette Birkhold[2], Norbert Strobel[3], Bernhard Egger[4], Srikrishna Jaganathan[1], Markus Kowarschik[2], Andreas Maier[1]

[1]Pattern Recognition Lab, FAU Erlangen-Nürnberg
[2]Siemens Healthcare GmbH, Forchheim
[3]Fakultät Elektrotechnik, HS für angewandte Wissenschaften Würzburg-Schweinfurt
[4]MIT - BCS, CSAIL & CBMM, USA
karthik.shetty@fau.de

Abstract. Many minimally invasive interventional procedures still rely on 2D fluoroscopic imaging. Generating a patient-specific 3D model from these X-ray data would improve the procedural workflow, e.g., by providing assistance functions such as automatic positioning. To accomplish this, two things are required. First, a statistical human shape model of the human anatomy and second, a differentiable X-ray renderer. We propose a differentiable renderer by deriving the distance travelled by a ray inside mesh structures to generate a distance map. To demonstrate its functioning, we use it for simulating X-ray images from human shape models. Then we show its application by solving the inverse problem, namely reconstructing 3D models from real 2D fluoroscopy images of the pelvis, which is an ideal anatomical structure for patient registration. This is accomplished by an iterative optimization strategy using gradient descent. With the majority of the pelvis being in the fluoroscopic field of view, we achieve a mean Hausdorff distance of 30 mm between the reconstructed model and the ground truth segmentation.

1 Introduction

Over the last decades, the amount of X-ray guided interventional procedures has increased steadily, raising the awareness for optimized procedural workflows and radiation-dose induced adverse effects. Assistance systems based on a 3D digital twin of the patient have the potential to speed up procedures and minimize the required radiation. However, precisely representing the individual human anatomy based on the commonly acquired 2D projection images is an ill-posed problem. Ehlke et al. showed that an accurate and fast 3D reconstruction of the human pelvis from 2D projection images is possible by learning its shape space in the form of tetrahedral mesh structures from a large set of pelvis scans including bone density information [1]. In theory, this approach can generate digital twins of patients from live fluoroscopic imaging and may support advanced assistance applications for interventions.

© Der/die Autor(en), exklusiv lizenziert durch
Springer Fachmedien Wiesbaden GmbH, ein Teil von Springer Nature 2021
C. Palm et al. (Hrsg.), *Bildverarbeitung für die Medizin 2021*,
Informatik aktuell, https://doi.org/10.1007/978-3-658-33198-6_70

The process of generating a 3D model from 2D projection images is known as inverse-rendering and has received considerable attention in computer vision [2, 3]. However, achieving this usually means solving an ill-posed problem, and rendering pipelines are not necessarily differentiable. This is usually overcome by softening the non-differentiabilities by soft-rasterization [2]. Usually, a 3D scene is represented by a polygon mesh, which can be expressed by a set of vertices and faces. Such a representation is usually chosen for statistical shape and pose modeling. Skinned Multi-Person Linear Model (SMPL) is an example of such a parameterized model, which is deformable and accurately represents a large variation of human shapes [4]. Employing such a model enables more precise and faster 3D reconstruction from a 2D projection image space due to the incorporation of prior knowledge [3]. To carry out the 3D reconstruction from X-ray projections, we need to calculate artificial X-ray projections from a 3D model, e.g., a Statistical Shape Model (SSM). Generation of transmission images from mesh structures has been previously proposed [1, 5]. For a viable reconstruction, we seek to optimize the shape β and pose θ parameters by minimizing a similarity function between the simulated image and the acquired image. To this end, we propose a framework to combine existing X-ray rasterization approaches with a differentiable rasterizer, to create a setup that can be iteratively optimized by gradient descent techniques. The proposed renderer enables end-to-end frameworks.

2 Methods

2.1 Differentiable rasterizer

A watertight manifold surface can be represented as a triangular mesh by a set of faces $f \in \mathbb{N}^{N_f \times 3}$ and vertices $v \in \mathbb{R}^{N_v \times 3}$, where the the object has N_f faces and N_v vertices. Given a projection matrix, it is possible to transform the mesh from world coordinates to detector coordinates while maintaining the actual depth of the vertex. In traditional rasterization of 3D scenes, each pixel P_{xy} on the screen is affected by only the face f_j nearest to the ray from the camera. This is usually achieved by storing the depth information for all the faces influenced by a given pixel in the form of z-buffer. However, in the case of transmission imaging we need to know the distance traveled by a ray through an object in the form of l-buffer [5]. For each face f_j, the normals $\overrightarrow{N}_{f_j}$ in the projective space are computed. The sign of the dot product $D_{f_j R_{xy}} = sign\left(\overrightarrow{N}_{f_j} \cdot \overrightarrow{N}_{view}\right)$ between the face normal $\overrightarrow{N}_{f_j}$ and detector plane normal $\overrightarrow{N}_{view} = (0,0,1)^T$ determines if the ray R_{xy} is either entering or exiting the object for a given face. Hence, the total path length L_{xy} traveled by a ray for a given object p from the source to the detector pixel position P_{xy} is visualized in Fig. 1 and can be formulated as

$$L_{xy} = \sum_{j=1}^{K} D_{f_j R_{xy}} Z_{xy f_j} \qquad (1)$$

Fig. 1. Visualization for the determination of the ray distance for a simplified structure. Here, total distance covered by the ray is $L_{xy}=d_1-d_2+d_3-d_4$.

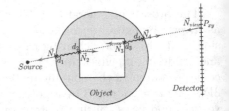

Z_{xyf_j} is the distance between the face f_j and the detector pixel position P_{xy}, while j and K represents the current valid intersection and the fixed number of mesh overlaps stored in the z-buffer, respectively. As a result, there is no substantial requirement for the elements of the z-buffer to be stored in a sorted manner. The only constraint is the number of faces K influencing a given pixel. To determine the gradients for the backward pass we follow the same procedure as implemented by Ravi et al [2], with an exception for the gradients for the z-buffer

$$\frac{\partial C}{\partial z_{xyj}} = \frac{\partial C}{\partial L_{xy}} D_{f_j R_{xy}} \tag{2}$$

Here, z_{xyj} represents the z-buffer distance from the pixel P_{xy} corresponding to face f_j with C as some cost function, e.g., the normalized gradient correlation (NGC) explained below.

It is generally assumed that the number of incoming rays for a given object is the same as the outgoing rays. However, artifacts occur when the face normal is perpendicular to the detector plane or in the presence of a non-manifold surface. The occurrence of such a situation can be determined when the summation over the pixel sign function $\sum_j^K R_{xyf_j}$ is non-zero. To overcome this, we set the image pixel value to a neighbouring pixel with zero sum and set the gradient for that particular pixel to zero.

2.2 X-ray rendering

The pipeline for generating the X-ray projection image for a human patient model is depicted in Fig. 2. Distance projection maps L_p are generated individually for air (L_{air}), body (L_{body}), bones (L_{bones}) and organs (L_{organs}). L_{air} represents the Euclidean distance from a detector pixel P_{xy} in world coordinates to the X-ray source. L_{body}, L_{bones} and L_{organs} are generated as described in Sec. 2.1 from individual meshes respectively. For ease of explanation, we describe L_{organs} as a single organ distance map, however it is a subset of lungs, heart, liver, kidney and spleen. As L_{air} is inclusive of L_{body}, we define the actual air distance map as $L_{\text{air}} - L_{\text{body}}$. For the body we proceed similarly as shown in Fig. 2.

The X-ray projection is generated using a primary signal I_{xy} for a pixel P_{xy} described using the Beer-Lambert law as shown in Eq. 3 with a photon energy E, X-ray energy $I_o(E)$, and linear attenuation coefficients $\mu(p, E)$ for objects p

$$I_{xy} = \sum_E I_o(E) e^{\sum_p (\mu(p,E) L_{pxy})} \tag{3}$$

Making use of the aforementioned distance maps L_p, the simulation can be extended for polychromatic X-ray beam spectra.

2.3   Application: inverse rendering

We build a statistical parametric model $M(\boldsymbol{\beta}, \boldsymbol{\theta}; \boldsymbol{\Phi})$, similar to SMPL [4] extended for internal anatomy using principal component analysis to characterize the human anatomy shape space from a large set of segmented whole-body CT scans. This makes it possible to generate realistic X-ray projections with the entire pipeline being differentiable in nature. Here, $\boldsymbol{\Phi}$ represents the learned parameters of the model. To reconstruct a 3D model from a projection image we fix the camera projection matrix of the simulation system as defined by the target along with an initial mean shape $\boldsymbol{\beta}_m$ and rest pose $\boldsymbol{\theta}_r$. A gradient descent based optimization with backpropagation is applied to the simulation model. NGC is used as a similarity measure [6], which is defined by the normalized cross-correlation of the image gradient between two images. The model is optimized until convergence to obtain the optimal pose $\boldsymbol{\theta}$ and shape $\boldsymbol{\beta}$ parameters.

For evaluation, we used the dataset provided by Grupp et al. made up of the hip anatomy from 6 patients [7]. For each patient, a 3D segmentation of the pelvis along with 14 landmarks and a total of 366 fluoroscopy images in varying orientations with their respective projection matrices are available.

3   Evaluation and results

The SSM is registered to each patient from the dataset. This resulted in a base score with an average Hausdorff distance of 17.79 mm and a mean landmark error of 11.81 mm. The rotation and translation parameters obtained are assumed as the ground truth irrespective of the shape parameters. The 2D-3D reconstruction is tested by applying a random translation in the range of [-10,10] mm and a rotation in the range of [-5,5]° on all three axes for the SSM. The randomization is small due to the nature of the loss function being sensitive to changes only around a small region, such precision of initialization could be either provided manually or achieved with a network learning those initialization parameters.

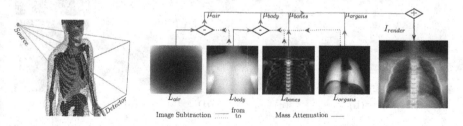

Fig. 2. Left: Projection performed around the thorax section from a mesh representation of a patient model. Right: Pipeline to generate a transmission image from the given mesh structures and projection matrix.

Table 1. Overview of the reconstruction and landmark error. All distances are measured in mm. The lower bound error is dependent on the shape model, with a mean Hausdorff distance of 17.79 mm and a mean landmark error of 11.81 mm.

Initial		Reconstructed	
Hausdorff distance	Landmark Error	Hausdorff Distance	Landmark Error
46.59 ± 4.64	30.00 ± 8.30	29.11 ± 4.56	22.06 ± 6.13

Fig. 3 shows sample outputs of our proposed method along with the quantitative results in Table 1. For evaluation, we consider only the images where the region of pelvis visible is greater than 50%.

4   Discussion and conclusion

We presented an approach for differential rendering and reconstructing a patient-specific 3D mesh model from a single 2D X-ray projection image. We demonstrated that using a deformable human model parameterized by shape and pose, we were able to approximately register patients to an X-ray projection. We found that given a visibility above 50% and an initialization of a generic model shape positioned close to the actual image, the 3D reconstruction error is significantly reduced with our optimization approach. The remaining error may be due to the simultaneous unconstrained optimization of shape and pose. This is because changes in shape and translation across depth, i.e., in z-direction, results in a large range of solutions causing the simulated image to appear similar to the target image. For now, we ignore the case when less than 50% of the pelvis is visible due to the intrinsic nature of the loss function being sensitive to the initial position. In general, the error could be reduced with an additional prior to determine a good initial pose [8].

As the registration is independent of the patient pose we can overcome possible pose mismatches resulting from employing preoperative CT scan for reg-

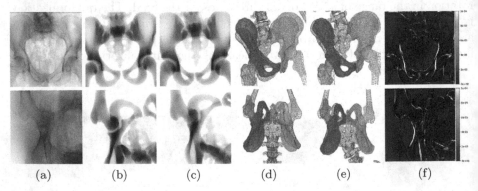

(a)   (b)   (c)   (d)   (e)   (f)

Fig. 3. Samples for 3D reconstruction from 2D projection images. (a) Target image, (b) Projection image with a random translation and rotation, (c) Projection image after registration, (d) Initial 3D overlay of template mesh, (e) 3D overlay of the meshes after registration, (f) NGC map after registration.

istration. Still, the pipeline has limitations. First, the X-ray simulation is an approximation of a real X-ray image, as it does not take into account any scattering mechanisms and other effects causing noise. This can be possibly improved by employing a deep learning model for predicting patient-specific scatter [9]. Second, the renderer assumes a constant density for any given material, resulting in a pseudo-realistic rendering. One way to overcome this problem would be to use a tetrahedral mesh with learned bone density distributions. Third, due to ambiguous depth information in fluoroscopy images, accurate registration becomes a challenging task. This error could be minimized with multi-view images or by using the table position as a constraint. To summarize, we proposed a differentiable renderer by deriving the distance travelled by a ray inside mesh structures. This was further extended to generate X-ray images from human models. Finally, we showed that it could be successfully used to reconstruct 3D models from 2D fluoroscopy images.

Disclaimer. The concepts and information presented in this paper are based on research and are not commercially available.

References

1. Ehlke M, Ramm H, Lamecker H, et al. Fast generation of virtual x-ray images for reconstruction of 3D anatomy. IEEE Trans Vis Comput Graph. 2013; p. 2673–2682.
2. Ravi N, Reizenstein J, Novotny D, et al. Accelerating 3d deep learning with pytorch3d. arXiv preprint arXiv:200708501. 2020;.
3. Liu S, Li T, Chen W, et al. Soft rasterizer: a differentiable renderer for image-based 3d reasoning. In: Proc IEEE Int Conf Comput Vis; 2019. p. 7708–7717.
4. Loper M, Mahmood N, Romero J, et al. SMPL: a skinned multi-person linear model. ACM Trans Graph (Proc SIGGRAPH Asia). 2015 Oct;34(6):248:1–248:16.
5. Vidal FP, Garnier M, Freud N, et al. Simulation of x-ray attenuation on the GPU. In: Tang W, Collomosse J, editors. Theory and Practice of Computer Graphics. The Eurographics Association; 2009. .
6. Penney GP, Weese J, Little JA, et al. A comparison of similarity measures for use in 2-D-3-D medical image registration. IEEE Trans Med Imaging. 1998;17(4):586–595.
7. Grupp RB, Unberath M, Gao C, et al. Automatic annotation of hip anatomy in fluoroscopy for robust and efficient 2D/3D registration. Int J Comput Assist Radiol Surg. 2020 May;15(5):759–769.
8. Bier B, Unberath M, Zaech JN, et al. X-ray-transform invariant anatomical landmark detection for pelvic trauma surgery. In: Med Image Comput Comput Assist Interv. Springer; 2018. p. 55–63.
9. Roser P, Zhong X, Birkhold A, et al. Physics-driven learning of x-ray skin dose distribution in interventional procedures. Med Phys. 2019;46:4654–4665.

Abstract: Are Fast Labeling Methods Reliable?
A Case Study of Computer-aided Expert Annotations on Microscopy Slides

Christian Marzahl[1,2], Christof A. Bertram[3], Marc Aubreville[1], Anne Petrick[3], Kristina Weiler[4], Agnes C. Gläsel[4], Marco Fragoso[3], Sophie Merz[3], Florian Bartenschlager[3], Judith Hoppe[3], Alina Langenhagen[3], Anne Katherine Jasensky[5], Jörn Voigt[2], Robert Klopfleisch[3], Andreas Maier[1]

[1]Pattern Recognition Lab, Department of Computer Science, Friedrich-Alexander-Universität Erlangen-Nürnberg (FAU), Germany
[2]R & D Projects, EUROIMMUN Medizinische Labordiagnostika AG
[3]Institute of Veterinary Pathology, Freie Universität Berlin, Germany
[4]Department of Veterinary Clinical Sciences, Clinical Pathology and Clinical Pathophysiology, Justus-Liebig-Universität Giessen, Germany
[5]Laboklin GmbH und Co. KG, Bad Kissingen, Germany
c.marzahl@euroimmun.de

Deep-learning-based pipelines have shown the potential to revolutionize microscopy image diagnostics by providing visual augmentations and evaluations to a pathologist. However, to match human performance, the methods rely on the availability of vast amounts of high-quality labeled data, which poses a significant challenge. To circumvent this, augmented labeling methods, also known as expert-algorithm-collaboration, have recently become popular. However, potential biases introduced by this operation mode and their effects on training deep neuronal networks are not entirely understood [1]. This work aimed to evualte this for three pathological pattern of interest. Ten trained pathology experts performed a labeling tasks without and with computer-generated augmentation. To investigate different biasing effects, we intentionally introduced errors to the augmentation. In total, experts annotated 26,015 cells on 1,200 images in this novel annotation study. Backed by this extensive data set, we found that the concordance of multiple experts was significantly increased in the computer-aided setting, versus the unaided annotation. However, a significant percentage of the deliberately introduced false labels was not identified by the experts.

References

1. Marzahl C, Bertram CA, Aubreville M, et al. Are fast labeling methods reliable? A case study of computer-aided expert annotations on microscopy slides. Proc MICCAI. 2020; p. 24–32.

Abstract: Time Matters

Handling Spatio-temporal Perfusion Information for Automated Treatment in Cerebral Ischemia Scoring

Maximilian Nielsen[1,3], Moritz Waldmann[2], Thilo Sentker[1,3], Andreas Frölich[2], Jens Fiehler[2], René Werner[1,3]

[1]Department of Computational Neuroscience, University Medical Center Hamburg-Eppendorf, Hamburg, Germany
[2]Department of Diagnostic and Interventional Neuroradiology, University Medical Center Hamburg-Eppendorf, Hamburg, Germany
[3]Center for Biomedical Artificial Intelligence (bAIome), University Medical Center Hamburg-Eppendorf, Hamburg, Germany
m.nielsen@uke.de

Although video classification is a well addressed task in computer vision (CV), corresponding CV methods have so far only rarely been translated to the automatic assessment of X-ray digital subtraction angiography (DSA) imaging. We demonstrate the feasibility of a respective method translation by making the first attempt on automatic treatment in cerebral ischemia (TICI) scoring. [1] In a clinical setting, the TICI score is used to evaluate the initial as well as the perfusion state after thrombectomy, i.e. the intervention success. Therefore, a medical expert assigns a TICI score based on the observed perfusion in the spatio-temporal DSA image information. This process is, however, known to be time consuming and subject to a high inter- and intrarater variability, making its application cumbersome in large clinical trials. Due to the complex data and perfusion dynamics, automatic TICI scoring has, for a long time, been considered beyond the scope of machine (deep) learning. In the present work, we create a first benchmark for automated TICI scoring. The backbone of our method is formed by a two-arm image encoder and a gated recurrent unit (GRU) architecture, combined with a custom loss function that reflects the high label uncertainty and ordinality of the TICI score. Furthermore, framewise pseudo-perfusion labels are generated and used as framewise annotations in addition to the expert TICI annotation during the GRU training. By increasing robustness and physiological plausibility of the training process, we achieve differences between predicted TICI scores and annotations in the order of literature-reported interrater variability of human experts during test time.

References

1. Nielsen M, Waldmann M, Sentker T, et al. Time matters: handling spatio-temporal perfusion information for automated TICI scoring. Proc MICCAI. 2020;part I:86–96.

© Der/die Autor(en), exklusiv lizenziert durch
Springer Fachmedien Wiesbaden GmbH, ein Teil von Springer Nature 2021
C. Palm et al. (Hrsg.), *Bildverarbeitung für die Medizin 2021*,
Informatik aktuell, https://doi.org/10.1007/978-3-658-33198-6_72

A Geometric and Textural Model of the Colon as Ground Truth for Deep Learning-based 3D-reconstruction

Ralf Hackner[1], Sina Walluscheck[1,2], Edgar Lehmann[3], Thomas Eixelberger[1], Volker Bruns[1], Thomas Wittenberg[1,2]

[1]Fraunhofer Institute for Integrated Circuits IIS, Erlangen
[2]Chair for Visual Computing, FAU Erlangen-Nürnberg
[3]E&L Medical Systems, Erlangen
ralf.hackner@iis.fraunhofer.de

Abstract. For endoscopic examinations of the large intestine, the limited field of vision related to the keyhole view of the endoscope can be a problem. A panoramic view of the video images acquired during a colonoscopy can potentially enlarge the field of view in real-time and may ensure that the performing physician has examined the entire organ. To train and test such a panorama-generation system, endoscopic video sequences with information about the geometry are necessary, but rarely exist. Therefore, we created a virtual phantom of the colon with a 3D-modelling software and propose different methods for realistic-looking textures. This allows us to perform a "virtual colonoscopy" and provide a well-defined test environment as well as supplement our training data for deep learning.

1 Introduction

One challenge in diagnostic colonoscopy being the endoscopic examination of the lower GI-tract (consisting of the rectum and the colon) is the limited 'field-of-view' of the colonoscope, also known as 'keyhole view'. During a colonoscopic examination, the flexible video-endoscope is advanced and navigated through the anus up the rectum, then the sigmoid-, descending-, transverse- and ascending colon, the cecum, and finally to the terminal cecum, and ultimately the terminal ileum (Fig. 1). During this insertion process, the endoscopist usually does not look for details on the colon walls, but rather concentrates on the fluent and painless insertion of the colonoscope into the lumen up to the terminal ilium.

The visual examination takes place in a second step, when the endoscope is slowly withdrawn through ascending, transverse, descending and sigmoid colon. During the withdrawal, the physician turns and bends the tip of the colonoscope for a closer examination of the colonoscopic tissue looking for possible adenomas. Even though in the past two decades, technological improvements in the field of endoscopic imaging have been proposed, such as HD, near-focus, wide-angle, or magnifying endoscopes, the limitations of the 'keyhole view' still remain. Thus, the endoscopist never perceives a complete view of the colon wall and must fuse the already seen scenes together in his/her mind in order to obtain a complete, so-called 'texture map' or 'image panorama' of the colon. This subjective 'visual impression' and the corresponding diagnostic findings are later transcribed textually in the clinical documentation or recited from memory in interdisciplinary conferences and councils.

1.1 Panorama endoscopy

The image-based documentation of the lower GI tract is currently limited to short videos (needing time for replay and viewing) or single images of observed lesions (usually not depicting the anatomical context). The mentioned "fused image information" of the physician is only available in his/ her mind and can hence not be used for documentation, interdisciplinary discussions or education.

In order to compensate the 'key-hole' effect during a colonoscopic examination, a mapping of the colon wall is desirable. Using the urinary bladder as an example of a hollow organ to be assessed with an endoscope, it has recently been shown, that it is possible to provide a so-called 'panorama' or 'map' of the bladder directly during the examination in real time [1, 2], which can afterwards be used for an image-based documentation. For the computation of real time panoramic images of the colon hardly any work is known. E.g, for the stomach Liu et al. [3] have proposed an approach using electromagnetic tracker mounted at the endoscope tip. Ali [2] suggested the computation of a panorama around the pyloric antrum using optical flow between successive image frames for tracking. Approaches to do an offline reconstruction of the geometry, what can be seen as closely related problem have been done by Widya et al. [4] and Freedman et al. [5].

1.2 Objective

As the colon—in contrast to the bladder—is an organ with a much more complex (partially tubular, partially flat, partially hemisphere) and dynamic geometry, a mapping of the colon wall is related to the use of 3D-reconstruction methods such as real-time panorama mapping pipelines (SLAM, PTAM) and "Structure from Motion" (SfM) or "visual odometry", making use of simultaneous localization and mapping of the hollow based on monocular views of the hollow. Nevertheless, for the development and extensive evaluation of such 3D-reconstruction from monocular colonoscopic image sequences, a known ground truth of the colon geometry is required. Thus, in this work, we propose the definition and application of a textured 3D phantom of the colon, in which random images with known geometry, controllable illumination, predefined textures, and even flat and sessile adenomas can be rendered as objective ground truth for 3D-reconstruction experiments.

2 Materials and methods

To model our phantom, we used the open-source 3D-modelling software *Blender*. As reference for the texture appearance we used colonoscopic video sequences from Malteser Waldkrankenhaus St. Marien, Erlangen.

The model was formed based on typical sizes [6] of a large intestine. An overview is given in Fig. 1. The average diameter is 5 centimeters, widening up to 7 cm in the cecum. The appendix is not modelled. The entire model has a total length of 1.5 m. Characteristic structures as haustra and taeniae were modelled manually.

Fig. 1. Geometry of the colon model.

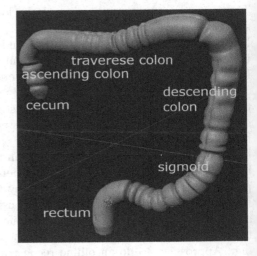

2.1 Model texture

The mucosa of the gastrointestinal wall is a complex structure of many tissue layers with different optical characteristics. Even a photorealistic rendering of ordinary skin is a complex task. In case of the colon mucosa, additional structures such as the intestinal villi create rough, light-scattering surface. Furthermore, the entire surface is coated by a thin layer of mucus.

We identified two primary components to mimic a surface, which is close to reality and especially contains all visual aspects expected to be important as features for the reconstruction of the structure from monocular views. A formative element of the mucosa are the vascular trees embedded in a widely ambient, slightly translucent, blood shaded surface. The second element is the mucus coating. This coat is glossy and typically causes specular highlights in endoscopic imaging, due to light source integrated in the device tip.

To create vessel-like structures, we evaluated two different approaches: The first approach was to use our existing panorama generation software "Endo-rama" [1] for cystoscopy to create a number of such panoramas of real human urinary bladders. The urinary bladder wall also contains similar vessel structures. We used a common image editing software to compose these panoramas to a texture patch of the size 279 × 4096. Bladder specific elements like *trigone* and *orifice* were removed. The texture can be seamlessly concatenated at its longer corner to allow a smooth loop closing, when mapping the texture to a cylindrical structure. The texture is large enough to use it without repeating, so that there is a unique vessel structure at every surface location. Subsurface rendering is used to simulate the blood shading of the tissue between the vessels.

The second approach was to generate random vessel-like structures. Inspired by an existing approach [7], we used random Voronoi textures to create vessel-like structures. Two independent textures simulating bluish and red blood vessels are combined. Musgrave textures (an algorithm, originally designed for modelling landscapes [8]) are used to slightly scatter the surface normales for a more natural look.

To simulate the mucus layer, we used a glass BSDF shader with an index of refraction corresponding to water.

2.2   Colonoscope tip, light and camera

A typical colonoscope is a flexible video endoscope with a diameter between 0.8 and 1.2 cm (E.g. common devices like Olympus GIF-IIQ Series [9] or Fujifilm [10]). Integrated in the tip of the endoscope is a tiny video sensor with a small fish-eye lens. A typical field of view has 140 degrees. The primary light source is outside the endoscope and glass fibers bundles are used to transport the light to the endoscope tip. A common arrangement are two fiber bundles with a distance of 0.5 cm, whose outlets are placed on each side of the sensor or slightly above. Correspondingly, we modelled a "virtual endoscope tip", using two point light sources with a power between 25 and 40 mW and placed them 0.25 cm aside of the virtual camera. The light sources are moved through the colon together with the camera. To create a realistic impression of an endoscope withdrawal, the camera is moved on a spiral-like manner through the virtual colon with different angles and varying speed.

3   Results

We rendered about 6000 single views based on our digital model with varying textures, camera positions, light intensity and shape variations of the colon. For every frame a corresponding depth map was generated. It contains the geometric information of the image, that can be used for purpose of training or testing a neural network. Some examples using a bladder-panorama texture can be seen in Fig. 2. Fig. 3 depicts the same frames featuring randomly generated Voronoi textures.

4   Discussion

The virtual phantom is designed for the training and testing of mosaicking applications, SLAMs and similar applications. These applications typically use surface patterns to register image tiles to each other in a correct way, where repeating patterns may lead to erroneous registrations. Thus, all patterns in both textures are strictly non-repeating as it is true for a real organ, either by using an image of sufficient size or random generated data. By providing different textures, we can also reduce the risk of on algorithm becoming too specific to the test data surface. Adding a glass shader to simulate the mucus coat created rather realistic highlights (Fig. 3(b)). For most image processing tasks these highlights are disruptive factors. For the application of depth estimation—that is a necessary step towards the geometry reconstruction—in contrast, these highlights might be useful information, since they indicate, that the surface normal is straight to the camera. The mapping between the panorama-based vessel texture is not perfect in all cases, sometimes leading to slightly stretched vessel structures (Fig. 2(b), bottom left corner). This happens especially, when the geometry has been changed without performing a manual correction. A varying resolution for all mapped regions would be necessary to create a perfect match. The randomly generated Voronoi texture has an advantage here, since it always

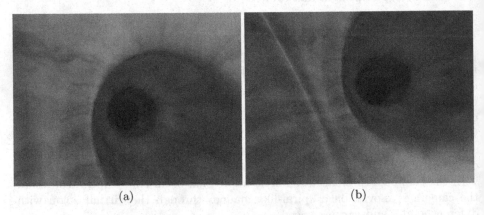

(a)   (b)

Fig. 2. Rendered images using the bladder-based texture.

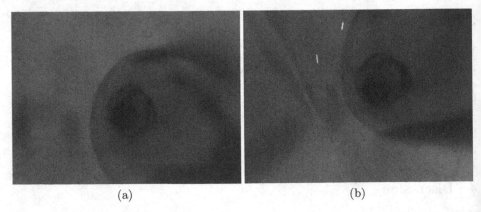

(a)   (b)

Fig. 3. Rendered images with random Voronoi textures (same positions as in Fig. 2).

fits the real surface and has no predefined shape or size. Images of with both textures were shown to an expert endoscopist. He preferred the panorama-based texture, because he judged the shading in the random texture as too dominant. Both textures were considered to look slightly "wax-like". It might be possible to reduce these flaws by fine-tuning some parameters of the shaders. When first panorama patches of the large intestine are available, it might be become possible to further improve the texture by using images of a real colon. On the long term, other fields of use might come into focus, like simulated, interactive training sessions for surgeons.

Acknowledgement. Parts of the research has been funded by the Bavarian Research Society (BFS) under the project GastroMapper (AZ-1349-18).

References

1. Bergen T. Real-time endoscopic image stitching for cystoscopy. Universität Koblenz Landau; 2016.
2. Ali S. Total variational optical flow for robust and accurate bladder image mosaicing. Université de Lorraine; 2016.
3. Liu J, Wang B, Hu W. Global and local panoramic views for gastroscopy: an assisted method of gastroscopic lesion surveillance. IEEE Trans Biomed Eng. 2015 Sep;62(9).
4. Widya AR, Monno Y, Imahori K, et al. 3D reconstruction of whole stomach from endoscope video using structure-from-motion. Proc IEEE EMB. 2019; p. 3900–4.
5. Freedman D, Blau Y, Katzir L, et al. Detecting deficient coverage in colonoscopies. IEEE Trans Biomed Eng. 2020 Nov;39(11).
6. Large intestine; 2020.
7. What is the best way to make a scene look like the inner of the colon? [online]; 2020.
8. Musgrave K. Methods for realistic landscape imaging. Yale University; 1993.
9. GIF-HQ190;.
10. Endoscopy mastercatalogue; 2018.

Deep Learning-basierte Oberflächenrekonstruktion aus Binärmasken

Carina Tschigor[1], Grzegorz Chlebus[1], Christian Schumann[1]

[1]Fraunhofer-Institut für Digitale Medizin MEVIS
christian.schumann@mevis.fraunhofer.de

Zusammenfassung. Die Darstellung anatomischer Strukturen auf Basis von Segmentierungsergebnissen in Form von Binärmasken ist eine grundlegende Aufgabe im Bereich der medizinischen Visualisierung. Hierfür werden meist polygonale Oberflächen genutzt. Bei Binärmasken fehlt jedoch die Information über die tatsächliche Oberfläche, wodurch die erzeugten Repräsentationen unter Artefakten leiden. Eine Glättung der Maske oder der polygonalen Repräsentation kann dies reduzieren, führt jedoch auch zu Ungenauigkeiten. Diese Arbeit beschreibt einen Ansatz zur Berechnung einer vorzeichenbehafteten Distanzfunktion für eine gegebene Binärmaske auf Basis eines neuronalen Netzwerkes. Diese lässt sich anschließend mit klassischen Methoden in eine Oberfläche überführen, deren Visualisierung glatt und artefaktfrei ist und nur minimale Abweichungen einführt.

1 Einleitung

Für Applikationen im Bereich der Diagnostik und vor allem der Therapieplanung ist eine qualitativ hochwertige Darstellung von segmentierten anatomischen Strukturen wünschenswert. Hierbei ist vor allem eine realistische Darstellung der Morphologie ohne störende Artefakte wichtig. Gleichzeitig sollte die Visualisierung nur minimale Ungenauigkeiten einführen. Durch die Segmentierung anatomischer Strukturen aus CT- oder MRT-Volumen werden typischerweise Binärmasken gewonnen, die jeden Voxel entweder als Teil der Struktur oder des Hintergrundes klassifizieren. Hierdurch geht der Partialvolumeneffekt verloren, wodurch die Erzeugung einer glatten Oberfläche durch gängige Polygonialisierungsverfahren wie den Marching Cubes Algorithmus [1] erschwert wird. Die Ergebnisse lassen sich teilweise durch Glättung verbessern, entweder angewendet auf die Binärmaske oder das Polygonialisierungsergebnis [2]. Die Reduktion aller Artefakte erfordert jedoch viele Iterationen oder große Nachbarschaften, worunter die Genauigkeit der Rekonstruktion leidet. Im Fall der nachträglichen Glättung der polygonalen Oberfläche kann das Ergebnis jedoch durch eine explizite Analyse der eingeführten Artefakte weiter verbessert werden [3, 4]. Ein naheliegender Ansatz für die Glättung der Binärmaske vor der Oberflächenextraktion ist die Nutzung eines Gauß-Filters. Dies kann in Einzelfällen zu akzeptablen Ergebnissen führen. Je nach Morphologie werden aber unterschiedlich große

Kernel benötigt. Somit ist eine Anwendung unter Erhaltung kleiner Strukturen bei gleichzeitig ausreichender Glättung sehr weitläufiger Treppenartefakte nicht möglich. Vielversprechender ist die explizite Rekonstruktion bzw. Optimierung einer vorzeichenbehafteten Distanzfunktion auf Basis der Binärdaten, welche die Extraktion einer glatten Oberfläche erlaubt. Einige Verfahren leiten hierbei auf Basis der Voxeldaten Punkte und assoziierte Normalenvektoren an der Oberfläche ab [5, 6], um gängige Punktwolken-basierte Oberflächenrekonstruktionsverfahren nutzen zu können, welche vorzeichenbehaftete Distanzfunktionen auf Basis der Punktwolken erzeugen, die in einem weiteren Schritt polygonalisiert werden können. Weitere Verfahren zur Erzeugung von Distanzfunktionen auf Basis von Punktwolken, wie KinectFusion [7] oder gar mit Hilfe von Deep Learning [8], wären hier denkbar, wurden aber noch nicht auf Voxeldaten angewendet. Eine direkte Optimierung einer Distanzfunktion auf Basis der Binärmaske wird zum Beispiel von Lempitzky vorgeschlagen [9]. Der hier präsentierte Ansatz, Neural Network Narrow Distance Function (N^3DF), verfolgt ein ähnliches Ziel, nutzt jedoch ein neuronales Netz, um aus der Binämaske eine Distanzfunktion abzuleiten, welche die Extraktion einer glatten Oberfläche ermöglicht.

2   Material und Methoden

Die grundlegende Idee des Ansatzes ist die Überführung der Binärmaske in eine vorzeichenbehaftete Distanzfunktion mit Hilfe eines trainierten neuronalen Netzes. Hierbei markiert die Eingabemaske Hintergrundvoxel mit -1 und Voxel innerhalb der Struktur mit 1. Analog zu der in der Bildverarbeitung verbreiteten Distanztransformation (DTF) nennen wir diese Umwandlung N^3DF. Im Unterschied zur klassischen Distanztransformation, die lediglich den Abstand zum nächstgelegenen Objekt-Voxel ausgibt, approximiert N^3DF die Entfernung zur ursprünglichen Oberfläche innerhalb einer kleinen Nachbarschaft der Oberfläche. Voxel innerhalb der Struktur erhalten den Wert 1, Voxel außerhalb den Wert -1. Voxel mit einem Abstand kleiner als 1 mm zur Oberfläche erhalten einen entsprechenden Gleitkommawert. Das Ergebnis der N^3DF ist somit eine beschnittene Distanzfunktion [7]. Sie kann anschließend mit einem Polygonalisierungsverfahren wie Marching Cubes in eine Oberfläche überführt werden unter Nutzung des Iso-Wertes 0 (Abb. 1).

Das Training des Netzes wird nicht mit realen Daten durchgeführt, da die Ground Truth für eine gegebene Maske nicht ermittelt werden kann. Stattdes-

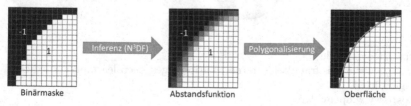

Abb. 1. Pipeline zur Erzeugung einer glatten Oberfläche aus einer binären Maske verdeutlicht an einem Ausschnitt einer 2D-Schicht.

sen werden künstliche Daten genutzt. Die grundlegende Idee ist hierbei, aus den glatten Oberflächen einfacher generischer Grundformen sowohl Binärmasken als auch Abstandsfunktionen abzuleiten und für das Training zu nutzen. Da hierbei die echte Geometrie bekannt ist, werden in den Trainigsdaten die echten Abstände gespeichert und für das Training genutzt. Ziel des Trainings ist somit, ein neuronales Netz zu erzeugen, das aus einer Binärmaske eine beschnittene Distanzfunktion ableiten kann, die den Abstand zu einer Oberfläche, die zu der Eingabemaske passen würde, darstellt. Es wird somit nicht direkt die Distanz zu der Grenze zwischen Vorder- und Hintergrund in der Maske wiedergegeben, wie dies bei gängigen Distanztransformationen der Fall ist, sondern der zu einer möglichen, glatten Oberfläche, die nahe dieser Grenze liegt.

Das trainierte Netz wird anschließend auf Binärmasken angewendet, die verschiedene Strukturen aus einem CT-Datensatz repräsentieren. Die resultierenden Distanzfelder werden mit Hilfe des Marching Cubes Algorithmus [1] in polygonale Oberflächen überführt. Die Experimente wurden in MeVisLab[1], einer integrierten Entwicklungsumgebung für medizinische Bildverarbeitung und Visualisierung durchgeführt. Hierbei wurde das integrierte Remote Deep Learning Framework (RedLeaf)[2] genutzt.

2.1 Trainingsdaten

Abb. 2 zeigt die verwendeten Grundformen für Training und Validierung des neuronalen Netzes. Um möglichst vielfältige Daten zu erhalten, werden die Grundformen in den drei Hauptachsen anisotrop skaliert und rotiert. Zusätzlich werden Kugeloberflächen mit kleinen Vertiefungen oder Erhebungen erzeugt, um auch kleine Details im Voxelbereich zu trainieren. Die Oberflächen werden unter Nutzung von OpenVDB[3] voxelisiert bei gleichzeitiger Berechnung der Distanzfunktion. Daraus wird mit Thresholding die Binämaske erzeugt, um so die benötigten Datenpaare zu erhalten. Die Binärmasken müssen hierbei analog zur Inferenz ebenfalls Hintergrundvoxel mit -1 und Voxel innerhalb der Struktur mit 1 markieren. Insgesamt werden so 1600 Datenpaare erzeugt, die in 70% Training, 10% Validierung und 20% Testen gesplittet werden.

Abb. 2. Für das Training verwendete Grundformen: Kugel, Ellipsoid, Torus und Zylinder.

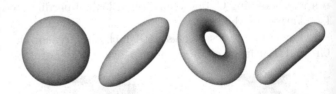

---

[1] https://mevislab.de
[2] https://www.mevis.fraunhofer.de/en/solutionpages/deep-learning-in-medical-imaging.html
[3] https://www.openvdb.org

2.2 Netzwerk Architektur

Die hier verwendete Architektur ist ein 3D U-net [10]. Dies findet Anwendung sowohl in der Klassifikation, als auch in der Regression von dreidimensionalen medizinischen Bilddaten. Es werden drei Auflösungsstufen und eine Filtergröße von 3x3x3 genutzt. Somit ergibt sich ein rezeptives Feld von 44^3. Die Outputfunktion tanh schränkt den Output auf den gewünschten Wertebereich von (-1,1) ein. Das Downsampling besteht aus je zwei aufeinanderfolgenden Faltungen und anschließenden Max Pooling (2x2x2). Zudem wird Batch Normalization verwendet. Beim Upsampling folgen auf eine transponierte Faltung (2x2x2) jeweils zwei Faltungen.

2.3 Training

Für das Training wird eine Patchsize von 64^3 sowie eine Batchsize von 2 verwendet. Eine Validierung erfolgt alle 250 Iterationen. Als Lossfunktion wird die mittlere quadratische Abweichung (MSE) gewählt. Die Lernrate ist auf 0.0001 gesetzt. Das Training hat eine Dauer von 200 Epochen. Anschließend wird das beste Modell verwendet, d.h. jenes, welches auf den Validierungsdaten den geringsten Fehler hat.

3 Ergebnisse

Aus einem CT-Datensatz eines Torsoausschnittes wurden fünf Binärmasken verschiedener Strukturen (Rippen, Leber, Lebergefäßbaum, Lunge und Haut) erzeugt und die Distanzfunktionen durch Inferenz des trainierten neuronalen Netzes erlangt (NVIDIA GeForce GTX 1050 Ti GPU mit 4GB Videospeicher). Hierbei kam eine Tilesize von 32^3 zum Einsatz. Als Beispiel werden hier die Ergebnisse für den Datensatz mit knöchernen Gewebe wie Rippen und Wirbelsäule gezeigt. Die Berechnung der N^3DF für die 333x267x169 große Binärmaske dauerte 91 s. Abb. 3 zeigt das Ergebnis der Oberflächenrekonstruktion mit

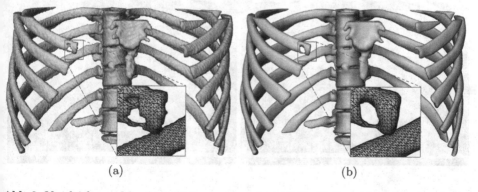

(a)   (b)

Abb. 3. Vergleich von Marching Cubes angewendet auf die Binärmaske (a) und auf das Ergebnis der N^3DF (b). Die Vergrößerung (rotes Quadrat) zeigt die Polygondichte sowie Abweichungen am Beispiel eines kleinen Loches.

Marching Cubes auf Basis der N^3DF im Vergleich zur Rekonstruktion auf Basis der Binärmaske. Zur quantitativen Bewertung wurde die Abweichung der N^3DF-Oberfläche von der Binärmaske berechnet. Die mittlere Abweichung beträgt 0,28 Voxeldiagonalen und ist somit sehr gering. Es wurde jedoch eine maximale Abweichung von 3,6 Voxeldiagonalen ermittelt. Solch starke Abweichungen treten vor allem bei sehr kleinen Strukturen oder Vertiefungen auf (Abb. 3).

Um die Glattheit der erzeugten Oberflächen objektiv beurteilen zu können, wurden Krümmungswerte in Form des Dihedralwinkels für die Oberflächenrekonstruktion mit Marching Cubes auf Basis der Binärmaske und der N^3DF berechnet und auf der Oberfläche visualisiert (Abb. 4). Die Polygongitter unterscheiden sich bzgl. ihrer Komplexität kaum voneinander. Die N^3DF-Oberfläche besteht aus 212902 Knoten und 425876 Polygonen, die Oberfläche basierend auf der Binärmaske aus 214865 Knoten und 429802 Polygonen.

4 Diskussion

Wir konnten zeigen, dass mit Hilfe eines neuronalen Netzes aus einer dreidimensionalen Binärmaske eine Distanzfunktion berechnet werden kann, die die Erzeugung einer glatt wirkenden Oberfläche erlaubt. Diese Glattheit resultiert daraus, dass hier nicht direkt die Distanz zu der Grenze zwischen Vorder- und Hintergrund berechnet wird, wie dies bei gängigen Distanztransformationen der Fall ist, sondern der Abstand zu einer möglichen, glatten Oberfläche, die nahe dieser Grenze liegt. Unseres Wissens nach ist N^3DF der erste Ansatz zur Berechnung einer solchen Distanzfunktion mit Hilfe von Deep Learning. Die Berechnung der Distanzfunktion nimmt dabei je nach Hardware eine nicht unerhebliche Zeit in Anspruch. Im Vergleich zu anderen Verfahren ist die Berechnungsdauer jedoch durchaus praktikabel und wir hoffen die Geschwindigkeit in Zukunft durch die Optimierung der Netzwerkarchitektur weiter steigern zu können. Desweiteren

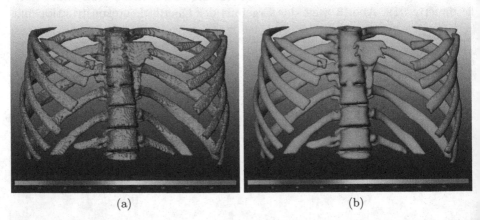

(a)   (b)

Abb. 4. Visualisierung des Dihedralwinkels für die Rekonstruktion auf Basis der Binärmaske (a) sowie auf Basis von N^3DF (b).

profitiert das Verfahren von der rasanten Entwicklung von Hardware, die speziell auf Deep Learning ausgelegt ist, wie zum Beispiel die hier genutzten GPUs von NVIDIA. Die Komplexität der entstandenen Oberflächen ist in Hinsicht auf die Polygonzahl vergleichbar mit der Anwendung von Marching Cubes auf Binärmasken. Die erzeugten Oberflächen sind jedoch weitaus glatter und geben die Morphologie der anatomischen Strukturen ohne störende Artefakte wieder. Allerdings können noch vor allem bei kleinen Strukturen und Vertiefungen nicht unerhebliche Fehler auftreten. Eine Überabtastung könnte hier zu einer Verbesserung führen und so auch die kleinsten Strukturen korrekt darstellen.

In zukünftigen Experimenten sollten auch Trainingsdaten genutzt werden, die aus anatomischen Datensätzen gewonnen wurden, um das neuronale Netz noch besser an solche Strukturen anzupassen. Desweiteren soll die Nutzung anderer Polygonalisierungsverfahren getestet werden um z.B. eine adaptive Polygongröße zu gewährleisten und somit die Komplexität der erzeugten polygonalen Oberflächen zu reduzieren.

Literatur

1. Lorensen WE, Cline HE. Marching cubes: a high resolution 3D surface construction algorithm. Comput Graph (ACM). 1987;21(4):163–169.
2. Taubin G. A signal processing approach to fair surface design. Proc Conf Comp Graph Interact Tech. 1995; p. 351–358.
3. Moench T, Gasteiger R, Janiga G, et al. Context-aware mesh smoothing for biomedical applications. Comput Graph. 2011;35(4):755–767.
4. Wei M, Wang J, Guo X, et al. Learning-based 3D surface optimization from medical image reconstruction. Opt Lasers Eng. 2018;103:110–118.
5. Schumann C, Oeltze S, Bade R, et al. Model-free surface visualization of vascular trees. Eurographics/ IEEE-VGTC Sym Vis. 2007; p. 283–290.
6. Wu J, Wei M, Li Y, et al. Scale-adaptive surface modeling of vascular structures. Biomed Eng Online. 2010;9(1):75.
7. Newcombe RA, Izadi S, Hilliges O, et al. KinectFusion: real-time dense surface mapping and tracking. Proc IEEE Int Sym Mix Augm Real. 2011; p. 127–136.
8. Park JJ, Florence P, Straub J, et al. Deepsdf: learning continuous signed distance functions for shape representation. Proc IEEE CVPR. 2019; p. 165–174.
9. Lempitsky V. Surface extraction from binary volumes with higher-order smoothness. Proc IEEE Comput Soc Conf Comput Vis Pattern Recognit. 2010; p. 1197–1204.
10. Çiçek Ö, Abdulkadir A, Lienkamp SS, et al. 3D U-Net: learning dense volumetric segmentation from sparse annotation. Proc MICCAI. 2016; p. 424–432.

A Novel Trilateral Filter for Digital Subtraction Angiography

Purvi Tripathi[1], Richard Obler[2], Andreas Maier[1], Hendrik Janssen[3]

[1]Pattern Recognition Lab, Friedrich-Alexander-University Erlangen-Nürnberg
[2]Department of Interventional Radiology, Advanced Therapies, Siemens Healthineers GmbH, Forchheim
[3]Institute for Neuroradiology, Center for Radiology and Neuroradiology, Hospital of Ingolstadt, Ingolstadt
purvi.tripathi@fau.de

Abstract. In this paper, we formulate a novel Trilateral Filter (TF) for denoising digital subtracted angiography (DSA) without losing any vessel information. The harmful effect of X-rays limits the dose resulting in degraded signal-to-noise ratio (SNR). A bilateral filter (BF) is often applied for edge-preserving denoising. However, for a low SNR image, the filter needs to be iterated with smaller spatial window to avoid over-smoothing of low-contrast vessels. The proposed TF combines the BF of wider spatial window with the Frangi vessel enhancement filter to denoise the DSA and to improve the vessel visibility without the need for iteration. The experimental results shows that our method provides better vessel preservation and greater noise reduction than the BF.

1 Introduction

X-ray angiography is one of the most common and widely practiced forms of interventional radiology. It is often used to produce fluoroscopic images while guiding within the blood vessels [1]. Despite being an effective non-invasive medical imaging technique, X-rays can cause significant damage to the human body. The ionizing radiation of X-rays is a high energy electromagnetic radiation that partially penetrates the tissues to produce images of inner structures [2]. Exposure to ionizing radiation can damage human tissues deterministically (radiation burn) and impair the DNA stochastically [3]. The latter may cause cancer or heritable effects, thus labeling X-rays as carcinogenic [4]. To ensure minimal exposure, all medical examinations are performed following the ALARA-principle (As Low As Reasonably Achievable) [5]. However, reducing the X-ray dose results in an image with a degraded signal-to-noise ratio (SNR).

It is well established that a clear and accurate vascular representation is an essential aspect of any angiographic imaging. A noisy medical image is not only visually frustrating but also perplexes the diagnosis and intervention. The image processing pipeline of an interventional radiology system applies various filters to enhance the visibility of clinically relevant aspects, such as vessel contrast and vessel edge definition. Since there is an on-going demand to further reduce the X-ray dose, which will consequently result in an image with even lower SNR, there is a strong need to further improve the performance of filters for angiographic images.

A bilateral filter is commonly used to denoise medical images while preserving edges. However, to avoid over-smoothing of low-contrast vessels in Digital Subtracted Angiography (DSA), the filtering is performed using a smaller spatial window leading to more number of iterations. In this paper, we propose novel trilateral filtering for DSA that can effectively reduce noise while preserving all the vessels without any iterations. The technique uses the Frangi vessel enhancement filter to identify the vessels and define the structural similarity. The structural similarity is integrated along with the geometric and photometric similarity of the BF to achieve vessel-preserving smoothing.

2   Materials and methods

2.1   Bilateral filter

A bilateral filter is an edge-preserving non-linear filter proposed by Tomasi et al [6] The main principle of a BF is that two pixels are considered neighbors not only when it is spatially close but also if it has similar photo-metric value. It is mathematically defined as

$$BF[I]_p = \frac{1}{W_p} \sum_{q \in S} G_{\sigma_s}(\| p - q \|) \cdot G_{\sigma_r}(\| I_p - I_q \|) I_q \qquad (1)$$

where I_p and I_q are pixel intensity at pixel location p and q, respectively. S is the spatial window around p, and W_p is a normalization factor given by

$$W_p = \sum_{q \in S} G_{\sigma_s}(\| p - q \|) \cdot G_{\sigma_r}(\| I_p - I_q \|) \qquad (2)$$

The amount of filtering in image I is controlled by parameters σ_s and σ_r. Equation (1) is a normalized weighted average where G_{σ_s} is a spatial Gaussian that regulates the effect of pixel-based on proximity, i.e., a closer pixel will result in more change to the center pixel p, and G_{σ_r} is a range Gaussian that decreases the effect of the pixel with higher intensity difference. It has been indicated in [7] that a BF with a wider kernel can lead to over-smoothing of the low-contrast vessel. To avoid that, the filter is often iterated increasing the computation time.

2.2   Frangi vessel enhancement filter

The vessel information is the most crucial aspect of interventional radiology. It is imperative to have a precise and clear vascular visualization and segmentation for clinical procedures. Frangi vesselness filter [8] is one of the most commonly used vessel enhancement techniques and is based on eigenvalue analysis of the Hessian matrix. The Hessian matrix is calculated by smoothing the image with a multiscale second order of the Gaussian (G_σ)

$$H_\sigma = G_\sigma * I = \begin{bmatrix} H_{xx} & H_{xy} \\ H_{xy} & H_{yy} \end{bmatrix} \tag{3}$$

The matrix is decomposed to calculate the two principle eigenvalues λ_1 and λ_2 [9]

$$\lambda_{1,2} = \frac{(H_{xx} + H_{yy}) \pm \sqrt{(H_{xx} - H_{yy})^2 + 4H_{xy}^2}}{2} \tag{4}$$

Analysis of the Hessian is performed to extract the principal local direction of curvature. The direction of curvature will be the smallest along the vessel. The pixels that are within the vessel will have a λ_1 close to zero and a large value for λ_2 [8]. A tubular structure is identified if it satisfies the following conditions:

$$\lambda_1 \approx 0 \tag{5}$$

$$\|\lambda_2\| \gg \|\lambda_1\| \tag{6}$$

Based on the second order ellipsoid, a ratio R_B is defined that describes blob-like structures or blobness. It is used to distinguish between line-like structure and plate-like structure and is given as

$$R_B = \frac{\|\lambda_1\|}{\|\lambda_2\|} \tag{7}$$

Further, a norm of Hessian matrix is used to measure the structureness, S. The structureness will be low for the region with low contrast and no structure. But in the region with high contrast, one of the eigenvalues will be large, and hence the value for S will be high [8]

$$S = \sqrt{\lambda_1^2 + \lambda_2^2} \tag{8}$$

Using R_B and S, the vesselness V_o is defined as

$$V_o(\sigma) = \begin{cases} 0, & \text{if } \lambda_2 > 0 \\ \exp(-\frac{R_B^2}{2\beta^2})(1 - \exp(-\frac{S^2}{2c^2})), & \text{otherwise} \end{cases} \tag{9}$$

where β, c are image-dependent parameters for blobness and structureness, respectively. For DSA images, the tubes are darker, and the lambda condition is reversed to $\lambda_2 < 0$. The σ used to calculate the Hessian matrix is used over a certain range, where the minimum σ depicts the detection of the smallest structure and maximum σ is for the biggest structure. For the cerebral DSA, we chose σ as 3, 5, and 7.

2.3   Trilateral filter

In this paper, we propose a novel trilateral filter as an extension of the BF to smooth a low-SNR DSA with wide kernel to maintain the denoising effect of a BF while preserving the low-contrast vessels. Along with the geometric and photometric similarity of a BF, the filter considers structural similarity (vesselness) as the third parameter, extracted using the Frangi vessel enhancement filter. The filter is mathematically defined as

$$TF[I]_p = \frac{1}{W_p} \sum_{q \in S} G_{\sigma_s}(\| p - q \|) \cdot G_{\sigma_r}(\| I_p - I_q \|) \cdot G_{\sigma_v}(\| V_p - V_q \|) I_q \quad (10)$$

where W_p is a normalization factor

$$W_p = \sum_{q \in S} G_{\sigma_s}(\| p - q \|) \cdot G_{\sigma_r}(\| I_p - I_q \|) \cdot G_{\sigma_v}(\| V_p - V_q \|) \quad (11)$$

The V_p and V_q are the normalized vesselness value drawn from the Frangi vesselness filter at a similar pixel location as that of the original image, and σ_v is the standard deviation for the vesselness. The principle of vessel preservation in the trilateral filter is similar to that of edge preservation. If the neighboring pixel has the same vesselness as that of the center pixel, its weight is higher than the pixel that is less similar. One of the features of the proposed filter is that for a region with no vessel, the vesselness is 0 resulting in vesselness Gaussian of 1. Therefore, the weight of the filter at those regions will be the same as the BF. Since the angiographic images are rarely flat, the vesselness difference between the vessel's pixels is mostly a non zero value, resulting in an additional smoothing within the vessel. The phenomenon together ensures controlled denoising and improves the visibility of low contrast vessels.

For our study, we selected wide kernel size of 21, with $\sigma_s = 6.0$, $\sigma_r = 15.0$, and $\sigma_v = 0.0005$. The filter first performs a Frangi vessel enhancement and stores the normalized vessel map as a new image. The original image and vessel map, along with the required parameter is passed for the trilateral filtering. For creating comparable results, we processed the image with both BF and TF with constant common parameters. Unlike the trilateral filtering approaches described by [10], with a favorable setting, this approach does not require iterations.

The DSA used in this study were acquired using ARTIS Biplane© (manufactured by Siemens Healthcare GmbH) at Center for Radiology and Neuroradiology, Hospital of Ingolstadt. To qualitatively evaluate the performance of the filter, we processed 15 DSA scenes of various dose levels using both the filters. The two filter techniques were ranked by four medical professionals based on the visual benefits. Quantitatively, we selected 10 high dose images and added Gaussian noise of standard deviation 7 and random Poisson noise to it. The images were then filtered and compared to the original image using two metrics: structural similarity index measure (SSIM), which is relevant for structural preservation, and peak signal to noise ratio (PSNR), relevant for noise reduction. The average of the 10 readings is accounted for the final comparison.

3   Results

As per the observer study conducted by the medical experts, the proposed TF shows a clear preference over the BF. For the 60 samples in study, the proposed TF was the preferred technique for 55 samples. A comparison of both filter approaches is shown in Fig 1. Fig 1(b) shows the over-smoothing effect of the BF. Also, the poor noise reduction around the bigger vessel reduces the visibility of the vessel. On the contrary, the TF in Fig 1(c) not only preserves the fine structures, but the additional smoothing within the vessels compensates for the contrast loss occurring due to bilateral filtering.

The quantitative comparison of the proposed TF with the BF is summarized in Table 1. The results show an increase in both SSIM and PSNR between BF and TF. With the selected parameter, the proposed filter performs the best for the reduction of Gaussian noise achieving an increase of 37% and 10% for SSIM and PSNR, respectively.

4   Discussion

In this paper, we proposed a combination of the BF and Frangi vessel enhancement filter to formulate the novel Trilateral filter for DSA, to perform vessel-preserving denoising. The proposed filter considers geometric, photometric, and

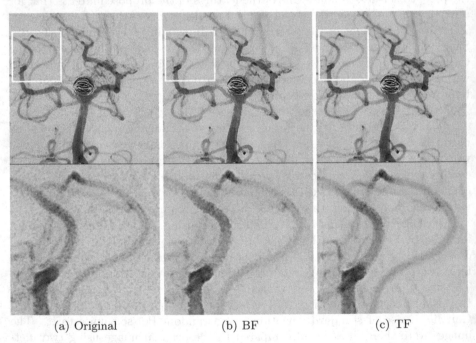

| (a) Original | (b) BF | (c) TF |

Fig. 1. Low-dose DSA. (a) Original image; denoised image with (b) Bilateral Filter and (c) Trilateral Filter. Source image courtesy: Center for Radiology and Neuroradiology, Hospital of Ingolstadt.

Table 1. SSIM and PSNR measure for low-dose DSA.

Noise	SSIM		PSNR	
	BF	TF	BF	TF
Gaussian	0.40	0.55	20.48	22.55
Poisson	0.27	0.31	17.55	18.32
Gaussian & Poisson	0.26	0.31	17.38	18.25

structural similarity in a wider neighborhood as a basis of filtering. The experiment with selected parameters shows an improvement in terms of noise reduction and vessel preservation both quantitatively and qualitatively. The results of the proposed TF are very promising, especially in accordance with the observer study.

Though the filter in its current state has no visible disadvantages, vessel like artifacts with very low-contrast are a potential drawback of the TF. Further research is necessary to explore this problem and improve the filter's efficiency by automatically adapting the parameters. We shall also investigate other vessel enhancement methods to be combined with the BF. The filter shall also be extended to process images from other modalities like MRI.

References

1. Grossman W, editor. Cardiac catheterization and angiography. 3rd ed. Philadelphia, Pa.: Lea & Febinger; 1986. P. 115-119.
2. Hirsch P, Howie A, Whelan M. On the production of X-rays in thin metal foils. Philos Mag Lett. 1962;7(84):2095–2100.
3. Zamanian A, Hardiman C. Electromagnetic radiation and human health: a review of sources and effects. High Frequency Electronics. 2005;4(3):16–26.
4. Herzog P, Rieger CT. Risk of cancer from diagnostic X-rays. The lancet. 2004;363(9427). P. 2192-2193.
5. Hendee W, Edwards F. ALARA and an integrated approach to radiation protection. Semin Nucl Med. 1986 05;16:142–50.
6. Tomasi C, Manduchi R; IEEE. Bilateral filtering for gray and color images. Proc IEEE ICCV. 1998; p. 839–846.
7. Choudhury P, Tumblin J. The trilateral filter for high contrast images and meshes. In: Rendering Techniques; 2003. p. 186–196.
8. Frangi AF, Niessen WJ, Vincken KL, et al. Multiscale vessel enhancement filtering. In: International conference on medical image computing and computer-assisted intervention. Springer; 1998. p. 130–137.
9. Fu W, Breininger K, Schaffert R, et al. Frangi-net. In: Bildverarbeitung für die Medizin 2018. Springer; 2018. p. 341–346.
10. Wong WC, Chung AC, Yu SC; IEEE. Trilateral filtering for biomedical images. Proc IEEE ISBI. 2004; p. 820–823.

Abstract: JBFnet
Low Dose CT-denoising by Trainable Joint Bilateral Filtering

Mayank Patwari[1,2], Ralf Gutjahr[2], Rainer Raupach[2], Andreas Maier[1]

[1]Pattern Recognition Lab, Friedrich-Alexander Universität Erlangen-Nürnberg
(FAU), Erlangen, Germany
[2]Siemens Healthcare GmbH, Forchheim, Germany
mayank.patwari@fau.de

Deep neural networks have shown great success in low dose CT denoising. However, most of these deep neural networks have several hundred thousand trainable parameters. This, combined with the inherent non-linearity of the neural network, makes the deep neural network difficult to understand with low accountability. In this study we introduce JBFnet, a neural network for low dose CT denoising. The architecture of JBFnet implements iterative bilateral filtering. The filter functions of the Joint Bilateral Filter (JBF) are learned via shallow convolutional networks. The guidance image is estimated by a deep neural network. JBFnet is split into four filtering blocks, each of which performs Joint Bilateral Filtering. Each JBF block consists of 112 trainable parameters, making the noise removal process comprehendable. The Noise Map (NM) is added after filtering to preserve high level features. We train JBFnet with the data from the body scans of 10 patients, and test it on the AAPM low dose CT Grand Challenge dataset. We compare JBFnet with state-of-the-art deep learning networks. JBFnet outperforms CPCE3D, GAN and deep GFnet on the test dataset in terms of noise removal while preserving structures. We conduct several ablation studies to test the performance of our network architecture and training method. Our current setup achieves the best performance, while still maintaining behavioural accountability. [1]

References

1. Patwari M, Gutjahr R, Raupach R, Maier A. JBFnet - low dose CT denoising by trainable joint bilateral filtering. Proc MICCAI. 2020:506–515. Available from: http://dx.doi.org/10.1007/978-3-030-59713-9_49.

Interactive Visualization of 3D CNN Relevance Maps to Aid Model Comprehensibility

Application to the Detection of Alzheimer's Disease in MRI Images

Martin Dyrba[1], Moritz Hanzig[1,2]

[1]German Center for Neurodegenerative Diseases (DZNE), Rostock, Germany
[2]Institute of Visual & Analytic Computing, University of Rostock, Germany
martin.dyrba@dzne.de

Abstract. Relevance maps derived from convolutional neural networks (CNN) indicate the influence of a particular image region on the decision of the CNN model. Individual maps are obtained for each single input 3D MRI image and various visualization options need to be adjusted to improve information content. In the use case of model prototyping and comparison, the common approach to save the 3D relevance maps to disk is impractical given the large number of combinations. Therefore, we developed a web application to aid interactive inspection of CNN relevance maps. For the requirements analysis, we interviewed several people from different stakeholder groups (model/visualization developers, radiology/neurology staff) following a participatory design approach. The visualization software was conceptually designed in a Model–View–Controller paradigm and implemented using the Python visualization library Bokeh. This framework allowed a Python server back-end directly executing the CNN model and related code, and a HTML/Javascript front-end running in any web browser. Slice-based 2D views were realized for each axis, accompanied by several visual guides to improve usability and quick navigation to image areas with high relevance. The interactive visualization tool greatly improved model inspection and comparison for developers. Owing to the well-structured implementation, it can be easily adapted to other CNN models and types of input data.

1 Introduction

Convolutional neural networks (CNN) achieved a high accuracy for the automated detection of disease patterns in MRI scans. Several relevance mapping algorithms have been proposed to generate heatmaps that indicate the influence of a particular image region on the decision of the CNN model [1, 2]. Two previous studies compared CNN relevance mapping algorithms with respect to brain regions driving the detection of Alzheimer's disease in structural T1-weighted MRI [3, 4]. These relevance maps were found to greatly improve CNN comprehensibility and identification of reasons why a model failed [1, 3]. Notably,

© Der/die Autor(en), exklusiv lizenziert durch
Springer Fachmedien Wiesbaden GmbH, ein Teil von Springer Nature 2021
C. Palm et al. (Hrsg.), *Bildverarbeitung für die Medizin 2021*,
Informatik aktuell, https://doi.org/10.1007/978-3-658-33198-6_77

these approaches generate 3D relevance maps for each single input image (=MRI scan). In addition, several post-processing steps are required in order to improve their visual appeal and information content. These steps include smoothing, color scale transformation, relevance score and cluster size thresholding, which are not implemented in the feature portfolio of common MRI viewers. Further, preparation of static images from a specific parameter set yields large amounts of output files, which is prone to loosing track of the particular parameter settings used to generating these files in explorative research with various CNN model and post-processing parameter combinations.

In this paper, we present an interactive visualization toolkit for the online generation, parameterization, and inspection of CNN relevance maps for individual MRI scans. In the following sections, we describe the conceptual considerations and implementation, followed by a demonstration of the realized user interface and use case.

2   Materials and methods

We used pretrained CNN models obtained from [4, 5], which were implemented in Keras 2.2.4 and Tensorflow 1.15. The CNN visualization library iNNvestigate 1.0.8 [2] was used to derive the relevance maps. After drafting a first prototype user interface for the visualization, we collected a list of key requirements from a range of stakeholders following a participatory design approach. Therefore, we interviewed two physicians trained in radiology/neurology, two experienced visualization developers, and two machine learning model developers. From their comments, we defined the list of requirements:

- Directly run in CNN modeling environment (Python)
- Optional: remote display for the case where data handling and model execution need to be run remotely
- Visualization as slice-based 2D plots, which clinical users are familiar with
- For regular users: interactive selection of MRI scans, adjustable relevance and cluster size thresholds
- For expert users: selection of alternative CNN models and relevance mapping algorithms

The Python visualization library Bokeh [6] met the requirements with respect to Python runtime environment and remote viewing instance in a web browser. It provides a Python server instance back-end and Javascript browser libraries front-end to remotely trigger Python function calls and return execution results to the web browser for displaying.

We divided the implementation into three components following the well-established Model–View–Controller design pattern. Fig. 1 provides an overview of implemented methods and Fig. 2 shows a sequence diagram of function calls being executed when selecting a new MRI scan. In addition to the key requirements, we implemented various visual guides in order to facilitate parameterization and quick navigation to brain regions with high relevance scores (Fig. 3).

Fig. 1. Class diagram illustrating core components and functions.

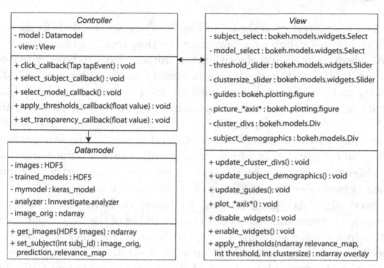

Among them are (a) a histogram providing the distribution of cluster sizes next to the cluster size threshold slider, (b) plots visualizing the amount of positive and negative relevance per slice next to the slice selection sliders, and (c) statistical information on the currently selected cluster. Further, assuming spatially normalized MRI data in MNI reference space, we added (d) atlas-based anatomical region lookup for the current cursor/cross-hair position and (e) the option to display the outline of the anatomical region to simplify visual comparison with the cluster location.

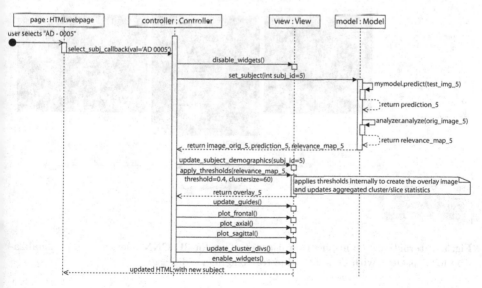

Fig. 2. Sequence diagram of functions being executed when loading a new MRI scan.

3   Results

The realized user interface is shown in Fig. 3. The source code is freely available on GitHub: https://github.com/martindyrba/DeepLearningInteractiveVis. The employed relevance mapping algorithm was initially fixed to layer-wise relevance propagation (LRP) as this method was already applied previously [3, 4]. The distribution and location of clusters with highest relevance scores varied between people with most consistent contributions from hippocampus, putamen and thalamus (Fig. 4). Notably, the highlighted regions mostly indicated actual gray matter atrophy as visible from the background images. This was confirmed by a quantitative comparison in which automatically derived hippocampus volume measures highly correlated with the aggregated relevance scores in the hippocampus region (Pearson's $r \approx -0.81$, see [5] for further details).

The used high-level programming interfaces of Keras, iNNvestigate, and Bokeh enabled a clean and structured programming of the web application. The complete application was realized in approximately 700 lines of code including view specification and program logic (model, controller). The app does not require a GPU to be available on the host, i.e. works smoothly on CPU. Loading of a new person currently takes ≈5 sec and loading a new model takes ≈15 sec. Adjusting the other sliders or directly clicking on the brain image/clusters updates the visualizations with a short latency of ≈200 ms. With the web page front-end, the visualization can also be run remotely on mobile devices such as tablets or smartphones without modification.

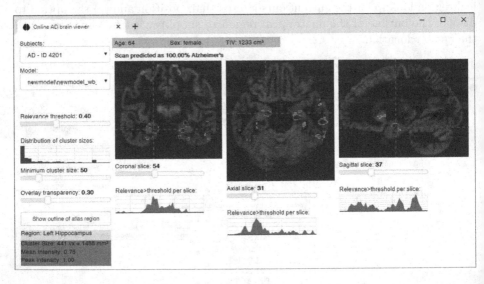

Fig. 3. Interactive web application user interface for 3D CNN relevance map visualization for a patient with dementia due to Alzheimer's disease.

4   Discussion

The presented visualization framework allows the inspection of CNN relevance maps for individuals and the assessment of drivers of the CNN decision. There-

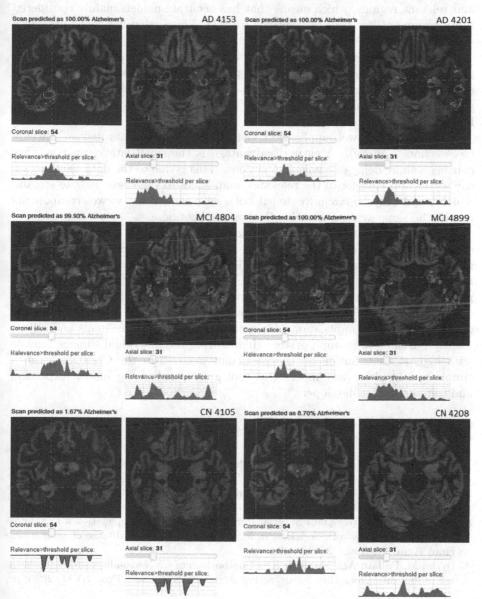

Fig. 4. Comparison of 3D CNN relevance maps for six randomly selected MRI scans. Top row: two patients with dementia due to Alzheimer's disease, middle row: two patients with mild cognitive impairment, bottom row: two controls with normal cognition.

fore, it contributed to model comprehensibility in the sense that it revealed the regional sensitivity of the CNN models, which is currently not assessed in the majority of papers with focus on model accuracy. As previously reported for other application domains [1], we found an association of model performance and relevant regions, which means that less accurate models mainly considered brain regions of low clinical relevance for AD. Thus, relevance maps provide a useful tool for CNN model 'debugging'.

Consulting experts from various disciplines for the requirements analysis greatly improved usability of the initial prototype application with many useful comments and recommendations such as adding the visual guides. The presented application was implemented as model- and data-agnostic tool such that it can be easily adjusted for other types of 3D input data.

The interactive web application met all the requirements defined initially (see section 2 above). A clear disadvantage is the small latency in reactivity causing a short delay of navigation actions. This is due to the data handling on the server and transfer of the relevance map slices to the client as byte stream, which could only be circumvented if both data model and viewer components run on the same system as native Python application.

For future work, there are ideas on additional features, for instance the import of new MRI scans, export for relevance maps, and 3D rendering view components. Further evaluation of the actual improvement of CNN comprehensibility for end users such as clinical staff is advised. Most importantly, more research is required to define evaluation metrics for relevance map quality and plausibility.

In summary, we presented a concept and implementation of an interactive online visualization application to inspect 3D CNN relevance maps and adjust display parameters as appropriate. Highlighting the individual's image regions with highest contribution on the particular decision of the CNN model in a simple and intuitive way makes this tool greatly enhancing model inspection and comparison for developers.

References

1. Samek W, Binder A, Montavon G, et al. Evaluating the visualization of what a deep neural network has learned. IEEE T Neur Net Lear. 2017;28(11):2660–2673.
2. Alber M, Lapuschkin S, Seegerer P, et al. iNNvestigate neural networks! J Mach Learn Res. 2019;20:1–8.
3. Böhle M, Eitel F, Weygandt M, et al. Layer-wise relevance propagation for explaining deep neural network decisions in MRI-based Alzheimer's disease classification. Front Aging Neurosci. 2019;11:194.
4. Dyrba M, Pallath AH, Marzban EN. Comparison of CNN visualization methods to aid model interpretability for detecting Alzheimer's disease. Proc BVM. 2020; p. 307–312.
5. Dyrba M, Hanzig M, Altenstein S, et al.. Improving 3D convolutional neural network comprehensibility via interactive visualization of relevance maps: evaluation in Alzheimer's disease; 2020. https://arxiv.org/abs/2012.10294.
6. Bokeh contributors. The bokeh visualization library; 2020. https://bokeh.org.

Abstract: VirtualDSA++

Automated Segmentation, Vessel Labeling, Occlusion Detection, and Graph Search on CT Angiography Data

Florian Thamm[1], Markus Jürgens[2], Hendrik Ditt[2], Andreas Maier[1]

[1]Pattern Recognition Lab, Department of Computer Science,
Friedrich-Alexander-Universität Erlangen-Nürnberg, Erlangen, Germany
[2]CT Pre-Development, Siemens Healthcare, Erlangen, Germany
florian.thamm@fau.de

Computed tomography angiography (CTA) is one of the most commonly used modalities in the diagnosis of cerebrovascular diseases like ischemic strokes. Usually, the anatomy of interest in ischemic stroke cases is the Circle of Willis and its peripherals, the cerebral arteries, as these vessels are the most prominent candidates for occlusions. The diagnosis of occlusions in these vessels remains challenging, not only because of the large amount of surrounding vessels but also due to the large number of anatomical variants. Having a good overview of all important vessels, would therefore ease the diagnosis of such cases We propose a fully automated image processing and visualization pipeline, which provides a full segmentation and modelling of the cerebral arterial tree for CTA data. The model itself enables the interactive masking of unimportant vessel structures e.g. veins like the sinus sagittalis, and the interactive planning of shortest paths meant to be used to prepare further treatments like a mechanical thrombectomy. Additionally, the algorithm automatically labels the cerebral arteries (middle cerebral artery left and right, anterior cerebral artery, posterior cerebral rtery left and right) and detects occlusions or interruptions in these vessels. The proposed pipeline does not require a prior non-contrast CT scan and achieves a comparable segmentation appearance as in a digital subtraction angiography (DSA) [1].

References

1. Thamm F, Jürgens M, Ditt H, et al. VirtualDSA++: automated segmentation, vessel labeling, occlusion detection and graph search on CT-angiography data. EG Workshop VCBM. 2020;.

© Der/die Autor(en), exklusiv lizenziert durch
Springer Fachmedien Wiesbaden GmbH, ein Teil von Springer Nature 2021
C. Palm et al. (Hrsg.), *Bildverarbeitung für die Medizin 2021*,
Informatik aktuell, https://doi.org/10.1007/978-3-658-33198-6_78

Interval Neural Networks as Instability Detectors for Image Reconstructions

Jan Macdonald[1], Maximilian März[1], Luis Oala[2], Wojciech Samek[2]

[1]Institut für Mathematik, Technische Universität Berlin
[2]Machine Learning Group, Fraunhofer HHI
macdonald@math.tu-berlin.de

Abstract. This work investigates the detection of instabilities that may occur when utilizing deep learning models for image reconstruction tasks. Although neural networks often empirically outperform traditional reconstruction methods, their usage for sensitive medical applications remains controversial. Indeed, in a recent series of works, it has been demonstrated that deep learning approaches are susceptible to various types of instabilities, caused for instance by adversarial noise or out-of-distribution features. It is argued that this phenomenon can be observed regardless of the underlying architecture and that there is no easy remedy. Based on this insight, the present work demonstrates, how uncertainty quantification methods can be employed as instability detectors. In particular, it is shown that the recently proposed *Interval Neural Networks* are highly effective in revealing instabilities of reconstructions. Such an ability is crucial to ensure a safe use of deep learning-based methods for medical image reconstruction.

1 Introduction

Deep learning has shown the potential to outperform traditional schemes for solving various signal recovery problems in medical imaging applications [1, 2]. Typically, such tasks are modelled as finite-dimensional linear inverse problems

$$\mathbf{y} = \mathbf{A}\mathbf{x} + \eta \tag{1}$$

where $\mathbf{x} \in \mathbb{R}^n$ is the unknown signal of interest, $\mathbf{A} \in \mathbb{R}^{m \times n}$ denotes the forward operator representing a physical measurement process, and $\eta \in \mathbb{R}^m$ is modelling noise in the measurements. Important examples include choosing $\mathbf{A}$ as a subsampled Fourier matrix (magnetic resonance imaging) or a discrete Radon transform (computed tomography). Solving the inverse problem (1) amounts to computing an approximate reconstruction of $\mathbf{x}$ from its observed measurements $\mathbf{y}$. The difficulty of this task is mainly determined by the strength of the noise and the degree of ill-posedness of (1), which is typically governed by the amount of undersampling in the measurement domain [3].

© Der/die Autor(en), exklusiv lizenziert durch
Springer Fachmedien Wiesbaden GmbH, ein Teil von Springer Nature 2021
C. Palm et al. (Hrsg.), *Bildverarbeitung für die Medizin 2021*,
Informatik aktuell, https://doi.org/10.1007/978-3-658-33198-6_79

In many cases, sparse regularization provides state-of-the-art solvers for (1), which are additionally backed up by theoretical guarantees, e.g. by compressed sensing [3]. However, it has been demonstrated that data-based deep learning methods are able to outperform their traditional counterparts in terms of empirical reconstruction quality and speed; see [2] for a recent overview.

In image classification, the susceptibility of deep neural networks to adversarial exploitation is well documented [4]. Recent works have reported similar instabilities for image reconstruction tasks [5, 6], which can be caused by visually imperceptible adversarial noise or features that have not been seen during training. The former can be found by solving a problem of the form

$$\underset{\mathbf{e}\in\mathbb{R}^m}{\text{maximize}} \|\text{Rec}(\mathbf{y}+\mathbf{e}) - \mathbf{x}\|_2 \quad \text{subject to} \quad \|\mathbf{e}\|_2 \leq \delta \qquad (2)$$

where Rec: $\mathbb{R}^m \to \mathbb{R}^n$ is a solution method for (1) and $\delta > 0$ is small. In other words, given measurements $\mathbf{y}$, the goal is to find a perturbation $\mathbf{e}$ that maximizes the error of a reconstruction algorithm.

Although there has been a first attempt to alleviate these shortcomings, [6] argues that such instabilities are in fact an unavoidable price for improvements in performance over classical methods. Hence, this work is motivated by the following premise: *if instabilities occur, we want to be able to detect them*. To that end, we demonstrate the potential of the recently proposed Interval Neural Network framework [7] as an instability detector. Its superiority over two other uncertainty quantification (UQ) methods [8, 9] is shown.

1.1 Overview and contributions

We consider a straight-forward approach to solving (1), which is based on post-processing a standard model-based inversion by a neural network [1]. Thus, the reconstruction is given by

$$\mathbf{x}_{\text{rec}} = \mathbf{\Phi}(\mathbf{A}^\dagger \mathbf{y}) \qquad (3)$$

where $\mathbf{\Phi}: \mathbb{R}^n \to \mathbb{R}^n$ denotes the prediction network (trained to minimize the loss $\|\mathbf{x} - \mathbf{\Phi}(\mathbf{A}^\dagger \mathbf{y})\|_2^2$) and $\mathbf{A}^\dagger$ symbolizes the non-learned model-based inversion. This scheme is studied for solving the severely ill-posed problem of limited angle computed tomography ($\mathbf{A}$ is a subsampled Radon transform), which has applications in dental tomography, breast tomosynthesis or electron tomography. We investigate the capacity of three UQ schemes (Sec. 2) to localize possible instabilities in the output of the prediction network $\mathbf{\Phi}$. As possible causes for such instabilities we consider: (i) adversarial noise on the input and (ii) imposed structural characteristics that have not been seen during training, i.e., out-of-distribution (OoD) features (Sec. 3). We believe that detecting OoD-instabilities is of particular importance in the context of medical imaging, since pathological changes are typically rare events in the training data. In summary, the contributions of this work are as follows:

a) We show that UQ can be utilized to detect the lack of robustness of deep learning-based image reconstruction methods.

b) Three UQ schemes for artificial neural networks are compared with respect to their capacity of revealing reconstruction instabilities.

c) We demonstrate that one UQ approach in particular, the so called Interval Neural Network, performs best as an instability detector.

2   Materials and methods

We briefly present three methods for UQ of neural network predictions and discuss the considered limited angle CT task.

2.1   Uncertainty quantification methods

In this work we consider only UQ methods that rely on the training of a single neural network and exclude computationally more costly approaches like ensemble learning or cross-validation.

2.1.1   Interval neural network. The recent work [7] has shown that by using interval arithmetic a baseline network $\boldsymbol{\Phi} \colon \mathbb{R}^n \to \mathbb{R}^n$ can be extended to an Interval Neural Network (INN) $\boldsymbol{\Phi}_{\text{INN}} \colon \mathbb{R}^n \to \mathbb{R}^n \times \mathbb{R}^n \times \mathbb{R}^n$, $\tilde{\mathbf{x}} \mapsto \left(\boldsymbol{\Phi}(\tilde{\mathbf{x}}), \underline{\boldsymbol{\Phi}}(\tilde{\mathbf{x}}), \overline{\boldsymbol{\Phi}}(\tilde{\mathbf{x}})\right)$, where $\underline{\boldsymbol{\Phi}}$ and $\overline{\boldsymbol{\Phi}}$ are mappings to lower and upper interval bounds for the prediction of the INN. Given training samples $(\tilde{\mathbf{x}}_i, \mathbf{x}_i) = (\mathbf{A}^\dagger \mathbf{y}_i, \mathbf{x}_i)$, the INN is trained by minimizing

$$\sum_i \| \max\{\mathbf{x}_i - \overline{\boldsymbol{\Phi}}(\tilde{\mathbf{x}}_i), 0\} \|_2^2 + \| \max\{\underline{\boldsymbol{\Phi}}(\tilde{\mathbf{x}}_i) - \mathbf{x}_i, 0\} \|_2^2 + \beta \| \overline{\boldsymbol{\Phi}}(\tilde{\mathbf{x}}_i) - \underline{\boldsymbol{\Phi}}(\tilde{\mathbf{x}}_i) \|_1$$

subject to constraints that guarantee $\underline{\boldsymbol{\Phi}}(\tilde{\mathbf{x}}) \leq \boldsymbol{\Phi}(\tilde{\mathbf{x}}) \leq \overline{\boldsymbol{\Phi}}(\tilde{\mathbf{x}})$ for all $\tilde{\mathbf{x}}$. Hence, the idea of INNs is to produce output intervals that contain the true labels with high probability, while remaining as tight as possible. The pixel-wise uncertainty estimate of an INN is then given by the width of the prediction interval, i.e., $\mathbf{u}_{\text{INN}}(\tilde{\mathbf{x}}) = \overline{\boldsymbol{\Phi}}(\tilde{\mathbf{x}}) - \underline{\boldsymbol{\Phi}}(\tilde{\mathbf{x}})$.

2.1.2   Monte Carlo dropout. In MCDROP proposed by [8], uncertainty scores are obtained through the sample variance of multiple stochastic forward passes on the same input data point. If $\boldsymbol{\Phi}_1, \ldots, \boldsymbol{\Phi}_T$ are realizations of independent draws of random dropout masks of the prediction network $\boldsymbol{\Phi}$, then the pixel-wise uncertainty estimate is given by $\mathbf{u}_{\text{MCDROP}}(\tilde{\mathbf{x}}) = \frac{1}{T-1}\left(\sum_{t=1}^T \boldsymbol{\Phi}_t(\tilde{\mathbf{x}})^2 - \frac{1}{T}\left(\sum_{t=1}^T \boldsymbol{\Phi}_t(\tilde{\mathbf{x}})\right)^2\right)$.

2.1.3   Mean and variance estimation. Another possibility is to double the number of outputs of the prediction network and train it to approximate the mean and variance of a Gaussian distribution. In [9], this is referred to as lightweight probabilistic networks (PROBOUT) $\boldsymbol{\Phi}_{\text{PROBOUT}} \colon \mathbb{R}^n \to \mathbb{R}^n \times \mathbb{R}^n$, $\tilde{\mathbf{x}} \mapsto (\boldsymbol{\Phi}_{\text{mean}}(\tilde{\mathbf{x}}), \boldsymbol{\Phi}_{\text{var}}(\tilde{\mathbf{x}}))$, trained by minimizing $\sum_i \| (\mathbf{x}_i - \boldsymbol{\Phi}_{\text{mean}}(\tilde{\mathbf{x}}_i)) / \sqrt{\boldsymbol{\Phi}_{\text{var}}(\tilde{\mathbf{x}}_i)} \|_2^2 + \| \log \boldsymbol{\Phi}_{\text{var}}(\tilde{\mathbf{x}}_i) \|_1$. The pixel-wise uncertainty score is given by $\mathbf{u}_{\text{PROBOUT}}(\tilde{\mathbf{x}}) = \boldsymbol{\Phi}_{\text{var}}(\tilde{\mathbf{x}})$.

2.2   Inverse problem, neural network and data

We consider a simulation of the noiseless Radon transform with a moderate missing wedge of 30° for the forward model (1). The non-learned inversion $\mathbf{A}^\dagger$ in (3) is based on the filtered backprojection algorithm (FBP). The underlying prediction network is a U-Net variant. Our experiments are based on a data set consisting of 512×512 human CT scans from the AAPM Low Dose CT Grand Challenge data [10].[1] In total, it contains 2580 images of 10 patients. Eight of these ten patients were used for training (2036 samples), one for validation (214 samples) and one for testing (330 samples).

3   Results

The code for our two experiments is at https://github.com/luisoala/inn.

3.1   Adversarial artifact detection (AdvDetect)

The AdvDetect experiment assesses the capacity of the considered UQ methods to capture artifacts in the output that were caused by adversarial noise. To that end, we create perturbed inputs for each measurement sample $\mathbf{y}$ in the test set by employing the box-constrained L-BFGS algorithm to minimize the function $\|\Phi(\tilde{\mathbf{x}}_{adv}) - \mathbf{x}_{adv.\ tar.}\|_2^2$ over the domain $\tilde{\mathbf{x}}_{adv} \in [0,1]^n$. Here, $\mathbf{x}_{adv.\ tar.}$ represents a corresponding adversarial target, which is created by subtracting 1.5 times its mean value from $\mathbf{x}_{rec}$ within a random 50×50 square, leading to clearly visible artifacts in the corresponding reconstructions (Fig. 1). It is arguable, whether the technical aspects of such an adversarial perturbation (i.e., attacking subsequently to a model-based inversion) is a realistic scenario in the context of inverse problems. However, for our purposes, such a simple setup ([5]) is sufficient.

In order to assess the adversarial artifact detection capacity, the different UQ schemes are then used to produce uncertainty heatmaps for the generated adversarial inputs. A quantitative evaluation is carried out by computing the mean Pearson correlation coefficient between the pixel-wise change in the uncertainty heatmaps $|\mathbf{u}(\tilde{\mathbf{x}}) - \mathbf{u}(\tilde{\mathbf{x}}_{adv})|$ and the change of reconstructions $|\mathbf{x}_{rec} - \Phi(\tilde{\mathbf{x}}_{adv})|$. The results are summarized in Tab. 1 and illustrated in Fig. 1. We observe that both INN and PROBOUT are able to detect the image region of adversarial perturbations. In particular INN highlights the effect of almost imperceptible input perturbations on the reconstructions. Overall, the uncertainty predictions of all three methods mostly emphasize boundary features in the image. While MCDROP shows fewer "False Positives", it also exhibits more "False Negatives" compared to INN and PROBOUT.

---

[1]   https://www.aapm.org/GrandChallenge/LowDoseCT/

3.2 Atypical artifact detection (ArtDetect)

The ArtDetect experiment is designed analogously to the setup described by [6], i.e., an atypical artifact, which was not present in the training data, is randomly placed in the input. We insert the silhouette of a peace dove in each image of the test set (Fig. 1). The simulation of the measurements and model-based inversions is carried out on the new test set as before.

In order to assess the atypical artifact detection capacity, the different UQ schemes are then used to produce uncertainty heatmaps on the resulting OoD inputs. A quantitative evaluation is carried out by computing the mean Pearson correlation coefficient between the change in the uncertainty heatmaps $|\mathbf{u}(\widetilde{\mathbf{x}}) - \mathbf{u}(\widetilde{\mathbf{x}}_{\text{OoD}})|$ and a binary mask marking the region of change in the inputs. The results are summarized in Tab. 1 and illustrated in Fig. 1. All three UQ methods are correlated with the input change, however INN achieves the highest correlation. This shows that UQ in general, and INNs in particular, can serve as a warning system for inputs containing atypical features that might otherwise lead to unnoticed and possibly erroneous reconstruction artifacts.

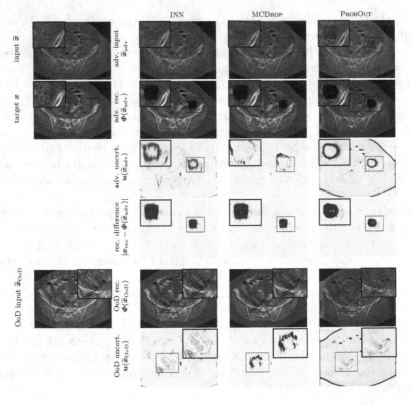

Fig. 1. Results of the three UQ methods for the AdvDetect and ArtDetect experiments for one exemplary slice. The plotting windows are slightly adjusted for better contrast.

UQ Method	AdvDetect	ArtDetect
INN	**0.56 ± 0.05**	**0.52 ± 0.03**
MCDROP	0.28 ± 0.02	0.26 ± 0.01
PROBOUT	0.48 ± 0.12	0.34 ± 0.04

Table 1. Mean Pearson correlation coefficients, averaged (± standard deviation) over three experimental runs, for both instability detection experiments.

4   Discussion

We demonstrated qualitatively and quantitatively that uncertainty quantification, in particular by INNs, bears great potential as a fine-grained instability detector. This was shown for limited angle CT as a prototypical example of a severely ill-posed inverse problem. The presented UQ methods are versatile and can be employed for various types of neural networks and other clinical applications. The implication and goal of this work is to ultimately move deep learning technology closer to a level of reliability that makes it a serious contender for integration in medical imaging workflows. If we want to harness the prowess of deep learning we will need to find strategies for accounting for its instabilities. Uncertainty quantification can be an important tool to that end.

Acknowledgement. We would like to thank Dr. Cynthia McCollough, the Mayo Clinic, and the American Association of Physicists in Medicine as well as the grants EB017095 and EB017185 from the National Institute of Biomedical Imaging and Bioengineering for providing the AAPM data.

References

1. Jin KH, McCann MT, Froustey E, et al. Deep convolutional neural network for inverse problems in imaging. IEEE Trans Image Process. 2017;26:4509–4522.
2. Arridge S, Maass P, Öktem O, et al. Solving inverse problems using data-driven models. Acta Numerica. 2019;28:1–174.
3. Foucart S, Rauhut H. A mathematical introduction to compressive sensing. Applied and Numerical Harmonic Analysis. Birkhäuser; 2013.
4. Szegedy C, Zaremba W, Sutskever I, et al. Intriguing properties of neural networks. In: International Conference on Learning Representations; 2014. .
5. Huang Y, Würfl T, Breininger K, et al. Some investigations on robustness of deep learning in limited angle tomography. Proc MICCAI 2018; p. 45–153.
6. Gottschling NM, Antun V, Adcock B, et al. The troublesome kernel: why deep learning for inverse problems is typically unstable?; 2020. ArXiv:2001.01258.
7. Oala L, Heiß C, Macdonald J, et al. Interval neural networks: uncertainty scores; 2020. ArXiv preprint arXiv:2003.11566.
8. Gal Y, Ghahramani Z. Dropout as a bayesian approximation: representing model uncertainty in deep learning. In: Balcan MF, Weinberger KQ, editors. Proceedings of The 33rd International Conference on Machine Learning; 2016. p. 1050–1059.
9. Gast J, Roth S. Lightweight probabilistic deep networks. 2018 IEEE/CVF Conf Comput Vis Pattern Recognit. 2018; p. 3369–3378.
10. McCollough CH. TU-FG-207A-04: overview of the low dose CT grand challenge. Med Phys. 2016;43(6 Part 35):3759–3760.

Invertible Neural Networks for Uncertainty Quantification in Photoacoustic Imaging

Jan-Hinrich Nölke[1,2], Tim Adler[1,3], Janek Gröhl[1], Thomas Kirchner[4],
Lynton Ardizzone[5], Carsten Rother[5], Ullrich Köthe[5], Lena Maier-Hein[1,3,6]

[1]Division of Computer Assisted Medical Interventions,
German Cancer Research Center, Heidelberg, Germany
[2]Faculty of Physics and Astronomy, Heidelberg University, Germany
[3]Faculty of Mathematics and Computer Science, Heidelberg University, Germany
[4]Institute of Applied Physics, University of Bern, Switzerland
[5]Visual Learning Lab, HCI, IWR, Heidelberg, Germany
[6]Medical Faculty, Heidelberg University, Germany
j.noelke@dkfz-heidelberg.de

Abstract. Multispectral photoacoustic imaging (PAI) is an emerging imaging modality that enables the recovery of functional tissue parameters such as blood oxygenation. However, the underlying inverse reconstruction problems are potentially ill-posed, meaning that radically different tissue properties may-in theory-yield comparable measurements. In this work, we present a new approach for handling this specific type of uncertainty using conditional invertible neural networks. We propose going beyond commonly used point estimates for tissue oxygenation and convert single-pixel initial pressure spectra to the full posterior probability density. This way, the inherent ambiguity of a problem can be encoded with multiple modes in the output. Based on the presented architecture, we demonstrate two use cases that leverage this information to not only detect and quantify but also to compensate for uncertainties: (1) photoacoustic device design and (2) optimization of photoacoustic image acquisition. Our in silico studies demonstrate the potential of the proposed methodology to become an important building block for uncertainty-aware reconstruction of physiological parameters with PAI.

1 Introduction

Photoacoustic imaging (PAI) is an emerging medical imaging modality that enables the recovery of optical tissue properties with a "light-in-sound-out" approach [1]: Tissue is illuminated using light pulses, which leads to the absorption of photons and subsequent heating of the tissue. The resulting thermoelastic expansion generates pressure waves, which can then be detected by broadband ultrasonic transducers. The initial pressure distribution p_0, determined for multiple wavelengths, can then be used to determine physiological tissue properties like blood oxygenation sO_2. However, the non-linear effect of the so-called light fluence makes the optical inverse problem ill-posed [2]. This can potentially lead to ambiguous solutions of the tissue properties. Prior work has addressed related problems with different approaches to uncertainty quantification [3, 4, 5, 6], yet explicitly representing ambiguities by full posterior distributions has not been attempted in the context of machine learning-based image analysis. In this work, we address this gap in the literature with conditional invertible neural networks (cINNs) [7]. In contrast to conventional neural networks, the INN architecture enables the computation of the full posterior density function (rather than a simple point estimate), which naturally enables the encoding of various types of uncertainty, including multiple solutions (modes). The contribution of this paper is two-fold: (1) We adapt the concept of cINNs to the specific problem of quantifying tissue parameters from PAI data. (2) We demonstrate the value of our approach with two use-cases, namely PAI device design and optimization of photoacoustic image acquisition.

2 Materials and methods

2.1 Virtual photoacoustic imaging environment

The virtual environment created for testing the proposed approach to uncertainty quantification is based on a digital PAI device. With it, 3D representations of the optical and acoustic properties of tissue can be generated, which are used to simulate synthetic PAI data for a given probe design, pose and ground truth tissue properties. The data is simulated using the Monte Carlo eXtreme framework [8]. For this study, each simulation is performed with 10^7 photons originating from a pencil-like source and a grid spacing of 0.34 mm. Each volume is simulated at 26 equidistant wavelengths between 700 nm and 950 nm.

2.2 Approach to uncertainty quantification

Our architecture builds upon the cINN architecture proposed in [7]. Based on a known forward process for converting tissue properties (here: pixel-wise tissue oxygenation x) to resulting measurements (here: pixel-wise initial pressure spectrum y), the task is to train a neural network to recover x from y while accounting for potential ambiguities. To this end, cINNs are leveraged as follows: Given training data consisting of (simulated) pairs (x, y), a cINN is trained to convert x to a Gaussian distributed latent space z, using y as conditioning input. This is achieved with maximum likelihood training. During inference time, because of the invertible architecture, we can sample the latent distribution and, given a new measurement y used as conditioning input y, generate a conditional probability distribution $p(x|y)$.

The architecture implemented in this work consists of 20 blocks, each with a random permutation and a conditional generative flow coupling block [9] (two fully connected layers of size 512 and rectified linear unit activations). During training, we apply normally distributed random noise with $\sigma = 0.001$ to the normalized input and $\sigma = 0.1$ to the conditioning input. The models are trained for 60 epochs with the AdamW optimizer and weight decay of 0.01. We start with a learning rate of 10^{-3} and reduce it by a factor of 10 after epoch 40 and 50.

To automate the detection of multimodal posteriors, we introduce a multimode score. We perform kernel density estimation on the posterior samples with 21 different bandwidths between 0.01 p.p. and 0.1 p.p. The score is then the fraction of estimates with more than one maximum relative to all estimates.

2.3   Experiments

The purpose of our experiments was to (1) validate the proposed approach to uncertainty quantification in PAI and to (2) showcase use cases that leverage the posteriors to not only detect and quantify uncertainties but to compensate for them. To this end, we generated four different settings.

2.3.1   S1: Single vessel, single illumination unit (IU).
Images (probabilistically) generated for this setting comprise a tube of muscle tissue with 2 cm diameter as background with blood oxygenation uniformly drawn between 0 and 1. In the center, a blood vessel with a radius uniformly drawn between 1 mm and 3 mm and oxygenation between 0 and 1 is placed. A single illumination source is used.

2.3.2   S2: Multiple vessels, single IU.
Setting S1 is enhanced by introducing an additional blood vessel randomly placed between the light source and the central vessel of interest. This vessel also has a radius between 1 mm and 3 mm and an oxygenation between 0 and 1. Fig. 1 illustrates the basic setup of the phantoms.

2.3.3   S2b: Multiple vessels, shifted single IU.
This setting is identical to S2, but the scene is illuminated from two additional angles ($\pm 45°$). We use the three different illumination setups as independent samples leading to a three times

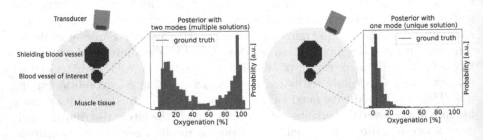

Fig. 1. *In silico* setting illustrating how slight changes in the PAI probe pose can resolve model ambiguity (training on S2b, sec. 2.3). Left: the posterior corresponding to a pixel of interest features two modes. Right: Owing to an improved acquisition pose, the same pixel features a uni-modal posterior.

bigger data set. This setting (S2b) was exclusively used to generate Fig. 1, i. e., to demonstrate the effect of probe position on the resulting posterior.

2.3.4 S3: Multiple vessels, multiple IUs. The setting uses the same data as S2b, but we concatenate the three spectra from the different illumination setups (thus simulating a complex device with three illumination units/detectors) which leads to a conditioning input dimension of $3 \cdot 26$. Fig. 2 gives an overview of the settings S1-S3.

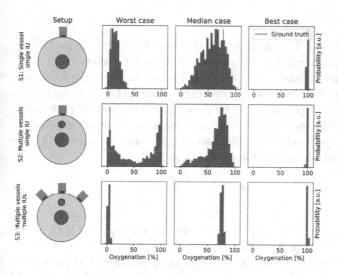

Fig. 2. Worst, median, and best case with respect to the IQR of S2 for three investigated settings. In contrast to a single vessel scenario (top), ambiguities are likely to occur in a multi-vessel scenario (middle) when using a single light source. These can be compensated for with multiple light sources (bottom).

We simulated 2,000 volumes for each of the settings and trained cINN models as described in Sec. 2.2 on each of them with 85% of the data. The remaining 15% of the data was used for testing. To validate the accuracy of the posteriors, we computed the calibration curves for scenarios S1-S3 as proposed in [10]. We processed the results to analyze the capability of our method to reveal ambiguous problems (multiple modes) and to determine the effect of device pose and design.

3 Results

As can be seen in Fig. 3 all calibration curves are close to the identity (median calibration error < 1.5 p.p.). This implies that the width of the posteriors is reliable. For the setting with a single vessel and single illumination (S1), the model is slightly underconfident.

In Fig. 4 we compare the distribution of IQRs, absolute errors, and the multi-mode score for the scenarios S1-S3 described in sec. 2.3. Our results demonstrate that not only the accuracy but also the likelihood for ambiguity of the problem depends crucially on the characteristics of the probe (e.g., number of illumination/detection units). For all three metrics, the performance for the setting with

Fig. 3. Calibration curves of the posterior distributions of the settings S1-S3 as described in sec. 2.3. Fraction of observations (left) and calibration error (right) as a function of the confidence interval on the test set.

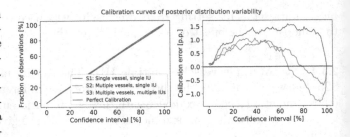

multiple vessels, but only one illumination (S2) is clearly the worst. In particular, this setting includes a non-negligible fraction of multimodal posteriors.

Fig. 1 and Fig. 2 further show that the accuracy at a given pixel depends crucially on the pose and the illumination geometry of the PAI device. Moreover, the ambiguity of the inverse problem can be potentially resolved by performing the acquisition from a different position/angle or by using a multiple illumination setting (S3). Our approach could thus serve as a basis for optimizing the measurement process and photoacoustic device design.

4 Discussion

To our knowledge, this is the first work exploring the concept of INNs in the context of PAI. Specifically, we have demonstrated the capabilities of cINNs to represent and quantify uncertainties in the context of physiological parameter estimation. Based on our initial experiments, we believe that our approach could serve as a basis for optimizing PAI probe design and image acquisition.

This work is similar to that proposed by Adler et al. [11] in the context of multispectral optical imaging. However, it differs in that we used cINNs instead of the original INN architecture, which comes along with several major advantages, including (1) no zero-padding needed, leading to smaller network size, (2) maximum likelihood training, and (3) no hyperparameters in the loss function.

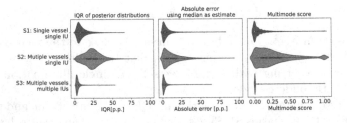

Fig. 4. The violin plots show the interquartile range (IQR) of the posterior distribution on the test set, the absolute error when using the median as an estimate, and the multimode score, introduced in sec. 2.2. We differentiate between the settings S1-S3 as described in sec. 2.3.

Our findings for device design are in line with Shao et al. [12] where a multi-illumination setup is suggested to improve image reconstruction. Our initial experiments indicate that our method may help in the optimization of the acquisition process. As a next step, our approach has to be extended such that it not only shows the current ambiguities but also proposes possible poses to resolve them. This might be achieved through the application of reinforcement learning.

In conclusion, we have demonstrated the potential of cINNs to reconstruct tissue parameters from PAI data while systematically representing and quantifying uncertainties.

Acknowledgement. This project has received funding from the European Union's Horizon 2020 research and innovation programme (grant agreement No. ERC2015-StG-37960 and No. 647769) and from the Federal Ministry of Education and Research of Germany project High Performance Deep Learning Framework (No. 01IH17002).

References

1. Zackrisson S, van de Ven SMWY, Gambhir SS. Light in and sound out: emerging translational strategies for photoacoustic imaging. Cancer Res. 2014;74(4):979 1004.
2. Yang C, Lan H, Gao F, et al. Deep learning for photoacoustic imaging: a survey. arXiv:200804221 [cs, eess]. 2020;.
3. Tarvainen T, Pulkkinen A, Cox BT, et al. Bayesian image reconstruction in quantitative photoacoustic tomography. IEEE Trans Med Imaging. 2013 Dec;32(12):2287–2298.
4. Tick J, Pulkkinen A, Tarvainen T. Image reconstruction with uncertainty quantification in photoacoustic tomography. J Acoust Soc Am. 2016;139(4):1951–1961.
5. Gröhl J, Kirchner T, Adler T, et al. Confidence estimation for machine learning-based quantitative photoacoustics. J Imaging. 2018;4(12):147.
6. Godefroy G, Arnal B, Bossy E. Solving the visibility problem in photoacoustic imaging with a deep learning approach providing prediction uncertainties. arXiv:200613096 [physics]. 2020;.
7. Ardizzone L, Lüth C, Kruse J, et al. Guided image generation with conditional invertible neural networks. arXiv:19070233092 [cs]. 2019;.
8. Fang Q, Boas DA. Monte Carlo simulation of photon migration in 3D turbid media accelerated by graphics processing units. Opt Express. 2009;17(22):20178–20190.
9. Kingma DP, Dhariwal P. Glow: generative flow with invertible 1x1 convolutions. arXiv:180703039 [cs, stat]. 2018;.
10. Ardizzone L, Kruse J, Wirkert S, et al. Analyzing inverse problems with invertible neural networks. arXiv:180804730 [cs, stat]. 2019;.
11. Adler TJ, Ardizzone L, Vemuri A, et al. Uncertainty-aware performance assessment of optical imaging modalities with invertible neural networks. Int J Comput Assist Radiol Surg. 2019;14(6):997–1007.
12. Shao P, Cox B, Zemp R. Estimating optical absorption, scattering, and Grueneisen distributions with multiple-illumination photoacoustic tomography. Appl Opt. 2011;50:3145–54.

Abstract: Inertial Measurements for Motion Compensation in Weight-bearing Cone-beam CT of the Knee

Jennifer Maier[1,2], Marlies Nitschke[2], Jang-Hwan Choi[3], Garry Gold[4], Rebecca Fahrig[5], Bjoern M. Eskofier[2], Andreas Maier[1]

[1]Pattern Recognition Lab, Friedrich-Alexander-Univeristät Erlangen-Nürnberg (FAU), Erlangen, Germany
[2]Machine Learning and Data Analytics Lab, Friedrich-Alexander-Univeristät Erlangen-Nürnberg (FAU), Erlangen, Germany
[3]College of Engineering, Ewha Womans University, Seoul, Korea
[4]Department of Radiology, Stanford University, Stanford, California, USA
[5]Siemens Healthcare GmbH, Forchheim, Germany
jennifer.maier@fau.de

The main cause of artifacts in weight-bearing cone-beam computed tomography (CT) scans of the knee is involuntary subject motion. Clinical diagnosis on the resulting images is only possible if the motion is corrected during reconstruction. Existing image-based or marker-based methods are time consuming in preparation or execution. We propose a motion correction using inertial measurement units (IMUs) attached to the leg of the subject to record the motion during the scan. The measured local acceleration and angular velocity are transformed to the global coordinate system in a multi-stage algorithm and used for a rigid motion compensation. To validate this novel approach, we present a simulation study using real motion of seven healthy standing subjects recorded with an optical 3D tracking system. With this motion, we animate a biomechanical model via inverse kinematics computation and simulate the measurements of a virtual IMU placed on the shank of the model. Furthermore, we non-rigidly deform the XCAT numerical knee phantom using the measured motion and simulate a CT scan leading to motion corrupted projection images. When applying our proposed correction approach to this data, motion artifacts in the reconstructed volumes are visibly reduced. The average structural similarity index and root mean squared error with respect to the motion-free reconstruction are improved by 13-21% and 68-70%, respectively, compared to the motion corrupted case. The comparison with a state-of-the-art marker-based method shows qualitatively and quantitatively comparable results. The presented study shows the feasibility of the proposed approach and is a first step towards a purely IMU-based motion compensation in C-arm CT. This work was published in [1].

References

1. Maier J, Nitschke M, Choi JH, et al. Inertial measurements for motion compensation in weight-bearing cone-beam CT of the knee. Proc MICCAI. 2020; p. 14–23.

© Der/die Autor(en), exklusiv lizenziert durch
Springer Fachmedien Wiesbaden GmbH, ein Teil von Springer Nature 2021
C. Palm et al. (Hrsg.), *Bildverarbeitung für die Medizin 2021*,
Informatik aktuell, https://doi.org/10.1007/978-3-658-33198-6_81

Abstract: Reduktion der Kalibrierungszeit für die Magnetpartikelbildgebung mittels Deep Learning

Ivo M. Baltruschat[1,2], Patryk Szwargulski[1,2], Florian Griese[1,2],
Mirco Grosser[1,2], Rene Werner[3], Tobias Knopp[1,2]

[1]Section for Biomedical Imaging, University Medical Center Hamburg-Eppendorf
[2]Institute for Biomedical Imaging, Hamburg University of Technology
[3]Department of Computational Neuroscience, University Medical Center
Hamburg-Eppendorf
ivo-matteo.baltruschat@tuhh.de

Die Magnetpartikelbildgebung (MPI) ist eine junge tomographische Bildgebungstechnik, die magnetische Nanopartikel mit einer hohen räumlichen und zeitlichen Auflösung quantitativ abbildet. Eine gängige Methode zur Rekonstruktion von MPI-Daten ist die Systemmatrix (SM)-basierte Rekonstruktion. Die komplexwertige SM wird in einer zeitaufwändigen Kalibrierungsmessung bestimmt. Die Anzahl der Voxel der SM beeinflusst direkt die Grösse des rekonstruierten Bildes, aber auch die Scanzeit – d.h. die Aufnahme einer 37^3 SM dauert etwa 32 Stunden im Vergleich zu einer 9^3 SM, die etwa 37 Minuten dauert. In unserer Arbeit [1] haben wir untersucht, ob Deep Learning (DL) eingesetzt werden kann, um die Ergebnisse für die SM-Vervollständigung zu verbessern. Wir haben dafür ein Framework entwickelt, welches drei zentrale Schritte umfasst. Zunächst messen wir einen SM mit niedriger Auflösung auf einem spezifischen Abtastraster. Wir nutzen danach ein Faltungsnetzwerk, das wir 3d-System-Matrix-Wiederherstellungsnetzwerk (3d-SMRnet) nennen, um die hochauflösende SM wiederherzustellen. Wir haben das Modell so anpassen, dass es mit 3d-Eingangsdaten arbeitet, und wenden es auf jede Frequenzkomponente der SM an. Um unser Model zu trainieren, setzen wir eine neuartige Erweiterung der Verlustfunktion zur Behandlung komplexer Zahlen ein. Das 3d-SMRnet wird anhand eines öffentlichen MPI-Datensatzes evaluiert und im Vergleich zum derzeitigen Goldstandard – d.h. Compressed Sensing – erreicht es bessere Ergebnisse bei der SM-Vervollständigung und den rekonstruierten Bildern. Unsere neuartige Methode, die auf einem 3d-SMRnet und einem ComplexRGB-Verlust basiert, kann die Kalibrierungszeit im MPI erheblich verkürzen – d.h. 64-mal weniger Messpunkte im Vergleich zur ursprünglichen hochauflösenden Systemmatrix.

Literatur

1. Baltruschat IM, Szwargulski P, Griese F, et al. 3d-SMRnet: achieving a new quality of MPI system matrix recovery by deep learning. Proc MICCAI. 2020; p. 74–82.

Autoencoder-based Quality Assessment for Synthetic Diffusion-MRI Data

Leon Weninger[1], Maxim Drobjazko[1], Chuh-Hyoun Na[2], Kerstin Jütten[2], Dorit Merhof[1]

[1]Imaging and Computer Vision, RWTH Aachen University
[2]Department of Neurosurgery, University Hospital RWTH Aachen
`leon.weninger@lfb.rwth-aachen.de`

Abstract. Diffusion MRI makes it possible to assess brain microstructure in-vivo. Recently, a variety of deep learning methods have been proposed that enhance the quality and utility of these acquisitions. For deep learning methods, a large amount of training data is necessary, but difficult to obtain. As a solution, different approaches to synthetic data creation have been published, but it is unclear which approach produces data that best matches the in-vivo characteristics. Here, a methodology to assess the quality of synthetic diffusion data which is based on denoising autoencoders is proposed. For this, the reconstruction errors of autoencoders trained only on synthetic data were evaluated. The more the synthetic data resembles the real data, the lower the reconstruction error. Using this method, we evaluated which of four different synthetic data simulation techniques produced data that best resembled the in-vivo data. We find that modeling diffusion MRI data with patient- and scanner specific values leads to significantly better reconstruction results than using default diffusivity values, suggesting possible benefits of precision medicine approaches in diffusion MRI analysis.

1 Introduction

MRI scans are used as a primary method in detecting diseases such as traumas, brain aneurysms, strokes, and tumors. Currently, medical professionals analyze these scans visually. However, deep learning could assist, e.g. by automatic detection of diseases, as deep learning approaches can notice subtle differences and patterns in data. In clinical research, deep learning methods have been established in a variety of diffusion MRI applications [1].

Deep learning approaches need a high amount of data to train on. Since the number of available MRI scans is always limited and groundtruth data is scarce, synthetic data can help to alleviate this problem. Software-based diffusion phantoms have been in use since several years [2]. However, if deep learning approaches are to be trained on synthetic data, the synthetic data needs to match the characteristics of in-vivo data as closely as possible. If the generating model of synthetic data only matches a subset of the characteristics of the in-vivo data, the trained algorithm will not be able to generalize to the complete range of in-vivo data. On the other hand, if the generating model induces too much variety, we hypothesize that a trained deep learning algorithm will perform suboptimally, as the neural network will lose specificity.

Different approaches for creating synthetic data exist, and it is not clear which one is optimally suited for deep learning models. The generating models need to be tested and compared in order to differentiate model qualities. We propose to assess the quality of synthetic diffusion data with an autoencoder, a network architecture originally designed for denoising [3]. Fitted on synthetic data and evaluated on real data, it can be used as an indicator for quality assessment. Better suited synthetic data will lead to better reconstruction performance on in-vivo data.

Our proposed autoencoder is self-adaptive to the shape of the input, i.e., to the number of diffusion directions, and was trained and evaluated on single-voxel data. Comparing the reconstruction performance on a local study dataset as well as on data from the Human Connectome Project (HCP), an open access dataset containing high quality diffusion MRI scans [4], the quality of 4 different synthetic diffusion data models was assessed.

2 Materials and methods

2.1 Data

Two different datasets were used: The freely available HCP dataset (isotropic voxel size of 1.25mm, three-shell b=1000,2000,3000 s/mm^2, 90 gradient directions per shell), as well as a dataset containing diffusion MRI scans (isotropic voxel size of 2.4mm, single-shell b=1000 s/mm^2, 64 gradient directions) of 28 healthy subjects acquired at the University Hospital Aachen. From the HCP dataset, all subjects of the "100 unrelated subjects" dataset were selected, and only the b=1000 s/mm^2 shell data was utilized. For the locally acquired data, all subjects have given written informed consent. The scans were approved by the ethics committee of the Medical Faculty of Aachen University (EK 294/15), and acquired according to the standards of Good Clinical Practice and the Dec-laration of Helsinki. The diffusion data of the local study were corrected for susceptibility induced and eddy current distortions with tools from FSL [5]. On the accompanying T1 image, the tissue was segmented into white matter (WM), gray matter (GM) and cerebrospinal fluid (CSF) with FSL Fast, and the seg-mentation map was transformed in diffusion space using an affine registration of the T1 and diffusion image. The HCP data was already preprocessed, and tissue segmentation maps were readily available.

2.2 Synthetic data creation

Four different synthetic data generating methods [6, 7, 8, 9], which were all previously used in deep learning settings by various groups, were evaluated.

For every subject, individual synthetic data was created. Three of the data generating techniques were multi-tensor simulations, for which only the settings for possible tensor eigenvalues differed. These multi-tensor simulations were made from up to three different single-fiber WM compartments with random main directions and random volume percentage, as well as possible GM and CSF compartments with a random compartment contribution from 0 to 100% each.

2.2.1 Syn. The first method, fully synthetic, further referred to as "Syn", is based on plausible pre-determined values for all compartments. The default values of the Dipy [6] diffusion simulation toolbox were used for the WM tensor eigenvalues, i.e. an axial diffusivity of $0.0015\,s/mm^2$, and a radial diffusivity of $0.0003\,s/mm^2$. The diffusivity was set to $0.0005\,s/mm^2$ for GM and to $0.003\,s/mm^2$ for CSF.

2.2.2 Sampled. Second, exemplary diffusion tensor eigenvalues were sampled from the subject in question using eroded tissue segmentation maps for all three tissues, which was similarly proposed in [7]. For WM, only single-fiber voxels, identified by an FA value larger than 0.7 were retained. Thus, the tensor eigenvalues follow the individual characteristics, and a variety of eigenvalues were employed. This method is further labelled "Sampled".

2.2.3 SampleAndMean. Third, eigenvalues were sampled for WM, but for CSF and GM the mean diffusivity values obtained from the subject were used. This method is thus referred to as "SampleAndMean", and was originally proposed in [8]. Taking the mean diffusivity instead of sampling GM and CSF was proposed in order to reduce noise in the synthetic data, as the diffusion signal can be especially noisy in CSF due to low signal levels.

2.2.4 RandomWM. Finally, [9] proposed to simulate the diffusivity of free water with $0.003\,s/mm^2$, and the diffusion attenuation of other microstructure compartments with a random variable per gradient following a uniform distribution $U(0,1)$. This synthetic diffusion data was originally employed to train a model that predicts the water compartment in a voxel, it was thus not intended to be a holistic simulation of diffusion signals. Nevertheless, it could be that such a model is also useful for other tasks, e.g., for neural network pretraining, and is thus also compared as "RandomWM" in the experiments.

2.3 Denoising autoencoder

With the denoising autoencoder, the diffusion data was reduced to a minimum size in the hidden layers, from which the original signal was reconstructed with the decoder part of the autoencoder. As single voxels were used as input, and a fully connected architecture was chosen, an automatically adjusting input size for different MRI scans was necessary. Two reducing and two increasing steps were chosen, and the reduction and increase of size was defined relatively to the previous layer size. The optimal reduction size was set to 1/8 of the input size, as experimentally determined by training and evaluating on real data. The intermediate layer size was set to 4/6, creating an hourglass-like shape. A batch size of 100, ReLU activation functions, a mean square error and an Adam optimizer with a learning rate of 0.0005 were chosen. 300,000 voxels were created for training, split into 25,000 voxels for training and 50,000 for validation. The neural network had to be trained for 50 epochs in order to reach convergence.

3   Results

The reconstruction performance of the autoencoders trained on the different synthetic datasets was compared using the raw diffusion attenuated signal, as well as metrics derived from fitted diffusion tensors.

First, to assess the reconstruction performance, the diffusion attenuated signal was used, i.e., the diffusion signal divided by the b0 measurement. The mean absolute deviation of the reconstructed signal on the brain MRI scans is shown in Fig. 1. Both, in the HCP as well as in the study data, the reconstruction performance for Syn, SampleAndMean and Sample was nearly identical with no statistically significant differences, while the RandomWM mode performed significantly worse. Meanwhile, the reconstruction performance between the HCP acquisitions and the study data was different. This effect can be explained by the acquisition settings: The MRI scanners used in the HCP and local study were similar, but the HCP used voxel sizes of 1.25mm, while 2.4mm were used in the local study, i.e., one voxel in the local data corresponds to $(\frac{2.4}{1.25})^3 \approx 7$ voxels in the HCP data. Thus, ignoring differences due to other acquisition settings and the preprocessing pipeline, a difference in signal-to-noise ratio (SNR) of $\sqrt{(\frac{2.4}{1.25})^3} \approx 2.66$ was expected between the two datasets. This falls exactly in line with the difference in raw reconstruction performance: The mean absolute

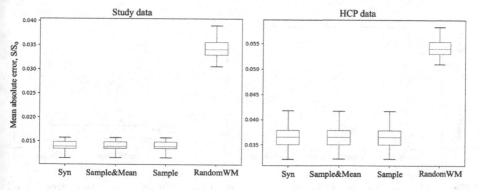

Fig. 1. Mean absolute error of the diffusion signal attenuation. Note the different y-axis between the two different datasets.

error for the three multi-tensor simulations was 0.014 on the local study data, and 0.037 for the HCP data.

Second, the reconstruction performance on metrics derived from fitted diffusion tensors was assessed. The difference in fractional anisotropy (FA) for the three multi-tensor modes Syn, SampleAndMean and Sample was negligible with a mean absolute error of 0.0075 for the three settings in local study data, and 0.0104 in the HCP data, while the RandomWM model was again significantly worse, with a mean absolute deviation of 0.17 on the local study data, and 0.22 on the HCP data.

However, significant differences between the multi-tensor modes could be observed for the reconstruction of the main fiber direction (Fig. 2). Especially, a strong difference between Syn and the WM sampling models could be observed, while the differences between the mean or sampling of GM and CSF diffusion attenuation did not affect the results as strongly. The performance of RandomWM (local study: $42.4 \pm 3.2°$, HCP: $42.7 \pm 2.8°$) was considerably worse than for the other techniques, it is not displayed for better visualization.

4 Discussion

In the analysis of raw signal reconstruction performance, the three different multi-tensor models had negligible difference, while the WM simulation with random values lead to worse results. This random value approach covers the largest variety in diffusion signals, but the autoencoder network, which needs to compress the data, is not able to distill the necessary information into the smaller latent space. Regardless of the task, modern deep learning approaches need to distill information at some point, which does not seem to be possible with a too unspecific data generation approach such as the method labeled RandomWM. Similar effects should occur when neural networks are trained on this synthetic data for other tasks, e.g. microstructure prediction or tractography.

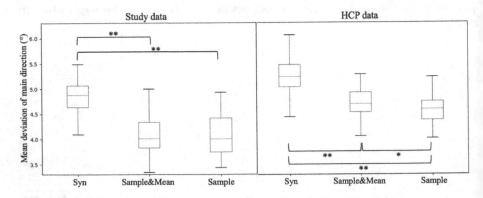

Fig. 2. Mean deviation of the main direction of the diffusion tensor in degree for all voxels with an fractional anisotropy (FA) value between 0.5 and 0.9. * statistically significant with $p<0.05$, ** significant with $p<10^{-8}$.

Multi-tensor models seem to be a good choice: The matching of SNR difference between the two datasets and reconstruction performance is an indicator for close-to-optimal reconstruction performance of the employed denoising autoencoder. How the diffusion tensor eigenvalues should be chosen depends on the application case: The simulation of multi-tensor data with pre-set tensor eigenvalues using openly available software is simple and fast, and the reconstruction performance on the raw signals and FA values is already good. Therefore, it is feasible to use such simulated data for quick and scanner-independent training or pretraining of neural networks, where the directionality of fibers is not relevant. If the application is dependent not only on raw signal values or FA, but instead on the direction of the WM fibers, the individual characteristics, depending on scanner and subject, should not be ignored. For example, in the application of deep learning to tractography [10], minor errors in fiber direction integrate over the whole fiber, possibly leading to major errors in the end region of the fiber. In such cases, a precision medicine approach is necessary: The diffusivity of WM and other compartments should be set to patient-specific values.

Acknowledgement. This work was funded by the German Research Foundation (DFG) – grant 269953372/GRK2150 and grant ME 3737/19-1.

References

1. Ravi D, Ghavami N, Alexander DC, et al. Current applications and future promises of machine learning in diffusion MRI. MICCAI Workshop on Computational Diffusion MRI (CDMRI). 2019; p. 105–121.
2. Neher PF, Laun FB, Stieltjes B, et al. Fiberfox: facilitating the creation of realistic white matter software phantoms. Magn Reson Med. 2014;72(5):1460–1470.
3. Goodfellow I, Bengio Y, Courville A. Deep learning. MIT Press; 2016.
4. Essen DCV, Smith SM, Barch DM, et al. The WU-minn human connectome project: an overview. NeuroImage. 2013;80:62–79. Mapping the Connectome.
5. Smith SM, Jenkinson M, Woolrich MW, et al. Advances in functional and structural MR image analysis and implementation as FSL. NeuroImage. 2004;23 Suppl. 1:S208–S219.
6. Garyfallidis E, Brett M, Amirbekian B, et al. Dipy, a library for the analysis of diffusion MRI data. Front Neuroinform. 2014;8:8.
7. Schultz T. Learning a reliable estimate of the number of fiber directions in diffusion MRI. Proc MICCAI. 2012; p. 493–500.
8. Weninger L, Koppers S, Na CH, et al. Free-water correction in diffusion MRI: a reliable and robust learning approach. MICCAI Workshop on Computational Diffusion MRI (CDMRI). 2019; p. 91–99.
9. Molina-Romero M, Wiestler B, Gómez P, et al. Deep learning with synthetic diffusion MRI data for free-water elimination in glioblastoma cases. Proc MICCAI. 2018; p. 98–106.
10. Poulin P, Cote MA, Houde JC, et al. Learn to track: deep learning for tractography. Proc MICCAI. 2017; p. 540–547.

Analysis of Generative Shape Modeling Approaches
Latent Space Properties and Interpretability

Hristina Uzunova[1], Jesse Kruse[1], Paul Kaftan[1], Matthias Wilms[2],
Nils D. Forkert[2], Heinz Handels[1], Jan Ehrhardt[1]

[1]Institute of Medical Informatics, University of Lübeck, Germany
[2]Department of Radiology, University of Calgary, Canada
uzunova@imi.uni-luebeck.de

Abstract. Generative shape models are crucial for many medical image analysis tasks. In previous studies, it has been shown that conventional methods like PCA-based statistical shape models (SSMs) and their extensions are thought to be robust in terms of generalization ability but have rather poor specificity. On the contrary, deep learning approaches like autoencoders, require large training set sizes, but are comparably specific. In this work, we comprehensively compare different classical and deep learning-based generative shape modeling approaches and demonstrate their limitations and advantages. Experiments on a publicly available 2D chest X-ray data set show that the deep learning methods achieve better specificity and similar generalization abilities for large training set sizes. Furthermore, an extensive analysis of the different methods, gives an insight on their latent space representations.

1 Introduction

The study of anatomical shapes is a fundamental process in medical image analysis. Generative shape modeling methods seek to capture as much information as possible to estimate the shape distribution of a population. Typically, a training set of shapes is used to train a model that is able to reproduce the training shapes and to generate new but similar shape instances. Applications of these models range from segmentation and registration, over data augmentation, to the detection and classification of diseases in medical images. A classical example of such generative models are PCA-based statistical shape models (SSMs) introduced by Cootes et al. in the early 1990s [1]. Since then, numerous extensions and modifications of these models have been proposed to alleviate problems and limitations regarding the linear nature of this approach [2], the need for 1-to-1 correspondences [3], or reduce the amount of training data required [4, 5]. More recently, the research focus has shifted towards deep learning-based generative modeling using approaches like autoencoders (AEs), variational autoencoders (VAEs), or generative adversarial networks (GANs). Although these approaches overcome major limitations of SSMs, they require even larger training data sets

© Der/die Autor(en), exklusiv lizenziert durch
Springer Fachmedien Wiesbaden GmbH, ein Teil von Springer Nature 2021
C. Palm et al. (Hrsg.), *Bildverarbeitung für die Medizin 2021*,
Informatik aktuell, https://doi.org/10.1007/978-3-658-33198-6_84

and their black-box nature makes them harder to interpret. Nevertheless, deep learning methods are successful, especially for the generation of synthetic images [6]. However, in the medical field training data is limited and only a few studies have examined the properties of generative models for this specific situation [7].

In a previous study [8], two conventional and two deep learning-based generative approaches for multi-organ shape modeling were compared. That study showed that approaches based on deep learning consistently show better results in terms of generalizability and specificity than classical PCA-based SSMs. Yet, it has been shown that extensions of classical SSMs [5] perform on par with and even outperform deep learning- based approaches in terms of generalizability, especially for smaller training sets. Moreover, deep learning approaches tend to model small or rare structures incorrectly when only few samples are available.

In this work, we extend [8] by (1) including other popular generative models, (2) investigating solutions for the incorrect generation of small structures in (V)AEs, and (3) examining the properties of the latent spaces of the models.

2   Materials and methods

2.1   Material

The generative shape models discussed in this paper use a publicly available 2D chest radiograph database [9]. We refrain from using 3D data here to avoid typical computational problems that would require special solutions for the deep learning approaches. The dataset contains 247 images with segmentations of five structures (left and right lung, left and right clavicle, and the heart). Segmentations are given as a set of 166 corresponding landmarks (input for the SSMs) and as binarized label images (input for the deep learning approaches; Fig. 1). We use the same fixed 123/124 images test/training split as in [9] to allow for a direct comparison of the results.

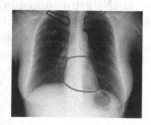 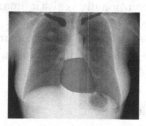

Fig. 1. Example shapes as contours (left) for the SSMs; and labels (right) for the CNNs.

2.2   Statistical shape models and locality-based multi-resolution SSMs

Statistical Shape Models (SSMs) use vectorized representations of landmark points that represent the shape of the object, typically the object contours. Principal Component Analysis (PCA) of a training set is used to create an orthonormal basis for projecting shape representations into a low-dimensional latent space or to reconstruct new shapes from latent representations [1]. In classical SSMs, the number of training samples influences the flexibility of the model, since the size of the latent space is limited by the size of the training set. Locality-based multi-resolution SSMs (LSSMs) [5] introduce additional flexibility by breaking global relationships and assuming that local shape variations have limited effects in distant areas. This idea can be integrated into the traditional SSM framework by manipulating covariances based on the distance between landmarks in a multi-resolution manner. LSSMs have been shown to perform on par or outperform other approaches like wavelet-based SSMs or Gaussian process models in terms of generalization and specificity [5, 10].

2.3   Autoencoders and variational autoencoders

Autoencoders (AEs) are neural networks consisting of an encoder $Q(X)$ that maps input data X to a low-dimensional latent vector $\mathbf{z}$, and a decoder $P(\mathbf{z})$ that attempts to reconstruct the input data X given $\mathbf{z}$. This is typically achieved by optimizing a reconstruction objective, s.t. $X \approx P(Q(X))$. Thus, unseen shapes can be reconstructed by forwarding them through a trained encoder and decoder. To generate new shapes, a random $\mathbf{z}$ can be sampled and propagated through a trained decoder [8].

However, AEs may simply learn an identity function and because of the unknown latent distribution, sampling a random $\mathbf{z}$ can cause the generation of implausible shapes. Those problems are addressed by variational autoencoders (VAEs), by restricting the latent space to a normal distribution. In practice, this is achieved by an additional Kullback-Leibler loss of the latent space [11].

2.4   Generative adversarial networks

Generative adversarial networks (GANs) can analogously be used as generative models. However, due to their adversarial training scheme, they are known to enable the generation of exceptionally realistic images. GANs learn to map a random noise vector $\mathbf{z}$ to an output image X_{fake} using a generator function $G : \mathbf{z} \to X_{fake}$ [6]. To ensure that the generator produces realistic images, an adversarial discriminator D is used during training, aiming at perfectly distinguishing real images and generated fake data.

2.5   Deformable autoencoders

AEs or VAEs often fail to reconstruct or generate small-sized structures, especially when trained on small datasets [8]. Deformable autoencoders (DAE) are an extension of VAEs that tackle this problem by representing shapes as the deformed version of a learned template image [12]. Rather than directly reconstructing the input, the DAE decoder generates a displacement field φ and implicitly learns a template T, which is deformed to match the input X s.t. $T \circ P(z) \approx X$. To ensure smooth displacement fields, a diffusion regularisation term is used as an additional penalty during model training.

3 Experiments and results

In this work, we focus on analyzing differences between the approaches presented in Sec. 2 with respect to specificity and generalization and also investigate the structure of each model's latent space. The experimental setup follows [8].

Specificity and Generalization: In this experiment, all methods are compared in terms of generalization and specificity for different training set sizes, where specificity describes the model's ability to generate new realistic samples and generalization denotes the ability to reconstruct unseen samples. As in [8], training set sizes ranging from 5 to 113 are used for a 5-fold-cross-validation. Average symmetric surface/contour distances (ASSD) are utilized to quantify the results.

The results for all methods are shown in Fig. 2. The deep learning methods show overall better results in terms of specificity. However, for small training set sizes (< 60), the LSSM model shows improved generalization abilities. For large training set sizes, the generalization abilities of the methods are roughly the same. While the deep learning methods seem to have similar generalization abilities, the DAE and GAN models achieve the best specificity.

Furthermore, for smaller training set sizes, VAEs and AEs are not able to reconstruct all labels, especially small labels like the clavicles. Thus, the percentage of images missing one or more labels is fairly high. This problem does not appear for the DAE model. However, the DAE seems to require larger training datasets to generate a proper template and consequently achieve a competitive generalization performance (Fig. 3).

Latent Space: The latent space of the methods presented here is crucial to their representation ability. The latent space size of the traditional methods lies in the ranges $[3, 14]$ (SSM) and $[4, 55]$ (LSSM) depending on the training set size. Compared to the deep learning methods with a fixed latent space of size

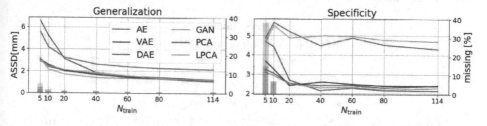

Fig. 2. Generalization and specificity of the models for varying training set sizes (lower values are better). The bars indicate the percentage of images with missing labels.

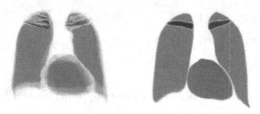

Fig. 3. The DAE learned templates with a different amount of training images. Left: $N = 5$; right: $N = 114$.

Table 1. Percent of non-normally distributed components of the latent vectors of all models determined by a Shapiro-Wilk test.

Method	Train	Test
VAE	10.1%	9.8%
DAE	15.1%	12.7%
GAN	19.7%	18.6%
AE	19.7%	18.0%
PCA	28.8%	32.7%
LPCA	27.9%	39.5%

512, the traditional methods have fairly compact latent spaces contributing to their interpretability. To further investigate the structure of the latent spaces, we linearly interpolate between the latent vectors of two randomly chosen images and project the interpolated vectors back to image space. In Fig. 4, examples for AE and DAE show that smooth interpolations are possible. However, AEs tend to generate artifacts and implausible shapes for smaller training sets. This is avoided in DAEs due to applying smooth deformations to a generated template.

Typically, a normal distribution is assumed for the latent space of the models when sampling new shapes. To verify this assumption, we apply a component-wise Shapiro-Wilk normality test on the latent encodings of the training and test data and calculate the percentage of non-normally distributed components (Tab. 1). Due to the explicit normalization of the latent spaces of the VAE and DAE, they have a small percentage of non-normally distributed components ($\sim 10\% - 15\%$). This value increases up to 40% for PCA and LPCA due to their linear nature, accounting for their worse specificity.

A further important property is that, in contrast to SSMs, neural networks do not guarantee that a reconstructed image is mapped to the same latent vector as the original image. We, therefore, calculate the distance between the encoding of the input image and the encoding of the reconstructed image averaged over all training data. To establish a consequent scheme, a Mahalanobis distance

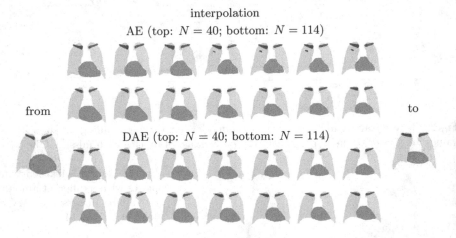

Fig. 4. Projected latent space interpolation between two shapes for different methods.

was used for all methods. As baseline (BL), we approximate the mean pairwise distance of the latent encodings. The values obtained are: VAE 0.01 (BL 0.41); AE 11 (BL 26.7); GAN 11 (BL 21.8); DAE 0.02 (BL 0.6). Those distances indicate an ambiguity and poor interpretability of the latent space, that is not present for the classical shape models.

4   Discussion and conclusion

In terms of generalization, the classical LPCA method is more robust for small training set sizes, whereas for large training set sizes, it is on par with the deep learning methods. Most deep learning methods fail to generate small structures when trained on small datasets, while deformable autoencoders cope with this problem, yet they require a considerable amount of training data to reach the generalization ability of the other approaches. In terms of specificity, the deep learning methods show significantly better results. The latent spaces of SSMs are much more compact and intuitive, however, their linear nature yields non-normally distributed latent spaces explaining their poor specificity. An interpolation experiment visualizes the smoothness of the latent spaces and shows the strengths of DAEs compared to AEs. Still, a rather large drawback of the deep learning methods is the ambiguity of their latent space.

References

1. Cootes TF, Taylor CJ, Cooper DH, et al. Active shape models-their training and application. Comput Vis Image Underst. 1995;61(1):38–59.
2. Kirschner M, Becker M, Wesarg S. 3D active shape model segmentation with nonlinear shape priors. Proc MICCAI. 2011; p. 492–499.
3. Krüger J, Ehrhardt J, Handels H. Statistical appearance models based on probabilistic correspondences. Med Image Anal. 2017;37:146–159.
4. Davatzikos C, Tao X, Shen D. Hierarchical active shape models, using the wavelet transform. IEEE Trans Med Imaging; p. 2003.
5. Wilms M, Handels H, Ehrhardt J. Multi-resolution multi-object statistical shape models based on the locality assumption. Med Image Anal. 2017;38:17–29.
6. Goodfellow I, Pouget-Abadie J, Mirza M, et al. Generative adversarial nets. In: Advances in Neural Information Processing Systems; 2014. p. 2672–2680.
7. Ruan X, Murphy RF. Evaluation of methods for generative modeling of cell and nuclear shape. Bioinformatics. 2018 12;35(14):2475–2485.
8. Uzunova H, Kaftan P, Wilms M, et al. Quantitative comparison of generative shape models for medical images. In: BVM; 2020. p. 201–207.
9. van Ginneken B, Stegmann MB, Loog M. Segmentation of anatomical structures in chest radiographs using supervised methods. Med Image Anal. 2006; p. 19–40.
10. Wilms M, Ehrhardt J, Forkert ND. A kernelized multi-level localization method for flexible shape modeling with few training data. Proc MICCAI. 2020; p. 765–775.
11. Kingma D, Welling M. Auto-encoding variational bayes. In: International Conference on Learning Representations; 2014. p. 1–10.
12. Shu Z, Sahasrabudhe M, Alp Güler R, et al. Deforming autoencoders: unsupervised disentangling of shape and appearance. Proc ECCV. 2018; p. 664–680.

Latent Shape Constraint for Anatomical Landmark Detection on Spine Radiographs

Florian Kordon[1,2,3], Andreas Maier[1,2,4], Holger Kunze[1,3]

[1]Pattern Recognition Lab, Universität Erlangen-Nürnberg (FAU), Erlangen
[2]Erlangen Graduate School in Advanced Optical Technologies (SAOT), Erlangen
[3]Siemens Healthcare GmbH, Forchheim
[4]Machine Intelligence, Universität Erlangen-Nürnberg (FAU), Erlangen
florian.kordon@fau.de

Abstract. Vertebral corner points are frequently used landmarks for a vast variety of orthopedic and trauma surgical applications. Algorithmic approaches that are designed to automatically detect them on 2D radiographs have to cope with varying image contrast, high noise levels, and superimposed soft tissue. To enforce an anatomically correct landmark configuration in presence of these limitations, this study investigates a shape constraint technique based on data-driven encodings of the spine geometry. A contractive PointNet autoencoder is used to map numerical landmark coordinate representations onto a low-dimensional shape manifold. A distance norm between prediction and ground truth encodings then serves as an additional loss term during optimization. The method is compared and evaluated on the SpineWeb16 dataset. Small improvements can be observed, recommending further analysis of the encoding design and composite cost function.

1 Introduction

Anatomical landmark localization is an important prerequisite in medical image processing. It mostly serves as a semantic prior for subsequent tasks which operate on single-point information and their spatial relationships [1, 2]. Traditionally, strategies to assess such a localization task either involve independent detection of a single landmark or incorporate information about relative positioning, spatial constraints, a priori knowledge, and characteristics of the local feature vicinity [2, 3]. In contrast to natural images, this additional information often presents itself as a natural choice to alleviate image-quality based ambiguities. This is due to anatomical landmarks following a rather rigid configuration constrained by the bio-mechanical range of motion of the human body.

A typical example of such a configuration can be observed for the localization of vertebral corner points on antero-posterior spine radiographs. On the micro level, the vertebrae within one spinal region are very similar to each other and describe a convex quadrilateral by their corner vertices. On the macro level, the vertical progression of all vertebrae on the X-ray image can be described by a plane curve. In the case of healthy patients, this curve approximates a straight line, and in cases of more severe scoliosis, it is more bent. If we want to translate these anatomical constraints for automatic localization methods using deep learning, we can distinguish between two basic approaches: (1) explicit constraints using domain knowledge, i.e. enforcing adjacency constraints or geometric rules [4], and (2) implicit constraints using a data-driven extraction of statistics about plausible and aberrant configurations [3, 5].

While using an explicit constraints scheme is an attractive approach, it is limited in its ability to generalize well to unseen data and to data that does not match the underlying geometric model. In contrast, a data-driven approach in theory can capture these variations, but presumes a sufficiently large training data corpus to do so. However, depending on the specific methodology such implicit constraints might require additional topological modifications to the learning model's architecture. To circumvent this additional computational effort during inference, [5] proposed a lightweight shape-aware method which they evaluated for segmentation and super-resolution tasks. The latent representation of an autoencoder is used to map both the ground truth as well as the neural network predictions onto a low-dimensional manifold. During optimization, the distance between both encodings serves as additional constraint to the cost function to pull back aberrant predictions onto anatomically accurate solutions.

Based on this idea, this study investigates an extension of this method for a joint coordinate representation of vertebral corner points. After estimating the spatial position for each of the 68 corner points using 2D heatmaps, normalized numerical coordinates are extracted using a differentiable spatial-to-numerical transform (DSNT) [6]. A shape representation of this coordinate set is then extracted as the latent encoding of a PointNet-Autoencoder and compared to the encoded shape of the corresponding ground truth. The influence of the proposed constraint is evaluated on the SpineWeb16 dataset [3].

2 Materials and methods

2.1 Geometric constraint via latent shape encoding

A common way to represent data as a set of discriminative and abstract features is the use of autoencoders. An autoencoder can learn to map the data features to a low-dimensional manifold in an unsupervised fashion by encoding and decoding a latent (vector) representation $h(\cdot)$ and measuring the quality of the input reconstruction. If we consider a set of representative landmark configurations of the vertebral corner points $\boldsymbol{y}$, such an autoencoder optimizes an abstraction of possible and anatomically correct spine shapes from which it can reconstruct all individual corner points. Consequently, if the distance between two latent vectors of a ground truth sample $h(\boldsymbol{y}_i)$ and a test sample $h(\tilde{\boldsymbol{y}}_i)$ is large, it can be assumed that the test sample describes a shape that is not suitable for decoding and anatomically aberrant (Fig. 1).

Fig. 1. Illustration of a low-dimensional shape manifold based on ground truth y and the learned mapping function $h(\cdot)$.

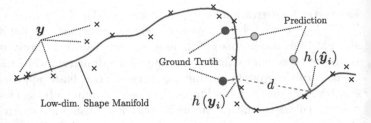

This idea of a latent distance measure naturally translates to an additional loss term within the cost function of an optimization problem [5]. Given the cost function for some optimization task $\mathcal{L}_{opt}$, a distance norm d (here L2-norm) on the latent vectors, and a weighting term λ, this can be described as $\mathcal{L}_{\text{total}} = \mathcal{L}_{\text{opt}} + \lambda \cdot d\left(h\left(y\right)\right), h\left(\tilde{y}\right)\right)$.

2.2 Architecture design variants

A popular way to estimate the position of 2D landmarks is to encode their spatial likelihood as heatmaps. This is achieved by placing a 2D Gaussian distribution with standard deviation σ and compact support $\pm 3\sigma$ on the landmark coordinates. The heatmaps are then estimated with a Fully-Convolutional Neural Network (FCN) and explicitly compared to the ground truth via image-to-image matching using a mean-squared error cost function (Fig. 2-A) [1, 7]. If we consider a computationally demanding task such as the prediction of a large set of corner points, the integration of the introduced shape constraint necessitates a comparably large autoencoder to encode all predicted heatmaps. To reduce this computational footprint, we employ a *spatial-to-numerical* transform [6] to map the heatmaps to normalized numerical coordinates. In contrast to a spatial argmax operation which is used to obtain the maximum response in case of heatmap matching, this transform is completely differentiable. This means that a cost functions can directly operate on the numerical coordinates while implicitly optimizing the heatmaps. Besides, using a numerical coordinate representation as input and target for the autoencoder allows for a lightweight autoencoder architecture (Fig. 2-B,C). To be able to find meaningful shape representations also in case of noisy label data, we propose to use a contractive autoencoder topology inspired by PointNet [8]. Given a landmark configuration in the form of a $(N, 2)$ tensor with N marking the number of landmarks, the input is first transformed to $(N, 1)$ using a number of convolutional blocks before a symmetry function is applied. Besides performing the final encoding step, this symmetry function (here max-pooling) makes the autoencoder invariant to the order of input landmarks. We assume this characteristic to aid in learning a global shape context and implicit geometric adjacency relations.

2.3 Data and experiment protocol

The comparison of the architecture variants is performed on the SpineWeb16 dataset which consists of 609 spinal antero-posterior radiographs [3] with la-

Fig. 2. Visualization of the model variants that are compared for the task of vertebral corner point detection. (A) Explicit heatmap prediction with subsequent spatial argmax. (B) Implicit heatmap prediction with *spatial-to-numerical* transform DSNT [6]. (C) Additional shape constraint penalizing the latent vector distance.

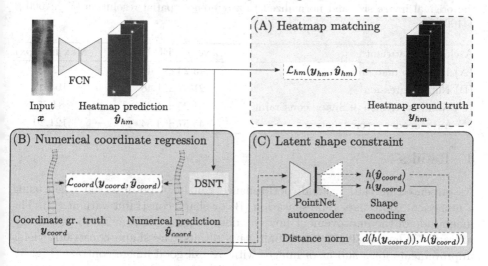

bels for 12 thoracic and 5 lumbar vertebrae, totaling 68 vertebral corner points. An initial semi-automatic screening of the annotation data revealed point and vertebrae permutations, shifting of upper and lower plates, as well as clinically implausible corners in areas of low contrast. A subset of 520 suitable images was selected after automatic and manual corrections of the annotation material. For all variants, we devised a 5(+1)-fold cross-validation scheme. The extra sixth fold was selected for an initial optimization of the shape constraint weight $\lambda \in [0.001, 0.003, 0.006, 0.010, ..., 1.000]$ and was used as additional training data in the subsequent cross-validation. As a main model for heatmap prediction we trained a single Hourglass module [7] with a feature root of 256 and additional instance normalization layers [1]. For the shape-constrained variant (C), a PointNet autoencoder was pre-trained for the corresponding fold configuration and included via an additional cost term with optimized weighting factor $\lambda = 0.003$ (Subsec. 2.1). For every architecture variant, the images were down-sampled and zero-padded to a common spatial resolution of [h:512 × w:192] px. Every image was processed with a homomorphic filtering operation to increase the image contrast in low-intensity areas and min-max normalized to the interval of $[0, 1]$. During training, an online augmentations scheme with randomized Gaussian blurring, contrast scaling, rotation, translation, scaling, and slight axis-aligned shrinking was applied. Training was performed for 250 epochs and the best model was selected based on the performance on the validation set[1].

---

[1] Curated annotations are available at doi:10.5281/zenodo.4413665.

Table 1. Cross-validation results for the three architecture variants ((A),(B),(C)) and autoencoder reconstruction (*). The average and max scores are reported across the five folds and are based on the individual mean/max of the Euclidean distance (ED) over all samples within the respective test fold. The reported scores are scaled w.r.t. the original image size and normalized to a reference spatial resolution of [h:1000 × w:1000] px.

Architecture variant	Average ED (px)	Max ED (px)
(A) Heatmap matching	23.23 ± 1.47	92.73
(B) Num. regression	21.67 ± 1.48	104.03
(C) Num. regression + Shape constraint	21.25 ± 1.24	84.55
(*) Autoencoder reconstruction	45.57 ± 4.84	121.20

3 Results

As presented in Tab. 1, small performance gains can be observed when using a numerical coordinate representation (B) or shape constraint variant (C). The magnitude of the improvement however does suggest the benefits to not be significant. When analyzing the qualitative results, the shape constraint yields improvements for a subset of images with overall good image contrast (Fig. 3). However, in case of more severe contrast differences and obscured image parts due to superimposed soft tissue, neither the DSNT variant nor the shape constraint approach benefit the landmark predictions. For such image characteristics in general, no model variant yields anatomically accurate landmark configurations. Interestingly, the autoencoder reconstruction frequently estimates much smoother landmark configurations at the cost of spatial precision.

4 Discussion

While the proposed shape constraint on average benefits the spinal shape, no consistent improvements w.r.t. the positional quality of the vertebral corner points

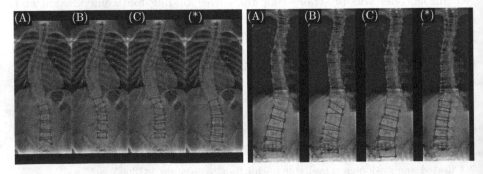

Fig. 3. Example predictions of a successful shape constraint (left) and a failure case (right). (*) marks the reconstruction obtained by the PointNet autoencoder. Red and blue coloring denotes the thoracic and lumbar spinal section respectively.

can be achieved, especially in the case of low-quality images. Based on the qualitative analysis, several potential problems can be identified. Although the quality of the autoencoder reconstruction indicates that a mapping function onto a meaningful shape manifold can be learned, the abstraction towards a probabilistic mean shape could be too strong to actually enforce geometrically meaningful landmarks. This assumption is supported by a small optimal weighting factor λ and a general pull back to a rectified spine shape (Fig. 3). Such behavior also relates to the observations by [3] who showcase that standard convolutional features do not warrant sufficiently accurate landmark positions. Also, a linear composition of the cost function might cause a suboptimal optimization and conflicting gradients, which could be solved by gradient manipulation [9] or adaptive weighting [1]. And lastly, adaptive pre-processing based on region-specific image statistics could help to alleviate image quality-based ambiguities, which often occur in the thoracic region. Hence, we seek to extend our evaluation and combine a data-driven approach with explicit shape constraints.

Acknowledgement. The authors gratefully acknowledge funding of the Erlangen Graduate School in Advanced Optical Technologies (SAOT) by the Bavarian State Ministry for Science and Art.

Disclaimer. The methods and information presented here are based on research and are not commercially available.

References

1. Kordon F, Fischer P, Privalov M, et al. Multi-task localization and segmentation for x-ray guided planning in knee surgery. In: Shen D, Liu T, Peters TM, et al., editors. Proc MICCAI. Springer; 2019. p. 622–630.
2. Urschler M, Ebner T, Štern D. Integrating geometric configuration and appearance information into a unified framework for anatomical landmark localization. Med Image Anal. 2018;43:23–36.
3. Wu H, Bailey C, Rasoulinejad P, et al. Automatic landmark estimation for adolescent idiopathic scoliosis assessment using BoostNet. In: Descoteaux M, Maier-Hein L, Franz A, et al., editors. Proc MICCAI. Springer; 2017. p. 127–135.
4. Imran AAZ, Huang C, Tang H, et al.. Bipartite distance for shape-aware landmark detection in spinal x-ray images; 2020. arXiv:2005.14330v1 [eess.IV].
5. Oktay O, Ferrante E, Kamnitsas K, et al. Anatomically constrained neural networks (ACNN): Application to cardiac image enhancement and segmentation. IEEE Trans Med Imaging. 2018;37(2):384–395.
6. Nibali A, He Z, Morgan S, et al. Numerical coordinate regression with convolutional neural networks. CoRR. 2018;abs/1801.07372.
7. Newell A, Yang K, Deng J. Stacked hourglass networks for human pose estimation. In: Leibe B, Matas J, Sebe N, et al., editors. Proc ECCV. Springer; 2016. p. 483–499.
8. Charles RQ, Su H, Kaichun M, et al. PointNet: Deep learning on point sets for 3D classification and segmentation. In: Proc IEEE Comput Soc Conf Comput Vis Pattern Recognit; 2017. p. 77–85.
9. Yu T, Kumar S, Gupta A, et al.. Gradient surgery for multi-task learning; 2020. arXiv:2001.06782v3 [cs.LG].

Autorenverzeichnis

Printed in the United States
By Bookmasters